FACIAL TRAUMA

FACIAL TRAUMA

edited by

SETH R. THALLER
W. SCOTT McDONALD

University of Miami School of Medicine
Miami, Florida, U.S.A.

informa
healthcare

Informa Healthcare USA, Inc.
52 Vanderbilt Avenue
New York, NY 10017

10 9 8 7 6 5 4 3 2

International Standard Book Number-13: 978-0-8247-4625-4 (Hardcover)

Visit the Informa Web site at
www.informa.com
and the Informa Healthcare Web site at
www.informahealthcare.com

PRINTED IN INDIA BY REPLIKA PRESS PVT.LTD.

Preface

Optimal management of patients who have sustained facial truma requires a collaborative interdisciplinary approach that incorporates the clinical expertise of a number of related specialties. This book reflects the efforts and the contributions to this field from eminent practitioners intimately involved in the challenging care and management of patients who have required reconstruction of both acute and established injuries to the facial hard and soft tissue. Although the treatment of facial injuries has made dramatic advances over the last decade due to our improved knowledge of wound healing, anatomy, diagnostic testing, and biomaterials, we trace our current refinements to the pioneering efforts of craniofacial surgery and the work of Dr. Paul Tessier of Paris, France. This book integrates the significant contributions made by basic science into the comprehensive care of this condition as well as the most recent clinical advances in the evaluation and management of facial injuries.

We give special thanks to our contributors, who willingly shared their own experience in order to expand our readers' knowledge base and improve our colleagues' final results in the care of their own clinical cases.

This book is dedicated to my wife, Pat, and children, Cody and Lexi Lee, who allow me the time to take care of my patients and educate our residents, and to my parents, who afforded me the opportunity to become a doctor.

Seth R. Thaller

I would like to thank all our contributors and acknowledge their advancements in the care of the trauma victim. In these most trying times for medicine it is comforting to know that these dedicated individuals have made the sacrifices to care for this world's unfortunate. I would especially like to thank my mother, Tommie, and my late father, Thomas E. McDonald, for all of their sacrifices to help me be who I am, and I dedicate this book to them.

W. Scott McDonald

Introduction

Despite society's ever-increasing concern for personal safety, trauma to the facial bones and enveloping soft tissue remains a relatively common occurence. While a significant percentage of these injuries are directly related to motor vehicle accidents, in urban trauma centers assault is also a common mode of wounding. In spite of recent progress in surgical technique, technology, and available biomaterials, the fundamental principles for achieving acceptable functional and aesthetic results remain constant. This is a comparatively young surgical specialty with an elegant history. Initially developed by general surgeons with a particular interest in this field, it has been refined by dentists, oral surgeons, otolaryngologists, and plastic surgeons.

The growth of tertiary trauma centers has had two important consequences: severely injured patients are now able to survive their initial physical insult and will require reconstruction of devastating facial injuries, and interdisciplinary teams can acquire greater experience with managing complex facial trauma. An additional benefit is that a dedicated craniomaxillofacial team not only improves quality of care, but can also be extremely cost-effective. Concentrated expertise and better technology have allowed us to answer previously controversial questions in this field. Arriving patients undergo radiological evaluation—generally CT scanning—that is aimed at precisely defining the location and magnitude of bony injury. Advances in managing severely injured patients have permitted early and definitive primary fracture treatment. Tessier's craniofacial techniques, including wide surgical exposure through extensive subperiosteal dissection and extensive primary bone grafting for replacement and reinforcement, are now commonly employed. It is now routine for patients to return to a productive life.

This book is the foundation for the comprehensive management of complex craniomaxillofacial trauma, and serves as the basis for discussing the evolution in care of the facially traumatized patient. Few areas in reconstructive surgery have undergone such a rapid transformation.

Alan Livingstone, M.D.
Professor & Chairman
Department of Surgery
University of Miami
Miami, Florida, U.S.A.

Contents

Contributors

Oleh M. Antonyshyn University of Toronto, Toronto, Ontario, Canada

Milton B. Armstrong Department of Clinical Surgery, Division of Plastic Surgery, University of Miami, Miami, Florida, U.S.A.

Steven R. Buchman Mott Children's Hospital, Ann Arbor, Michigan, U.S.A.

Mark Cockburn University of Miami, Miami, Florida, U.S.A.

Stephen M. Cohn UM Department of Surgery, University of Miami, Miami, Florida, U.S.A.

Steven R. Cohen Sharp Childrens' Hospital, San Diego, California, U.S.A.

Paul J. Donald Davis Medical Center, University of California, Davis Medical Center, Sacramento, California, U.S.A.

Danny J. Enepekides Davis Medical Center, University of California, Davis Medical Center, Sacramento, California, U.S.A.

Tony D. Fang School of Medicine, Stanford University School of Medicine, Stanford, California, U.S.A.

Kenton D. Fong School of Medicine, Stanford University School of Medicine, Stanford, California, U.S.A.

Jose I. Garri University of Miami School of Medicine, Miami, Florida, U.S.A.

Mutaz B. Habal The Tampa Bay Craniofacial Center, University of South Florida and University of Florida, Tampa, Florida, U.S.A.

Alan S. Herford Loma Linda University Medical Center, Loma Linda, California, U.S.A.

William Y. Hoffman University of California at San Francisco, San Francisco, California, U.S.A.

Ralph E. Holmes Sharp Childrens' Hospital, San Diego, California, U.S.A.

Igor Jeroukhimov University of Miami, Miami, Florida, U.S.A.

Leonard B. Kaban Massachusetts General Hospital, Boston, Massachusetts, U.S.A.

Henry K. Kawamoto, Jr. UCLA School of Medicine, Los Angeles, California, U.S.A.

Kevin J. Kelly Craniofacial Surgery Center, Vanderbilt University, Nashville, Tennessee, U.S.A.

Chen Lee McGill University, Montreal, Quebec, Canada

Michael T. Longaker Department of Surgery, Stanford University School of Medicine, Stanford, California, U.S.A.

Paul Manson Baltimore, Maryland, U.S.A.

Mark Martin McGill University, Montreal, Quebec, Canada

Robert E. Marx Department of Surgery, University of Miami, Miami, Florida, U.S.A.

W. Scott McDonald University of Miami School of Medicine, Miami, Florida, U.S.A.

Seung-Jun O Medical University of South Carolina, Charleston, South Carolina, U.S.A.

David A. O'Donovan Department of Surgery, University of Miami and Jackson Memorial Hospital, Miami, Florida, U.S.A.

Anil P. Punjabi Loma Linda University School of Medicine and Riverside County Regional Medical Center, Loma Linda, California, U.S.A.

Samuel T. Rhee Mott Children's Hospital, Ann Arbor, Michigan, U.S.A.

Bernard G. Sarnat Division of Oral Biology & Medicine, School of Dentistry and Division of Plastic Surgery, University of California and Cedars-Sinai Medical Center, Los Angeles, California, U.S.A.

HanJoon M. Song School of Medicine, Stanford University School of Medicine, Stanford, California, U.S.A.

Mark Stevens Department of Surgery, University of Miami, Miami, Florida, U.S.A.

Peter J. Taub New York Medical College, Valhalla, New York, U.S.A.

Seth R. Thaller University of Miami School of Medicine, Miami, Florida, U.S.A.

Lawrence Tong Mott Children's Hospital, Ann Arbor, Michigan, U.S.A.

Maria J. Troulis Department of Oral and Maxillofacial Surgery, Massachusetts General Hospital, Boston, Massachusetts, U.S.A.

Stephen M. Warren School of Medicine, Stanford University School of Medicine, Stanford, California, U.S.A.

S. Anthony Wolfe University of Miami, Miami, Florida, U.S.A.

Corinna E. Zimmermann Department of Pediatric Oral and Maxillofacial Surgery, Massachusetts General Hospital, Boston, Massachusetts, U.S.A.

FACIAL TRAUMA

1

Facial Trauma: Overview of Trauma Care

Igor Jeroukhimov, Mark Cockburn, and Stephen Cohn
University of Miami, Miami, Florida, U.S.A.

I. OVERVIEW

In the United States, trauma constitutes the third major cause of death of all age groups and the leading cause of death among persons less than 44 years old (1). Currently, more than 400 people die of injuries in the United States every day (2) and 50% of these deaths occur prior to hospital arrival. The major causes of trauma-related death are devastating injury of the central nervous system (50%) and uncontrolled hemorrhage (35%) (3). In addition to fatal injuries, 37 million people are treated in emergency departments each year, accounting for 37% of all emergency department visits; 2.6 million of these require hospitalization after injury (2). The total cost associated with injuries is estimated to be more than 250 billion dollars per year.

Satisfactory outcomes for injured patients are strongly influenced by the initial care delivered, particularly in the so-called "golden hour" following admission to the hospital emergency department (4). For some patients, this period may be only minutes (patients requiring a definitive airway), but for others, it may be measured in hours (unstable bleeding, pelvic fracture). Approximately 60% of all trauma-related hospital deaths occur during this crucial 1-h period. Inadequate assessment and resuscitation contributes to a preventable death rate of as high as 35% (5). Upon review of more than 500 patient deaths after admission to our center, 80% of those who succumbed to their injuries in the first hour after arrival did so within the first 15 min.

A schematic approach for the treatment of severely injured patients consists of triage, primary survey, resuscitation, secondary survey, monitoring, and evaluation, and transfer to definitive care (6).

The primary survey is performed to identify immediately life-threatening injuries.

1. Airway control with cervical spine protection
2. Breathing and ventilation
3. Circulation with hemorrhage control
4. Disability: neurological status
5. Exposure/environment control

The primary survey and resuscitation are performed simultaneously. The secondary survey consists of obtaining a complete history and a "head to toe" examination following the primary survey. Frequent reevaluation is performed to recognize and treat any deterioration in the patient's condition.

Although often dramatic in appearance, maxillofacial injuries by themselves are rarely life-threatening. Patients with maxillofacial injury often have significant associated injuries which confer increased mortality. These include airway obstruction, head and cervical spine injury, and cavitary organ injury with ongoing hemorrhage (7). A thorough understanding of the basic management principles of the multi-injured trauma patient is therefore essential.

II. AIRWAY MANAGEMENT IN THE TRAUMA SETTING

The first priority in treatment of the trauma patient is assessment of airway patency, adequate oxygenation, ventilation, and protection from aspiration (see Table 1). Airway compromise can occur insidiously and rapidly as a result of facial injury. The upper airway may be obstructed by the tongue or dislodged teeth. Blood, vomitus, a foreign body, or swollen tissues may also compromise the airway. If the obstruction is due to tissue laxity or posterior displacement of the tongue, a simple jaw thrust or chin lift maneuver may quickly alleviate the problem. However, if the blockage is due to a foreign body, distorted tissue, or vomited material, evacuating the airway becomes crucial.

Important information regarding previous difficult intubations; major comorbid diseases; medications; allergies; drug or alcohol use; and oropharyngeal, laryngeal, or dental diseases is not available in the trauma setting. Dysphonia, nasal or pharyngeal intonation, and other speech abnormalities noted during the initial examination may suggest either laryngeal injury or nasoethmoid or basilar skull fracture, with retropharyngeal or parapharyngeal edema (8). The subtle signs of airway compromise include agitation (hypoxia) and obtundation (hypercarbia). The use of the accessory muscles of ventilation may provide additional evidence of airway difficulties. Noisy breathing such as snoring, gurgling, and crowing sounds (stridor) may be caused by partial obstruction of the pharynx or larynx. Hoarseness (dysphonia) implies functional laryngeal obstruction. Edema and/or hematoma of the neck is a harbinger impending airway loss and should lead to early intubation.

At the scene of injury, if intubation is not necessary, the cervical spine should be immobilized. Administration of supplemental oxygen and relief of airway obstruction by manual removal or suction of mucus, blood, and debris from the mouth and oropharynx, followed by insertion of a well-lubricated oral airway. This action may allow time for the transport of injured patients to the hospital. One should remember that a nasal airway is contraindicated if midface fractures are suspected; furthermore, a forcefully placed nasal airway may cause nasal bleeding. Oral airway placement can cause retching and vomiting in the semiconscious patient. This may induce movement of the cervical spine or increased intracranial pressure lead to evacuation of intraocular contents in a patient with open-eye injury (9). The gastric emptying of trauma victims may be delayed by \pain, intoxication, or head injury (10–12), leading to an increased risk of aspiration.

A laryngeal mask airway (LMA) device may be inserted with the head secured in neutral position without use of muscle relaxants (13,14). Airway and cervical muscle tone are preserved when a secure airway is provided and right mainstem bronchus intubation can be avoided. The incidence of aspiration using the LMA during anesthesia in fastened patients is approximately two in 100,000 cases (15), but no study has demonstrated that a properly placed LMA is better protection from aspiration than bag/mask ventilation in the setting of trauma.

The most commonly used device for supporting ventilation is the bag-valve mask (BVM). BVM ventilation is extremely effective, but requires careful attention to maintain a tight mask seal, airway patency, and delivery of adequate tidal volume. The BVM device should be attached to high-flow supplemental oxygen with delivery of at least 15 L/min to avoid hypoxia. Even in skilled hands, BVM ventilation requires continuous monitoring of mask seal, airway patency, tidal volume, foreign material, and gastric insufflation. In patients with severe midface injury, a mask seal may be difficult to maintain. If adequate ventilation is unsuccessful with the BVM device, immediate intubation or surgical airway should be performed.

Table 1 Immediate Need for Definitive Airway

Suspect cervical spine injury
↓
Oxygenate/ventilate
↓
Severe maxillofacial injury
↓
Orotracheal intubation with in-line manual cervical immobilization
↓
Unable to intubate
↓
Surgical airway

III. INDICATIONS FOR INTUBATION

In spontaneously breathing patients, simple skills such as the removal of foreign bodies, airway suctioning, and chin-lift jaw-thrust maneuver can establish airway patency and restore adequate respiration. Intubation is reserved for those patients who continue to show signs of inadequate respiration after basic interventions or in those whom these interventions alone are not likely to sustain appropriate respiration (16).

A. Absolute Indications for Intubation

1. Airway obstruction unrelieved with basic interventions
2. Apnea or near apnea
3. Respiratory distress
4. Severe neurological deficit or depressed consciousness [i.e., focal deficit or Glasgow coma scale (GCS) rating less than 9] due to head trauma or any other cause

B. Urgent Indications for Intubation

1. Penetrating neck injury (with any signs of airway compromise or expanding hematoma)
2. Persistent or refractory hypotension, especially due to active hemorrhage
3. Chest wall injury with respiratory dysfunction
4. Less severe but moderate altered mentation, especially after head trauma, including both combative and mildly obtunded patients

C. Relative Indications for Nonemergent Intubation

1. Oromaxillofacial injury
2. Impending respiratory failure
3. Need for diagnostic or therapeutic procedures (e.g., computer tomography or angiography) in patients with risk for deterioration or those unable to remain motionless during the examination
4. Potential respiratory failure after sedative-analgesic use

D. Direct Orotracheal Intubation

All victims of blunt trauma undergoing urgent intubation should be regarded as having a cervical spine injury until proven otherwise. Preoxyenation should be performed in trauma patients prior to intubation. Oral endotracheal intubation with manual in-line stabilization of the cervical spine is the most rapid and reliable method to secure the airway of the apneic patient. This approach is superior to blind nasal intubation in terms of safety, success rate, time to intubation, and number of attempts required. Manual in-line stabilization of the cervical spine has been shown to significantly reduce extension and rotation of the cervical spine during laryngoscopy (17). In the optimal situation, three people are necessary to perform a successful intubation: one to perform laryngoscopy and intubation, the second to provide cervical spine immobilization, and the third to apply cricoid pressure. Suction devices should be readily available prior to an attempt at intubation whenever possible. Pharmacological agents may be given as part of an organized approach to these patients including sedatives, analgesics, and muscle relaxants.

E. Nasal Intubation

Nasal intubation is performed in a "blind" fashion and should not be used in the presence of head and neck injuries. The success rate for this procedure is significantly lower (65%), and requires more time than orotracheal intubation (18). Two cases of death from airway obstruction after nasal intubation have been reported (19). Nasal intubation can only be performed on patients who are breathing spontaneously and is therefore contraindicated in apneic patients. It is also contraindicated in those with midfacial, nasal, or basilar skull fractures. This technique is limited by operator experience and the frequent development of sinusitis after more than 48-hr duration. Nasal intubation has no advantages over oral intubation, may be technically more difficult, and should not be performed in trauma patients.

IV. SURGICAL AIRWAY

A surgical airway is required when basic interventions or intubation does not succeed (e.g., in cases of severe anatomical distortion of upper airway from middle or lower facial trauma) (16). At our center with excellent anesthesiology support services, we rarely have needed to perform a surgical airway (0.3% of trauma intubations).

A. Cricothyroidotomy

Cricothyroidotomy is the surgical airway of choice because it is simple, easy to perform, and relatively safe in the trauma setting. One must first identify anatomical landmarks (i.e., palpation of the thyroid cartilage and cricothyroid membrane). A vertical incision is made from the thyroid cartilage to the cricoid cartilage. The cricothyroid membrane is identified and a 1.5–2-cm transverse incision is made through the membrane followed by introduction of an endotracheal tube (usually size 6 mm) into the airway. The complication rate of cricothyroidotomy in the trauma setting approaches 39% (19) and includes minor hemorrhage, hypoxia secondary to prolonged procedure time, misplacement, esophageal perforation, laryngeal fracture, thyroid bleeding, and emphysema. Care must be taken to avoid lateral dissection and low incision. There are anecdotal reports that subglottic stenosis may develop after cricothyroidotomy. This has been postulated to result from prolonged insertion time resulting in ischemia or from error in surgical technique. Because of the smaller size and greater soft-tissue compliance of the pediatric airway, as well as the greater importance of the cricoid cartilage in maintaining patency of the tracheal lumen, this procedure is relatively contraindicated in pediatric trauma patients. Particularly in children 12 years old or younger, needle cricothyroidotomy with later conversion to tracheostomy is typically utilized to avoid subglottic stenosis (20).

B. Percutaneous Translaryngeal Catheter Insufflation

A large-bore (12–14 gauge) needle may be inserted into the relatively avascular cricothyroid membrane, which is located between the shield-shaped thyroid cartilage and the interiorly located ring-shaped cricoid cartilage. This can serve as a temporary measure to oxygenate a patient prior to establishing a definitive airway.

Severe hypercarbia may develop if the jet insufflation extends beyond 40 min. High-pressure or jet insufflation may lead to serious complications (subcutaneous emphysema, pneumathorax, pneumomediastinum, and neck hematoma from injured thyroid vessels) and should never be used in the trauma setting.

C. Tracheostomy

Tracheostomy is a poor choice of procedure for emergent airway control. The trachea lies deep in the neck surrounded by an extensive vascular supply and the isthmus of thyroid gland. Tracheostomy may be required in patients with acute laryngeal trauma in whom placement of a tube through the cricothyroid may complicate existing laryngeal injury.

V. AIRWAY MANAGEMENT IN THE PRESENCE OF MAXILLOFACIAL TRAUMA

Maintenance of the airway in the setting of significant maxillofacial injuries is mandatory. Death may occur from early airway obstruction, particularly in patients with mandibular fracture or combined maxillary, mandibular, and nasal fracture (21,22). When the patient is in the supine position, the "horseshoe" configuration of the mandible suspends the tongue. Loss of this suspensory arch causes the tongue to fall posteriorly and completely obstruct the airway. In addition, soft-tissue swelling around injured oronasal structures, especially when combined with decreased mentation, can result in loss of airway patency (23). Nasotracheal intubation is contraindicated because of possible midface instability and the potential that the tube will be inserted into the brain through the cranium. Swelling and hemorrhage within the hypopharynx may rarely make endotracheal intubation impossible. Under these circumstances, a surgical airway should be created to prevent asphyxia. The incidence of tracheotomies in maxillofacial injuries varies between 0.9 and 12.3% (24–26). At our center, only three surgical airways were performed in 1003 trauma patients requiring intubation during the last 2 years. Acute airway obstruction with failed endotracheal intubation or planned prolonged intubation is considered to be an indication for tracheotomy (27). Fiberscopic intubation is not routinely performed in patients with maxillofacial injury owing to the presence of blood in the upper airway limiting visibility.

VI. BREATHING AND VENTILATION

Four major pathological conditions affecting ventilation should be recognized during the primary trauma assessment: tension pneumothorax, open pneumothorax, massive hemothorax, and flail chest. Tension pneumothorax is a clinical diagnosis characterized by chest pain, signs of respiratory compromise, tachycardia, hypotension, absence of unilateral breath sounds, and later, tracheal deviation and neck vein distention. Treatment consists of immediate large-bore-needle decompression of the pleural cavity in the second intercostal space, midclavicular line followed by chest tube insertion. Open pneumothorax results from a traumatic defect of the chest wall large enough to permit air to enter into the pleural cavity. If the opening in the chest wall exceeds two-thirds the diameter of the trachea, air passes preferentially through the chest defect with every respiratory effort; the so-called "sucking chest wound." Initial management includes prompt occlusion of the wound with a large dressing, overlapping the wound's edges, and taping securely on three sides to provide a flutter-type valve effect. A chest tube should be placed remote from the wound. In patients with a flail-chest injury, an unstable segment of the normally rigid chest wall moves "paradoxically," in an opposite direction from the rest of the thoracic cage during the respiratory cycle. While a relatively unusual injury seen in 5–13% of the patients with chest trauma (28,29), flail chest is a marker for other significant injuries, specifically underlying lung contusion. Pulmonary contusion accompanies about one half of flail-chest injuries and appears to be the major cause of hypoxia in these patients. Diagnosis of flail chest is based on clinical findings of a paradoxically moving segment of the chest wall accompanied by rib crepitus and local pain, and is confirmed with chest x-ray. More than 70% of patients with flail chest have pneumothorax and/or hemothorax (30,31). Massive hemothorax results from the rapid accumulation of more than 1500 mL of blood in the pleural cavity. Clinically, massive hemothorax is usually associated with symptoms of hypovolemic shock, absent breath sounds, and dullness to percussion over the hemothorax. Treatment consists of simultaneous decompression of the involved pleural cavity and restoration of circulating blood volume.

VII. ASSESSMENT OF CIRCULATORY STATUS AND HEMORRHAGE CONTROL

After proper airway control and respiratory management, initial assessment of the circulatory status is required. The initial diagnosis of shock (inadequate delivery of oxygen to the tissues) is based on clinical signs, not laboratory data. Signs of hypoperfusion lead to immediate investigation into the source of blood loss. Most trauma patients in shock are experiencing bleeding resulting in hypovolemia. Rarely these patients may present to the hospital after trauma with neurogenic, cardiogenic, or even septic shock. Organ hypoperfusion does not result from isolated brain injury but can result from spinal cord injury, resulting in the loss of sympathetic tone. Cardiogenic shock may rarely result from direct myocardial injury, but more likely from an acute ischemic event. Septic shock is very unusual except in patients whose arrival has been delayed for many hours or days.

Hemorrhage is therefore the most common cause of shock in trauma patients. Thirty-five percent of all trauma-related deaths in the prehospital setting occur from uncontrolled hemorrhage. Profound hemorrhagic shock can be easily recognized because of obvious signs of inadequate perfusion of the central nervous system, skin, and kidneys. Hypotension is not manifested until more than 25% of the blood volume (20 mL/kg body weight (BW) or 1500 mL in a 70-kg patient) is lost. Therefore, subtle signs of occult hemorrhage such as agitation and mild increase of heart rate should be recognized as possible early signs of blood loss. Base deficit should be assessed with arterial blood gas analysis upon arrival and serially to aid in the diagnosis of metabolic acidosis secondary to hypovolemia. Two large-bore venous catheters should be placed to achieve efficacious access for fluid resuscitation.

The patient's response to initial fluid resuscitation is the key determinant guiding further therapy. A rough guideline of the total amount required for crystalloid resuscitation is to replace every milliliter of blood lost with 3 mL of crystalloid fluid, thus allowing replenishment of plasma volume and accounting for loss to the interstitial and intracellular spaces. The decision to start the infusion of blood is based on the patient's failure to respond to the initial fluid bolus. The primary purpose of blood administration is to provide additional oxygen-carrying capacity and to restore circulating volume. Fully cross-matched blood is preferred, but cross matching requires 45 min to complete. Type-specific blood can be provided within 10 min and this blood is compatible with ABO and Rh blood types. When type-specific blood is unavailable, type O packed red blood cells are utilized for unstable patients with life-threatening hemorrhage. Thus, the initial management goals in the care of the trauma victim with hemorrhagic shock include identification of the source of bleeding, achieving hemostasis, and resuscitation. Significant hemorrhage in a trauma patient may occur at multiple locations including: external bleeding; intracavitary hemorrhage into the pleural space or peritoneal cavity; bleeding into muscle and subcutaneous tissue from contusions and fractures; and bleeding into the retroperitoneum.

External hemorrhage from wounds is usually obvious and can be controlled by direct pressure. Sometimes bleeding from extremity wounds must be controlled by application of a tourniquet. Tourniquet time longer than 1 h should be avoided. External bleeding from lacerations (e.g., scalp) or vascular injuries may be quiescent until blood volume is restored.

Bleeding into the pleural cavity from large vessels like the aorta or pulmonary vessels is universally fatal. Bleeding from smaller vessels (intercostals or internal mammary) or from the lung's parenchyma can produce a hemothorax, which can be easily diagnosed by clinical examination and chest x-ray. Less than 10% of patients with traumatic hemothorax require thoracotomy. The remainder can be treated by thoracostomy tube drainage alone.

Substantial intra-abdominal blood loss can occur without obvious clinical signs. Hemoperitoneum may be easily diagnosed by abdominal ultrasonography or diagnostic peritoneal lavage. Only stable patients are able to undergo abdominal computed tomography (CT). Patients in shock with hemoperitoneum require urgent laparotomy.

The amount of blood loss into extremities or muscle layers of the torso is frequently underestimated (32–33). The blood loss from a femoral shaft fracture may reach 1–2 L. Pelvic fractures, renal injuries, and disruption of lumbar vessels might be the source of severe -retroperitoneal injury. Patients in shock with suspected arterial bleeding from a pelvic fracture should have diagnostic CT-angiography followed by angiographic embolization of the bleeding vessel.

Reassessment of the adequacy of resuscitation is essential to prevent organ dysfunction. Persistence of significant base deficits, uncorrectable lactic acidosis, and oliguria are all indicators of inadequate resuscitation. The initial goal in volume resuscitation should be restoration of organ perfusion rather than increased blood pressure. Serial examinations should be performed to identify evidence of ongoing hemorrhage, such as hypothermia, coagulopathy, and metabolic acidosis. Patients must be maintained in a warm environment and all infused solutions heated to 39°C before administration. Transfusion of coagulation factors, fresh-frozen plasma, and platelets is guided by clinical coagulation status supplemented by laboratory tests. Certainly, all efforts should be directed toward controlling hemorrhage rather than treating its complications.

VIII. LIFE-THREATENING BLEEDING FOLLOWING MAXILLOFACIAL TRAUMA

Life-threatening bleeding following maxillofacial trauma is rarely related exclusively to facial injuries. The occurrence of severe bleeding from facial trauma is found in 1–11% of patients (34–36). The origin of bleeding is complex because the vascular supply of the face involves branches of both internal and external carotid arteries. In addition, several anastomoses exist between the external and internal carotid branches. Traumatic facial bleeding originates from both hard-soft-tissue sources, adding to the difficulty of determining the exact source of bleeding (36). The origin of bleeding in maxillofacial trauma is usually the internal maxillary artery and its intraosseous branches. The course of the maxillary artery passes within the borders of common complex facial fractures. In addition, branches of the external carotid artery, such as the lacrimal, zygomatic, and ethmoidal arteries, may play a major role in the origin of bleeding (27).

Different methods for the control of bleeding of maxillofacial in origin have been described. Rapid resuscitation followed by posterior nasal packing is sufficient to control most bleeding. Immediate reduction of fractures is mandatory to control bleeding from the intraosseous branches. Ligation of the external carotid artery has been suggested, but this procedure is rarely successful owing to the collateral blood supply. Angiography with selective embolization of bleeding vessels is often helpful (37–39).

IX. ASSESSMENT OF NEUROLOGICAL STATUS (DISABILITY)

A rapid neurological assessment is performed as a part of the primary trauma survey. Level of consciousness, pupillary size and reactivity, and motor response are evaluated. Alcohol and other drugs may impact on the sensorium. Injury to the central nervous system must be excluded as a primary reason for neurological changes concurrent with the restoration of oxygenation and circulation. Hypoxemia and hypovolemia (secondary insults) worsen the morbidity and mortality associated with brain injury. Patients with severe head injury (GCS < 9) should undergo immediate intubation with mechanical ventilation irrespective of respiratory status at that time. As clinical examination of the abdomen in patients with severe brain injury is not possible, abdominal ultrasound or diagnostic peritoneal lavage should be performed in the early stages of management of the hypotensive patient with apparent brain injury.

Completion of the neurological examination is performed during the secondary survey and serial evaluations of the level of consciousness are mandatory. We perform a brain CT scan in every patient with known loss of consciousness, a GCS score of less than 15, or evidence of injury above the clavicles. Even using these strict criteria, the positive CT scan rate has been shown to be as low as 6% (40,41). The incidence of brain injury in patients with maxillofacial trauma varies from 15 to 48% (42). The risk of serious brain injury is particularly high with upper facial injury.

X. CERVICAL SPINE

Cervical spine injuries occur in 1.5–3% of blunt trauma victims, 25–75% of which are unstable (43–45). Patients with clinically significant head trauma may have a greater risk of cervical spine injury (4.9 vs. 1.1% without head injury), and the incidence increases to 7.8% in trauma victims with a GCS score less than 8 (46). Neurological deficit is present in 30–70% of patients with a significant cervical spine fracture and is most commonly associated with fracture dislocation of C5–C7 (47). Below the level of C5, the vertebral canal is narrower and bilateral facet dislocation and wedge fractures can result in subluxation of over 50% of vertebral bodies with spinal canal or cord injury. The diagnostic sensitivity of the combination of cross-table lateral, anteroposterior, and odontoid radiographs of the cervical spine is 92%; however, 7–20% of all cervical spinal injuries occur at the level of C7–T1 (48). The optimal visualization of these vertebrae may be difficult to obtain despite shoulder retraction (swimmer's view) and the use of cervical spine CT scan, which may be needed to rule out cervical spine injury (49). Despite widespread use of cervical-spine immobilization, delay in the diagnosis of spine fractures still occurs in 10–14% of patients. In patients with unrecognized injuries, secondary neurological injury is 7.5 times greater than in patients in whom cervical injury is recognized early (50–51). For that reason, during tracheal intubation, all trauma patients should be managed as if they had a cervical spine injury. We have added a cervical-spine CT scan to every head CT scan performed (which is required in all patients with significant maxillofacial injury). This procedure adds little time or cost and we feel that it improves accuracy and early identification of injuries in complex patients.

Patients with injuries usually arrive to the hospital with spine protection in place, including cervical collar and spinal board. These protective devices should not be removed before injury to the spine is excluded clinically or radiographically. Multicenter studies have confirmed a very low probability of cervical-spine injury if the patient meets none of the five following clinical criteria: midline cervical tenderness, focal neurological deficit, altered sensorium, painful injury, or distracting injury (sensitivity 99%, negative predictive value 99.8%) (61). Patients who meet one of the criteria should undergo radiological tests to exclude injury of the spine.

Maxillofacial trauma is often associated with cervical spine injury. The incidence of cervical spine fracture varies from 2 to 6% (52,53). Spinal injuries associated with mandibular fractures typically involve the first or second cervical vertebra, whereas middle or upper facial trauma typically is associated with injuries of the lower cervical spine (54). Prompt diagnosis of cervical-spine injury in patients with maxillofacial trauma is imperative for two reasons. First, the presence of cervical trauma in association with maxillofacial injury makes airway management more difficult. Second, traditional methods of treatment for maxillofacial trauma may require specific alterations in management related to the care of specific cervical-spine fractures and associated neurological compromise (55,56).

XI. COMPLETION OF ASSESSMENT AND MANAGEMENT OF THE TRAUMA PATIENT

Reassessment of vital signs, complete history of the mechanism of injury, past medical history, and a meticulous head-to-toe examination must be obtained in every trauma victim following an appropriate response to the initial resuscitation. Every trauma patient should be treated as if he has a "full stomach." Nasogastric or orogastric tubes should be used for stomach decompression in all patients with an altered level of consciousness, who require intubation, or who have associated abdominal injuries.

Baseline laboratory tests should include only an arterial blood gas with hematocrit and a type and cross matching. Other laboratory tests are not useful in the typical trauma victim. Base deficit obtained as a part of blood gas analysis has considerable clinical significance. The magnitude of a metabolic acidosis has prognostic value (57). In patients with a normal GCS, mortality exceeds 50% if base deficit is more than 20 (58–60). A persistent metabolic acidosis reflects a state of ongoing hypoperfusion.

XII. RADIOLOGICAL EVALUATION

The two diagnostic radiological studies that must be performed early in the care of the trauma patient with significant blunt trauma are the anteroposterior view of the chest and pelvis. Abdominal ultrasound has proved to be very sensitive in determining intraperitoneal as well as intrapericardiac fluid and has almost replaced the diagnostic peritoneal lavage (62–64). The limitations of ultrasound include its low sensitivity in detecting retroperitoneal injuries or hollow-viscus injuries in the early stages of trauma when no intraperitoneal fluid exists. Lavage is more sensitive in detecting hollow-viscus injury and diaphragmatic injuries than ultrasound but it is more time consuming, requires special equipment and surgical skill, and has an approximately 1% major complication rate.

CT scanning is an extremely helpful diagnostic method, particularly for assessing solid-organ injury and retroperitoneal injury. Organ injury scales based on CT findings combined with the patient's clinical condition permit safe, nonoperative management of some injuries. The presence of vascular "blush" (area of increased enhancement) in solid organs or pelvic vessels diagnosed by CT may be controlled by angiographic embolization. CT provides sufficient information about injuries to retroperitoneal organs (pancreas, adrenals, kidneys, and retroperitoneal parts of the colon and duodenum). It is also very sensitive for the diagnosis of spine and pelvic fractures. There are two major limitations of CT scanning in trauma patients. First, unstable patients cannot be transferred to the CT room, and second, the diagnosis of hollow-viscus injury lacks reliability.

The role of interventional radiology in the management of trauma patients is currently evolving. Spiral CT-angiography has largely replaced conventional angiography in many trauma centers; however, diagnostic angiography is still the procedure of choice in many hospitals around the world. The angiographic signs of hemorrhage or vascular injury include: (1) extravasation of contrast; (2) outpouching of the arterial wall that contains contrast, which represents the rupture of the intima and media but not adventitia of the vascular wall (pseudoaneurysm); (3) abrupt cutoff of a vessel; and (4) arteriovenous fistula, seen as an early filling of the venous system from an injured arterial wall. Angiography is not only an extremely sensitive diagnostic test, but can also be an excellent treatment modality. Different embolic materials are used for bleeding control in trauma patients with a high success rate. Angioplasty and stent placement can also be appropriate in the trauma patient. Partial occlusion or flow-limiting dissection in situations where surgical repair is not feasible may be managed by placement of an intravascular stent with improvement of blood flow. Other imaging modalities such as magnetic resonance imaging are still under investigation and are not routinely used in the acute-trauma setting.

XIII. CONCLUSION

In summary, the critical importance of establishing a definitive airway and maintaining adequate respiratory function and circulation cannot be understated. The recognition that traumatic brain injuries account for 50% of trauma-related deaths is key. Secondary hypoxic and, more importantly, hypotensive insults must be avoided. The various diagnostic modalities that help in identifying injuries to the head, chest, abdomen, and pelvis must be utilized in a rapid and efficient manner while observing the patient's response to resuscitation. Finally, those patients who become hemodynamically unstable or fail to respond to resuscitation belong either in the operating room (intracavitary bleeding) or in the angiography suite (bleeding from pelvic fracture).

REFERENCES

1. Fingerhut LA, Warner M. Injury chartbook. Health, United States, 1996–97, Hyattsville, MD, National Center for Health Statistics, 1997.
2. MacKenzie EJ, Fowler CJ. Epidemiology. In: Mattox KL, Feliciano DV, Moore EE, eds. Trauma. New York: McGraw-Hill, 2000:2:22.
3. Sauaia A, Moore FA, Moore EE, Moser KS, Brennan R, Read RA, Pons PT. Epidemiology of trauma deaths: a reassessment. J Trauma 1995; 38(2):185–193.
4. Trunkey DD. Trauma Sci Am 1983; 249:28.
5. Cales RH, Trunkey DD. Preventable trauma deaths: a review of trauma system development. JAMA 1985; 254(8):1059–1063.
6. American College of Surgeons Committee on Trauma. Resources for the Optimal Care of the Injured Patient. Chicago: American College of Surgeons, 1993.
7. Gwynn PP, Carraway JH, Horton CE et al. Facial fractures-Associated injuries and complications. Plast Reconstr Surg 1971; 47:225.
8. Nicolaou D, Kelen GD. Airway management for the trauma patient. In: Cameron JL, ed. Current Surgical Therapy. St. Louis: Mosby, 1998:911–917.
9. Robinson JS, Muddler DS. Airway control. In: Mattox KL, Feliciano DV, Moore EE, Trauma. New York: McGraw-Hill, 2000:173–188.
10. Simpson KH, Stakes AF. Effect of anxiety on gastric empting in preoperative patients. Br J Anaest 1987; 59(5):540–544.
11. Kao CH, ChangLai SP, Chieng PU, Yen TC. Gastric empting in head-injured patients. Am J Gastroenterol 1998; 93(7):1108–1112.
12. Zaricznyj B, Rockwood CA Jr, O'Donoghue DH, Ridings GR. Relationship between trauma to the extremities and stomach motility. J Trauma 1977; 17:920.
13. Pennant JH, Pace NA, Gajraj NM. Role of laryngeal mask airway in the immobile cervical spine. J Clin Anesth 1993; 5(3):226–230.
14. Logan A. Use of laryngeal mask in a patient with unstable fracture of cervical spine. Anaesthesia 1991; 46:987.
15. Berry A, Brimacombe J. Risk of aspiration with the laryngeal mask. Br J anaesth 1994; 73(4):565–566.
16. Vukmir RB, Rinnert KJ, Krugh JW. Trauma airway management. In: Peitzman AB, Schwab CW, Yealy DM, eds. The Trauma Manual. Philadelphia: Lippincott-Raven, 1998:91.
17. Majernick TG, Bieniek R, Houston JB, Hughes HG. Cervical spine movement during orotracheal intubation. Ann Emerg Med 1986; 15(4):417–420.
18. Shearer VE, Giesecke AH. Airway management for patients with penetrating neck trauma: a retrospective study. Anesth Analg 1993; 77(6):1135–1138.
19. Standards and guidelines for cardiopulmonary resuscitation (CPR) and emergency cardiac care (ECC). JAMA 1980; 244:453.
20. Brantigan CO, Grow JB Sr. Subglottic stenosis after cricothyroidotomy. Surgery 1982; 91(2):217–221.
21. Manson PN. Some thoughts on the classification and treatment of Le Fort fractures. Ann Plast Surg 1986; 17(5):356–363.

22. Gruss JS. Complex craniomaxillofacial trauma: evolving concepts in management: a trauma unit's experience. J Trauma-Injury Infect Crit Care 1990; 30(4):377–383.
23. Seyfer AE, Hansen JE. Facial trauma. In: Mattox KL, Feliciano DV, Moore EE, eds. Trauma. New York: McGraw-Hill; 2000:415–435.
24. Schultz RC. Facial injuries from automobile accidents: a study of 400 consecutive cases. Plast Reconstruct Surg 1967; 40(5):415–425.
25. Markowitz BL, Manson PN, Sargent L, Vander Kolk CA, Yaremchuk M, Glassman D, Crawley WA. Management of the medial canthal tendon in nasoethmoid orbital fractures: the importance of the central fragment in classification and treatment. Plast Reconstruct Surg 1991; 87(5):843–853.
26. Manson PN, Ruas EJ, Iliff NT. Deep orbital reconstruction for correction of posttraumatic enophthalmos. Clin Plast Surg 1987; 14(1):113–121.
27. Ardekian L, Rosen D, Klein Y, Peled M, Michaelson M, Laufer D. Life-threatening complications and irreversible damage following maxillofacial trauma. Injury 1998; 29(4):253–256.
28. Nakayama DK, Ramenofsky ML, Rowe MI. Chest injuries in childhood. Ann Surg 1989; 210(6):770–775.
29. LoCicero J, Mattox KL. Epidemiology of chest trauma. Surg Clin North Am 1989; 69:15.
30. Ciraulo DL, Elliott D, Mitchell KA, Rodriguez A. Flail chest as a marker for significant injuries. J Am Coll Surg 1994; 178(5):466–470.
31. Freedland M, Wilson RF, Bender JS, Levison MA. The management of flail chest injury: factors affecting outcome. J Trauma-Injury Infect Crit Care 1990; 30(12):1460–1468.
32. Pedowitz RA, Shackford SR. Non-cavitary hemorrhage producing shock in trauma patients: incidence and severity. J Trauma-Injury Infect Crit Care 1989; 29(2):219–222.
33. Mullins R. Management of shock. Mattox KL, Feliciano DV, Moore EE, eds. Trauma. New York: McGraw-Hill; 2000:212.
34. Frable MA, El-Roman N, Lenis A, Hung JP. Hemorrhagic complications of facial fractures. Laryngoscope 1974; 84(11):2051–2057.
35. Gwyn PP, Carraway JH, Horton CE, Adamson JE, Mladick RA. Facial fractures—associated injuries and complications. Plast Reconstruct Surg 1971; 47(3):225–230.
36. Ardekian L, Samet N, Shoshani Y, Taicher S. Life-threatening bleeding following maxillofacial trauma. J Cranio-Maxillo-Facial Surg 1993; 21(8):336–338.
37. Solomons NB, Blumgart R. Severe late onset epistaxis following Lefort I osteotomy: angiographic localization and embolization. J Laryngol Otol 1988; 102:260.
38. Olley SF. An aid to rapid nasal and post-nasal packing. Br J Oral Surg 1978; 16(2):179–182.
39. Cooke ET. An evaluation and clinical study of severe epistaxis treated by arterial legation. J Laryngol Otol 1985; 99(8):745–749.
40. Haydel MJ, Preston CA, Mills TJ, Luber S, Blaudeau E, DeBlieux PM. Indications for computed tomography in patients with minor head injury. N Engl J Med. 2000; 343(2):100–105.

41. Miller EC, Holmes JF, Derlet RW. Utilizing clinical factors to reduce head CT scan ordering for minor head trauma patients. J Emerg Med 1997; 15(4):453–457.
42. Miller EC, Derlet RW, Kinser D. Minor head trauma: is computed tomography always necessary?. Ann Emerg Med 1996; 27(3):290–294.
43. O'Malley KF, Ross SE. The incidence of injury to the cervical spine in patients with craniocerebral injury. J Trauma 1988; 28(10):1476–1478.
44. Ross SE, Schwab CW, David ET, Delong WG, Born CT. Clearing the cervical spine: initial radiologic evaluation. J Trauma 1987; 27(9):1055–1060.
45. Bayless P, Ray VG. Incidence of cervical spine injuries in association with blunt head trauma. Am J Emerg Med 1989; 7(2):139–142.
46. Hills MW, Deane SA. Head injury and facial injury: is there an increased risk of cervical spine injury? J Trauma 34(4):549–553; discussion 553–554, 1993.
47. Black P. Injuries of the spine and spinal cord: management in the acute phase. In: Zuidema G, Rutherford R, Ballinger W, eds. The Management of Traumas. Philadelphia: WB Saunders, 1979; :226–253.
48. Nichols CG, Young DH, Schiller WR. Evaluation of cervicothoracic junction injury. Ann Emerg Medic 1987; 16(6):640–642.
49. Woodring JH, Lee C. Limitation of cervical radiography in the evaluation of acute cervical trauma. J Trauma 1993; 34(1):32–39.
50. Rosen P, Wolfe RE. Therapeutic legends of emergency medicine. J Emerg Med 1989; 7(4):387–384.
51. Reid DC, Henderson R, Saboe L, Miller JD. Etiology and clinical course of missed spine fractures. J Trauma 1987; 27(9):980–986.
52. Merritt RM, Bent JP, Porubsky ES. Acute laryngeal trauma in pediatric population. Ann Otol Rhinol Laryngol 1998; 107(2):104–106.
53. McCabe JB, Angelos MG. Injury to the head and face in patients with cervical spine injury. Am J Emerg Med 1984; 2(4):333–335.
54. Lewis VL, Manson PN, Morgan RF, Cerullo LJ, Meyer PR. Facial injuries associated with cervical fractures: recognition, pattern and management. J Trauma 1985; 25(1):90–93.
55. Haug RH, Wible RT, Likavec MJ, Conforti PJ. Cervical spine fractures and maxillofacial trauma. J Oral maxillofacial Surg 1991; 49(7):725–729.
56. Ardekian L, Gaspar R, Peled M et al. Incidence and type of cervical spine injuries associated with mandibular fractures. J Cranio-Maxillofacial Trauma 1997; 3:18.
57. Siegel JH, Rivkind AI, Dalal S, Goodarzi S. Early physiologic predictors of injury severity and death in blunt multiple trauma. Arch Surg 1990; 125(4):498–508.
58. Rutherford EJ, Morris JA Jr, Reed GW, Hall KS. Base deficit stratifies mortality and determines therapy. J Trauma-Injury Infect Crit Care 1992; 33(3):417–423.
59. Davis JW, Parks SN, Kaups KL, Gladen HE, O'Donnell-Nicol S. Admission base deficit predicts transfusion requirements and risk of complications. J Trauma 1996; 41(5):769–774.

60. Mizock BA, Falk JL. Lactic acidosis in critical illness. Crit Care Med 1992; 20(1):80–93.
61. Hoffman JR, Mower WR, Wolfson AB, Todd KH, Zucker MI. Validity of a set of clinical criteria to rule out injury to the cervical spine in patients with blunt trauma. National Emergency X-Radiography Utilization Study Group. N Engl J Med 2000; 343(2):94–99.
62. Rozycki GS, Ochsner MG, Schmidt JA, Frankel HL, Davis TP, Wang D, Champion HR. A prospective study of surgeon-performed ultrasound as the primary adjuvant modality for injured patient assessment. J Trauma 1995; 39(3):492–498.
63. Dolich MO, McKenney MG, Varela JE, Compton RP, McKenney KL, Cohn SM. 2,576 ultrasounds for blunt abdominal trauma. J Trauma 2001; 50(1):108–112.
64. McKenney KL, McKenney MG, Cohn SM, Compton R, Nunez DB, Dolich M, Namias N. Hemoperitoneum score helps determine need for therapeutic laparotomy. J Trauma 2001; 50(4):650–654.

2

Microsurgical Options in Facial Trauma

Milton B. Armstrong
University of Miami, Miami, Florida, U.S.A.

I. INTRODUCTION

Facial injuries are commonplace in today's society. Motor vehicle accidents, accidental injuries, and falls (1) comprise the majority of causes for complex facial wounds. Basic trauma principles are utilized during initial stabilization of patients. This requires careful airway management, cervical spine stabilization, and evaluation of concomitant injuries. With complex wounds of the head and face neurological, craniomaxillofacial, and vascular injuries have to be managed in a systematic fashion. All traumatic facial injuries require readiographic assessment, usually in the form of computed tomography (2,3). After completion of these preliminary portions of the patient's management, definitive surgical care can then be addressed. The following discussion will be limited to treatment of large defects of soft tissue and bone requiring microsurgical intervention.

II. SCALP/SKULL

Loss of larger portions of the scalp (greater than one quarter) often requires complex reconstruction. The loss of this significant an amount of soft tissue will require the addition of distant tissues. The majority of large scalp defects are the result of extirpation of cutaneous carcinomas as seen in multiple studies (4–8). The latissimus dorsi and rectus abdominis muscle flaps have proven to be great adjuncts in reconstruction of large scalp defects (4–7), as have scapular cutaneous flaps with or without bone for composite defects (8). The muscle will cover defects up to $490\,cm^2$ (5). For scalp defects, the flap is best utilized as a muscle-only flap with a skin graft to the surface. Myocutaneous flaps tend to have too much bulk for the scalp (4,5). The muscle can be debulked at the time of inset to improve the contour. Muscle atrophy combined with skin graft construction, typically leads to an acceptable contour.

The latissimus dorsi and rectus flaps are relatively easy to dissect and have large-caliber blood vessels for microsurgery (usually greater than 2 mm in size). The omentum can also be used to cover large soft-tissue defects of the scalp (9,5); however, the added morbidity of an intraperitoneal incision with its concomitant risk of complications makes this a less attractive option in most situations. Scalp avulsions, alone, with intact vascular pedicles may be replanted with good outcomes (10).

In situations in which microsurgical reconstruction of large scalp defects is performed with the latissimus dorsi muscle flap, the superficial temporal vessels are most commonly used for anastomosis (4,5). Other vessels, such as the occipital arteries and the larger carotid and jugular vessels, are also good options depending on the anatomical requirements for the reconstruction.

III. UPPER AND MIDFACE

Upper and midfacial defects requiring free tissue transfers generally are devastating injuries with loss of contents from skull and scalp, orbital and nasal elements. Tumor ablation with loss of orbital contents, palate, and nasopharynx often requires 5 complex reconstructions (8,11,12), but can also be seen with massive trauma (8). The important principle to adhere to is separation of the perinasal sinuses from the central nervous system and ablation of dead space.

Orbital defects are a combination of loss of the globe and bony support. Again, this situation is more commonly seen in cases of resection for a malignant process, but can be seen in major trauma. The rectus abdominis muscle or myocutaneous flap are useful options for this type of reconstruction (11). The muscle flap provides adequate bulk to fill the space while the myocutaneous flap provides a skin paddle that can be used for external skin coverage (11).

Other flaps include latissimus dorsi muscle, latissimus dorsi myocutaneous and osteomyocutaneous flaps, the scapular cutaneous flap, and the scapular osteocutaneous flap. These combination flaps are bulky enough to fill extensive dead space and provide bone support for the orbital floors and palate.

IV. LOWER FACE MANDIBLE

Facial defects of the lower face, particularly of the mandible, are usually the result of penetrating trauma. These patients have generally suffered gunshot wounds to the face, most being self-inflicted (14). Shotguns are commonly used for suicide attempts. Because of the combination of wide distribution of shotgun pellets, close-range injury, and expanding gases at the site of the blast, the wound is extensive (14). Pellets tend to tract deep into the wound, necessitating aggressive debridement to remove contaminants (14,15). Large-caliber pistol injuries may also create larger, more complex facial wounds, nearly as destructive as shotgun wounds (16).

Shotgun wounds generally correspond to four patterns best classified by regional tissue loss. The four patterns are (1) the lateral mandible (34%), (2) the central face (26%), the lateral midface and orbit (28%), and the lateral cranium and orbit (17). Lower facial distribution was more common as a result of suicide attempts in 76% of patients sustaining gunshot wounds in study by Clark et al. (17). The placement of the muzzle of the gun helps in defining the nature of the soft-tissue injury. Muzzles placed below the mandible tend to create devastating mandibular bone and soft-tissue losses. The patient usually also has a variety of oronasal and orbital injuries, as a result of the angle of the muzzle in the mouth. In a study of 27 patients over a 10-year period, one third of the patients lost at least one eye from the blast injury (14).

Treatment for these devastating injuries always beings with the ABC's of trauma care, with particular attention being paid to airway management (18) and evaluation of cervical spine problems. Radiographic studies are needed after airway stabilization. These include plain roentgenographs to show extent and severity of injury such as projectiles and bone fragments, chest radiographs to detect aspiration, and computer tomography (CT), which shows intracranial damage and gives an accurate assessment of fractures and bony defects of the face (14,18).

Clark et al. present a comprehensive discussion of classification and an algorithm for treatment of high-energy ballistic and avulsive facial injuries. Their 17-year experience with 250 gunshot wounds and 53 shotgun wounds shows four general anatomical patterns for gunshot and shotgun wounds. They also separate the injuries into four general anatomical zones: the cranium, the orbit and upper midface, the lower midface, and the mandible.

Complications involving the skin and bone were minimal in the cranium and upper midface in the series. Comminuted mandible fractures, however, had 35% of patients with complications for immediate reconstruction (17). These included sepsis, persistent fistula, or wound breakdown requiring bone debridement.

The lower facial defects are complex and can consist of loss of mandibular segments, parts of the lip, anterior parts of the mouth base, and tongue (13). Providing adequate soft-tissue coverage and providing bony support are the key principles for reconstruction (16). Free tissue transfers for soft-tissue replacement is frequently necessary and can be accomplished with various flaps. The radial forearm flap is a versatile flap for intraoral and moderate-sized external defects and has proven useful for these complex problems (14,19). Other soft-tissue flaps may provide healthy, vascularized tissue with varying amounts of bulk for reconstruction of these facial defects. These flaps include the free scapular flap (8), the rectus abdominis myocutaneous free flap (11), the latissimus dorsi myocutaneous flap (7,14,23), the serratus free flap (7), and in limited case the omental free flap (9).

Loss of portions of the mandible will require reconstruction using a combination to plate fixation with bone grafts or vascularized bone flaps. The size and location of the missing bone segment(s) determine the need for bone graft versus bone flap for these complicated situations. Small defects of the mandible, less than 4 cm, may be amenable to plate reconstruction with bone grafts (14). Lateral defects may also have reasonably good reconstruction using plate fixation alone: adequate soft tissues are available to cover the plate (20). Most mandibular defects resulting from gunshot wounds, however, require vascularized bone flaps (4,16,17). Vascularized bone flaps available for mandibular reconstruction include: iliac crest (20), scapula (8), radius (21) and fibula (14,20). The fibula is by far the most versatile flap because of its abundant bone stock for placement of osteointegrated implants and its significant length. The fibula can be used to reconstruct the entire mandible from condyle to condyle (22). It can also carry a small to moderate sized skin paddle to aid in repair of some floor-of-the-mouth defects and lower-lip or chin skin losses. Blood supply to the fibula comes from the peroneal artery with perforators through the intermuscular septum or direct cutaneous branches that supply the skin paddle; 241/2 to 26 cm of bone (21) can be safely harvested for reconstructive purposes. Care should be taken to preserve ankle stability by leaving the distal 61/2 to 8 cm of bone. The proximal osteotomy should be approximately 8 cm distal to the fibular head to minimize risk to the superficial peroneal nerve. Multiple osteotomies can be performed in the bone for shaping, as long as the soleus muscle cuff with periosteum is preserved (21).

Table 1 Flaps Used to Reconstruct Facial Trauma

Flap	Blood supply	Tissue type
Latissimus dorsi	Thoracodorsal artery/vein	Muscle/musculocutaneous/ osteomyoctaneous
Rectus abdominis	Deep inferior epigastric artery/vein	Muscle or musculocultaneous
Scapula/parascapular	Subscapular artery/ circumflex scapular/ vein	Cutaneous or osteocutaneous
Radial forearm	Radial artery/vena comitantes or cutaneous veins	Cutaneous or osteocutaneous
Fibula	Peroneal artery/vein	Osseous or osteocutaneous

Staged sequential reconstruction of these complex scalp through lower-face defects has been replaced by earlier, more comprehensive replacement of missing tissues with free-tissue transplants of missing structures. Single-tissue replacements, such as skin-free flaps, can be used for soft-tissue-only losses versus composites of skin, muscle, and/or bone for more complicated wounds. Early reconstruction with free flaps appear to lessen the amount of distortion by limiting scar contraction. It also allows these patients to get back to work and school faster owing to the ability to promote more rapid dental restoration and other prosthetics onto stable frameworks. Overall, early reconstruction with free-tissue transplants save time and money as well as providing a more aesthetic and stable result.

REFERENCES

1. Sastry SM, Santry CM, Paul SK, et al. Leading causes of facial trauma in the major trauma outcome study. Plast Reconstruct Surg 1995; 95:196–197.
2. Rohrich RJ, Shewmake KB. Evolving concepts of craniomaxillofacial fracture management. Clin Plast Surg 1992; 19:1–10.
3. Levine RS, Grossman RI. Head and Facial Trauma. Symposium on emergency department radiology. Emerg Med Clini North Am 1985; 3(3):447–473.
4. Ford Jones N, Hardesty RA, Swartz WM, Ramasastry SS, Heckler FR, Newton ED. Extensive and complex defects of the scalp, middle third of the face, and palate: The role of microsurgical reconstruction. Plast Reconstruct. Surg 1988; 82(6):937–950.
5. Pennigton DG, Stern, HS, Lee KK. Free-flap reconstruction of large defects of the scalp and calvarium. Plastic and Reconstructive Surgery April 1989; 83(4):655–661.

6. Borah GL, Hidalgo DA, Wey PD. Reconstruction of extensive scalp defects with rectus free flaps. Ann Plast Surg 1995; 34(3):281–287.
7. Furnas H, Lineaweaver WC, Alpert B, Buncke HJ. Scalp reconstruction by microvascular free tissue transfer. Ann Plas Surg 1990; 24(5):431–436.
8. Robb GL. Free scapular flap reconstruction of the head and neck. Clini Plast Surg 1990; 24(5):431–443.
9. Irons GB, Witzke, DJ, Arnold PG, Wood MD. Use of the omental free flap for soft-tissue reconstruction. Ann Plast Surg 1983; 11(6).
10. Juri J, Irigaray A, Zeaiter C. Reimplanation of scalp, Case Report: Juri et al: Reimplantation of Scalp. Ann Plast Surg 1990; 24(4):354–361.
11. Kroll SS, Reece GP. Aesthetically successful mandibular reconstruction with a single reconstruction plate. Clini Plast Surg 2001; 28(2):273–282.
12. Funk GF, Laurenzo JF, Valentino J, McCulloch TM, Frodel JL, Hoffman HT. Free-tissue transfer reconstruction of midfacial and cranioorbito-facial defects. Arch Otolaryngol Head Neck Surg 1995; 121:293–303.
13. Burt JD, Burns AJ, Muzaffar AR, Byrd S, Hobar PC, Beran SJ, Adams WP, Kenkel JM. Total soft tissue reconstruction of the middle and lower face with multiple simultaneous free flaps in a pediatric patient. Plast Reconstruct Surg 2000; 105(7):2440–2447.
14. Suominen E, Tukianinen E. Close-range shotgun and rifle injuries to the face. Clini Plast Surg 2001; 28(2):323–337.
15. Frensilli, JA, Kornblut, AD, Tenen C. Reconstruction of a mandible after shotgun trauma: report of case. Clini Rep JADA 1985; 110:49–51.
16. Denny AD, Sanger JR, Matloub HS, Yousif NJ. Self-inflicted midline facial gunshot wounds: the case for a combined cranofacial and microvascular team approach. Ann Plast Surg 1992; 29(6):564–570.
17. Clark N, Birley B, Manson PN, Slezak S, Vander Kolk C, Robinson B, Crawley W. High-energy ballistic and avulsive facial injuries: classification, patterns, and an algorithim for primary reconstruction. Plastic Reconstruct Surg 1995; 98(4):583–601.
18. Thorne CH. Gunshot wounds to the face. Clini Plast Surg 1992; 19.
19. Sanger JR, Yousif J, Matloub HS, Larson DL, Sewall SS. Reconstruction of lower third of face with three simultaneous free flaps. Plast Reconstruct Surg 1994; 94(5):909–913.
20. Kroll SS, Baldwin BJ. Head and neck reconstruction with the rectus abdominis free flap. Clin Plast Surg 1994; 21(1):97–105.
21. Swartz WM, Banis JC. Mandible reconstruction. Swarts WAY, Banis JC.Head and Neck Microsurgery. Baltimore: Williams and Wilkins 1992:187–224.
22. Yuen JC, Zhou A, Shewmake K. Staged sequential reconstruction of a total lower lip, chin, and anterior mandibular defect. Ann Plasti Surg 1998; 40(3):297–301.
23. Shestak, KC. Soft-tissue reconstruction of craniofacial defects. Clini Plast Surg 1994; 21(1):107–111.

3

Synopsis of Dental Guidelines for Management of Facial Injuries

Kevin J. Kelly
Vanderbilt University, Nashville, Tennessee, U.S.A.

I. OVERVIEW OF DENTAL ANATOMY

The oral cavity and the dentition are situated at the center of the maxillofacial complex. Thorough understanding of the dental and occlusal anatomy with its surrounding structures is paramount for the diagnosis and management of facial injuries in both the adult and pediatric population.

A. Cross-Sectional Anatomy of Gingiva, Periodontal Membrane, and Supporting Bone and Nerve Supply

In humans the teeth are complicated living organs with a pulp chamber at the core, which continues as the pulp canal in the root (Fig. 1). This pulp tissue furnishes a rich network of nerves and blood vessels to each individual tooth through the apical foramen. The size of the pulp chamber and the widths of the root canals vary according to age. In the developing teeth, the pulp chamber and the root canals are wide, especially at the apex of the root. As the development of the tooth progresses, the apex of the root narrows.

An individual tooth has three subunits:

1. The *crown* is the portion one sees in the oral cavity, assuming a healthy periodontium. It is covered with an ectodermal derivative "enamel."

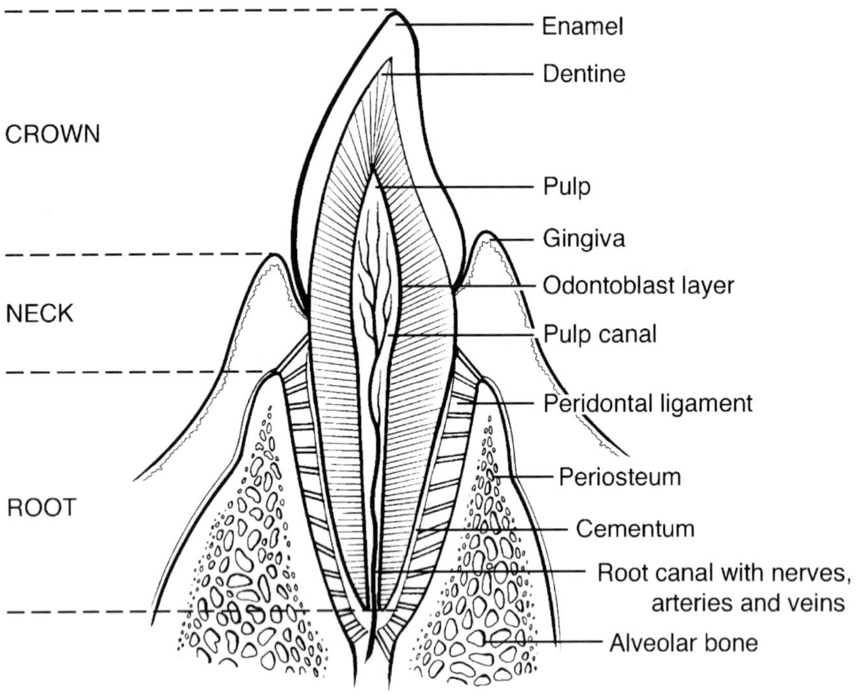

Figure 1 Cross-sectional anatomy of a tooth.

2. The *root* is the portion of the tooth embedded in the bony walls of the alveolar socket. It is covered by a mesodermal derivative "cementum." A much softer substance than enamel, it surrounds the outer portion of the neck and root of the tooth, providing connective-tissue attachments to the adjacent alveolar bone via the periodontium.
3. The *neck* starts from the junction between the cementum and the enamel and submerges beneath the periodontium extending down to the alveolus.

The bulk of the tooth consists of "dentin" that is present beneath the enamel and cementum encompassing the pulp chamber and canal. The interior alveolar branch of the mandibular division of the trigeminal nerve is the only nerve supplying the mandibular teeth. The maxillary teeth are supplied by the maxillary division of the trigeminal nerve. This nerve divides into the anterior, middle, and superior alveolar branches. The blood supply to the mandibular teeth is through the inferior alveolar branch of the internal maxillary artery while that of the maxillary teeth is via the posterior superior alveolar and infraorbital branches of the same artery.

B. Description of Teeth (Deciduous vs. Permanent), Occlusal Anatomy, Mean Lengths

The development and eruption of teeth occur through primary (deciduous) and secondary (permanent) dentition phases. The normal pediatric dental arch contains 20 teeth, 10 in each arch. There is one central incisor, one lateral incisor, one cuspid (canine), and two deciduous molars in each quadrant (Fig. 2). As the primary teeth exfoliate they are replaced by

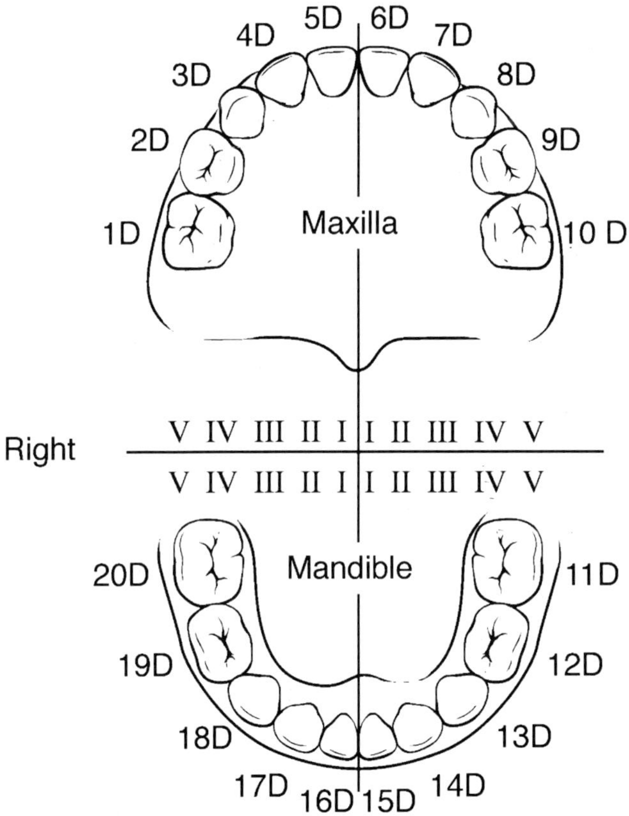

Figure 2 Normal pediatric dental arches.

permanent teeth. This would therefore lead the adult dental quadrant to contain eight teeth, totaling 32 in both arches (Fig. 3). The primary teeth have a close resemblance to their permanent successors. They, however, have shorter root lengths and smaller crowns. Tooth position and surfaces are described relative to an imaginary line drawn between the central incisors in the mandibular or the maxillary arches. The "mesial" surface of a tooth faces toward this midline, whereas the "distal" surface faces away from the midline. The "lingual" surface of all teeth faces the tongue. The "buccal" surfaces of teeth indicate areas that face the cheek. However the anterior six teeth (central incisor through cuspid on each side) have a "labial" surface since they are adjacent to the lips (Fig. 4).

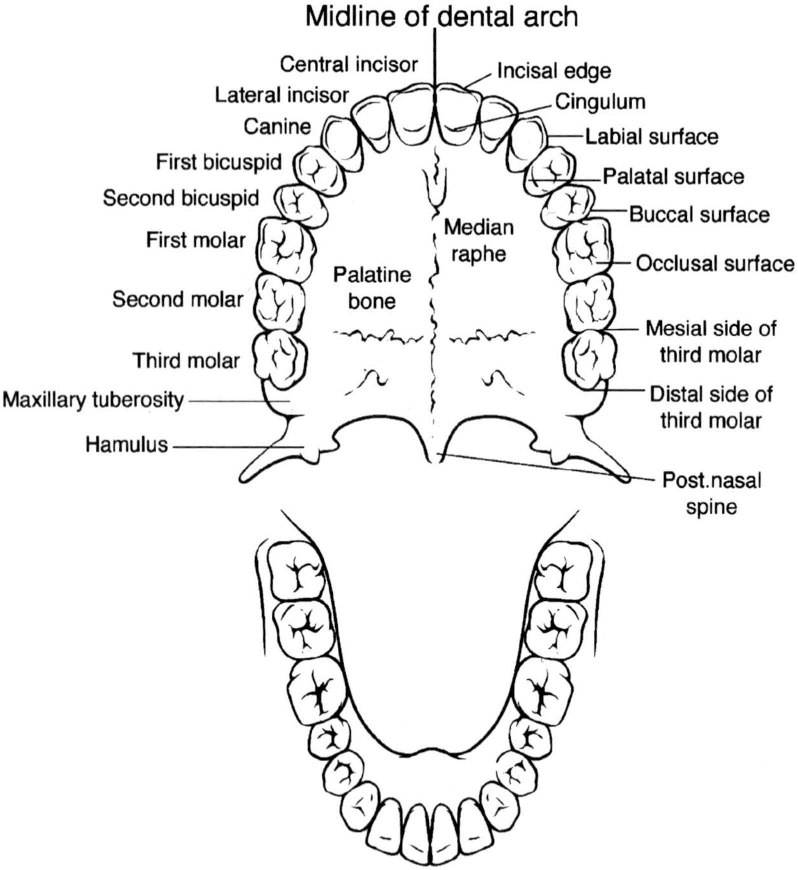

Figure 3 Normal adult dental arches.

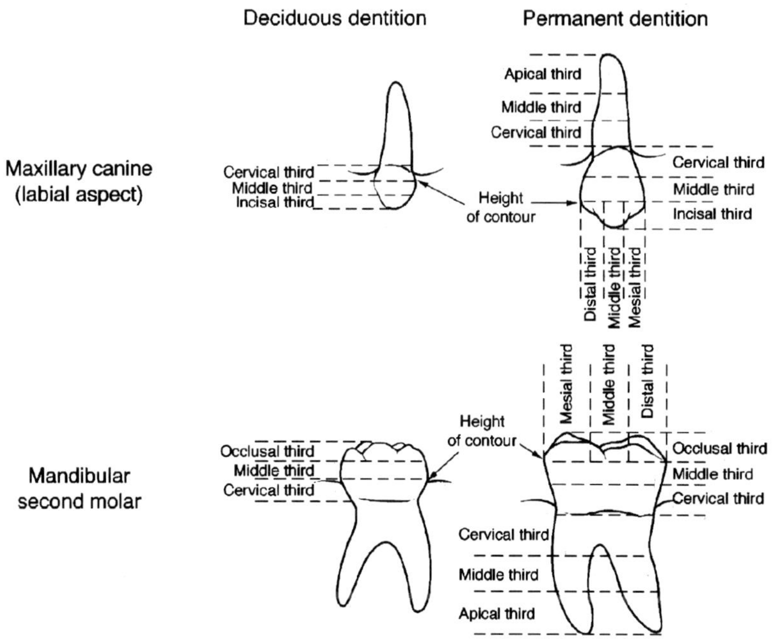

Figure 4 Tooth anatomy.

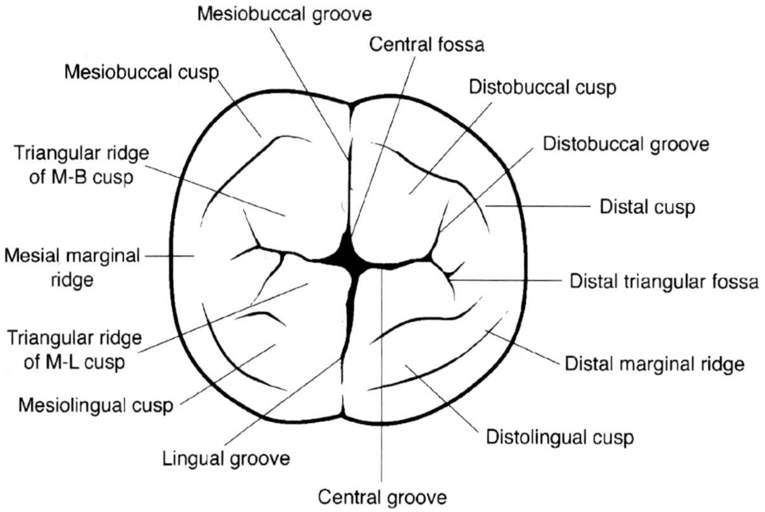

Figure 5 Occlusal anatomy of mandibular second molar.

The chewing and biting surfaces of teeth are worthy of note. These are referred to as the "incisal surface" for the incisors and cuspids and the "occlusal surface" for molars. The incisal edge of cuspids has a sharp labial point or cusp and a short blunted lingual cusp or cingulum. The bicuspids, as their name indicates, have two cusps, a buccal and a lingual. The mandibular permanent molars have five cusps, three buccal and two lingual. The buccal cusps are separated by the mesiobuccal and distobuccal grooves whereas the lingual cusps are separated by the lingual groove (Fig. 5). The mandibular second and third permanent molars' occlusal surfaces are similar to the first molar's with the exception of having only two buccal cusps. The maxillary permanent first molars are rhomboid-shaped with four cusps, two buccal and two palatal. The second and third maxillary molar teeth are similar to the first with the exception of only one palatal cusp. There is a large individual variability in the size of teeth: however, mean lengths as described by Sicher and Harry (2) may be helpful (Fig. 6).

C. Nomenclature of the Dentition (Deciduous and Permanent)

The most common notation system for permanent teeth is the universal, or military system, where the maxillary teeth are numbered from 1 to 16,

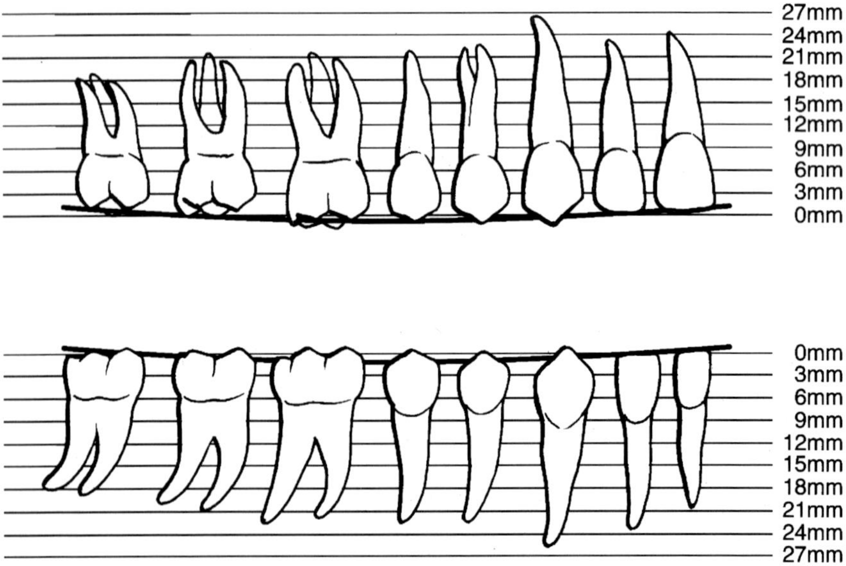

Figure 6 Root and crown anatomy and lengths of maxillary and mandibular teeth.

starting with the upper right third molar (#1), advancing around the arch to the upper left third molar (#16) (Fig. 3). The mandibular teeth are numbered from 17 to 32, starting with the lower left third molar (#17), preceding to the lower right third molar (#32) (e.g., the mandibular right central incisor is #25).

	1	2	3	4	5	6	7	8	9	10	11	12	13	14	15	16	
Right	- - -	- - -	- - -	- - -	- - -	- - -	- - -	- - -	- - -	- - -	- - -	- - -	- - -	- - -	- - -	- - -	Left
	32	31	30	29	28	27	26	25	24	23	22	21	20	19	18	17	

The 20 primary teeth are noted in similar fashion. Letters A to T are used instead (e.g., the mandibular right central incisor is P).

	A	B	C	D	E	F	G	H	I	J	
Right	- - -	- - -	- - -	- - -	- - -	- - -	- - -	- - -	- - -	- - -	Left
	T	S	R	Q	P	O	N	M	L	K	

This can also be done with numbers for the primary teeth by just adding a "D" (for deciduous) after the number depicting each tooth:

1D	2D	3D	4D	5D	6D	7D	8D	9D	10D
Right	- - -	- - -	- - -	- - -	- - -	- - -	- - -	- - -	Left
20D	19D	18D	17D	16D	5D	14D	13D	12D	11D

D. Eruption Sequence

Knowledge of the eruption sequence of teeth is imperative for the physician treating patients with either traumatic or congenital deformities of the dentofacial skeleton. The first deciduous teeth, the incisors, erupt at about 6 months of age (Fig. 7). While the incisors are developing, the molars being to erupt, followed by the cuspids. Understanding root development of teeth is important when securing a patient into maxillomandibular fixation (the first step in reduction of fractures involving tooth-bearing bone segments). From 3 to 6 years of age there is adequate primary tooth root developed to provide good tooth stability and facilitate arch bar placement using circumdental wires without avulsing these teeth. Similarly, after age 12, the adult dentition has erupted and root formation has matured enough to support an arch bar and maxillomandibular fixation. A combination of adult and primary teeth is present in the oral cavity between 6 and 12 years of

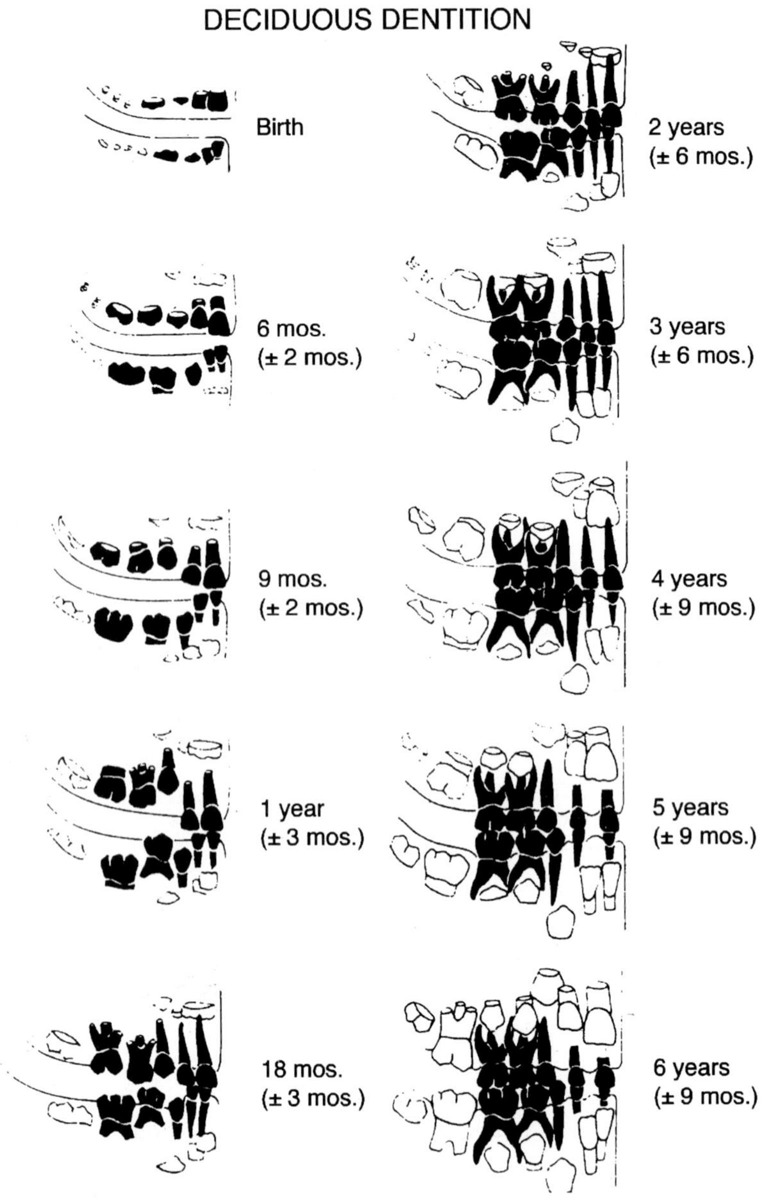

Figure 7 The eruption sequence of deciduous, mixed, and permanent dentition. (Courtesy of W.B. Saunders, from *Orthodontics, Principles, and Practice*, 3rd ed. Copyright 1972, Elsevier Science, USA.)

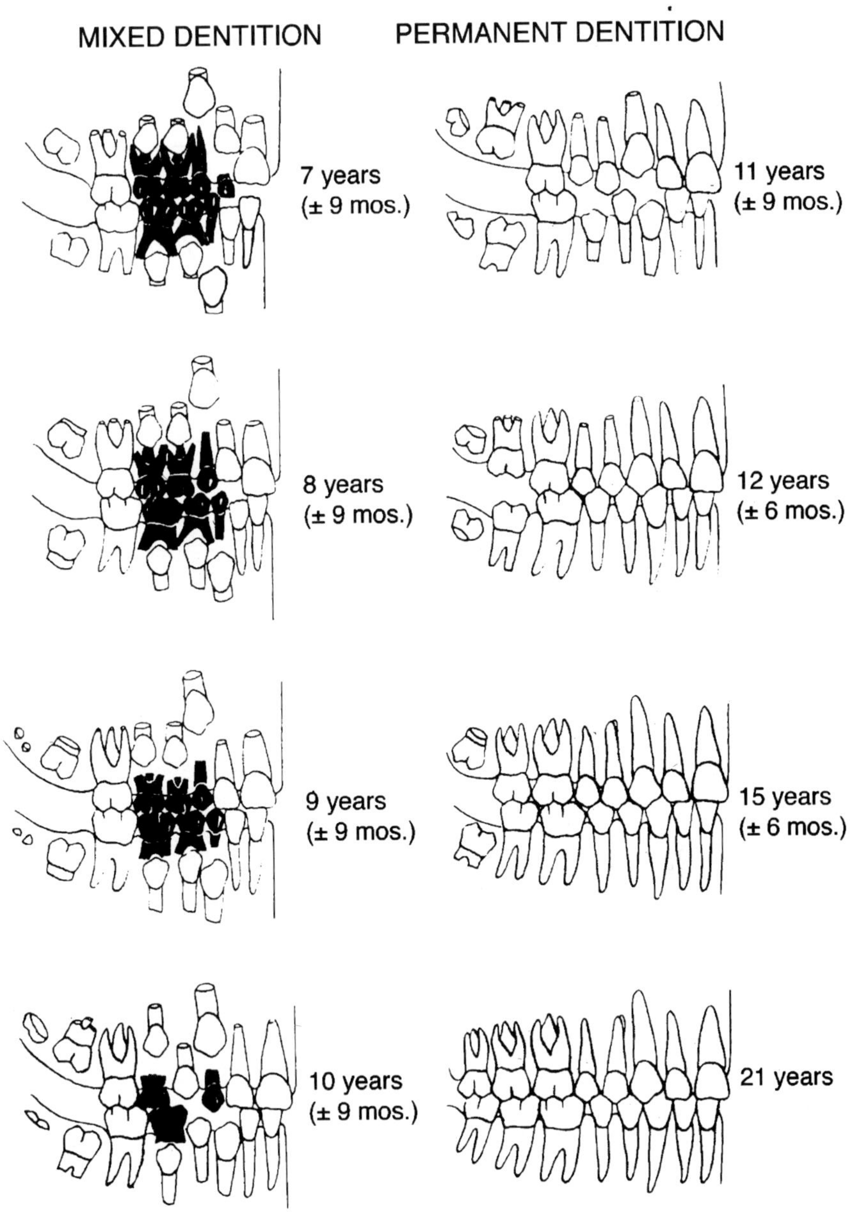

Figure 7 *(continued)*

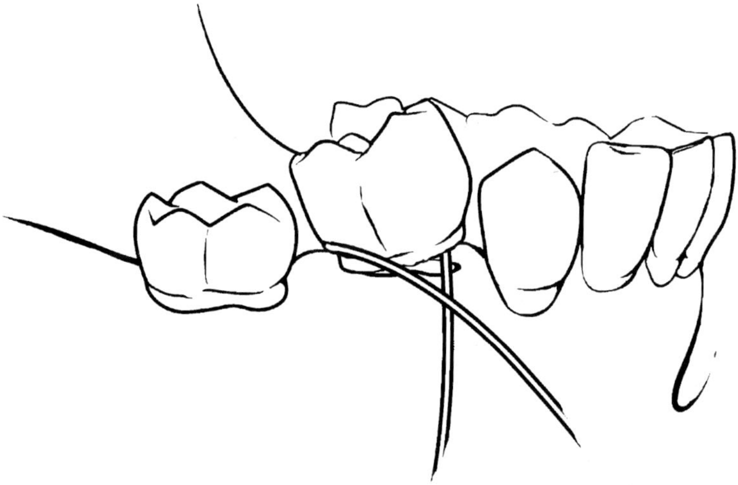

Figure 8 Deciduous teeth with advanced root resorption may get avulsed during ligation with a wire.

age. It is during this "mixed dentition" stage that obtaining support for an arch bar to place a patient in maxillomandibular fixation may become very difficult. In this stage the roots of the deciduous teeth are resorbing while the roots of the permanent teeth are not yet fully formed. Therefore, placement of wires around such teeth may lead to their inadvertent avulsion (Fig. 8). Therefore, during the mixed-dentition stage it may be necessary to use a dental splint and circumbone wire fixation to stabilize the splint to achieve maxillomandibular fixation.

It is very difficult to recall the exact configuration of each tooth root at each age. It will be very helpful to use an x-ray such as a Panorex to evaluate the dentition for each individual patient. A Panorex can be very helpful to evaluate the development of primary and permanent dentition prior to the application of maxillomandibular fixation and/or open reduction and internal fixation. This will also allow the physician to predict the location of the developing adult tooth buds prior to placement of ridged fixation if necessary (Fig. 9a and b).

II. OCCLUSION

Occlusion is the functional relationship of the maxillary to the mandibular teeth. It has a physiological and functional component, interrelating the dentition, muscles of mastication, temporimandibular joint, and complete

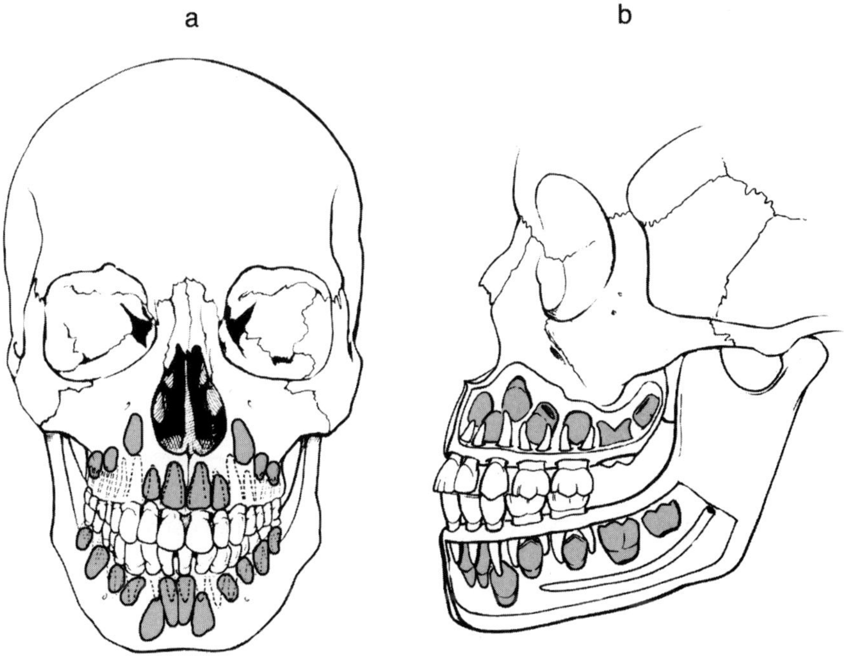

Figure 9 Frontal (a) and lateral (b) diagrams of the primary dentition with developing tooth limbs in the bone of a child.

masticatory system into a balanced pain-free state. The knowledge and determination of a proper occlusal relationship are paramount for the reduction of maxillofacial fractures to restore normal function.

A. Curve of Spee, Angulation of Teeth

When observing the interdental occlusion from the buccal surface, an anteriorly positioned curve called "curve of Spee" (3) is noted (Fig. 10). This is a concave curve of the mandibular teeth with a reciprocal convex curve in the maxilla teeth. The curve of Spee may range from a slight to a pronounced arc. It permits the maximum utilization of tooth contacts during function that would not be possible with a flat occlusal plane. The angulation and positioning of the teeth are an adaptation to a balanced occlusion where their long axis is best suited for optimal resistance to the maximal forces of the muscles of mastication. The teeth are not in continual contact in normal individuals. A mandibular "rest position" exists where the patient is erect and the muscles of mastication are relaxed. In this position a space of

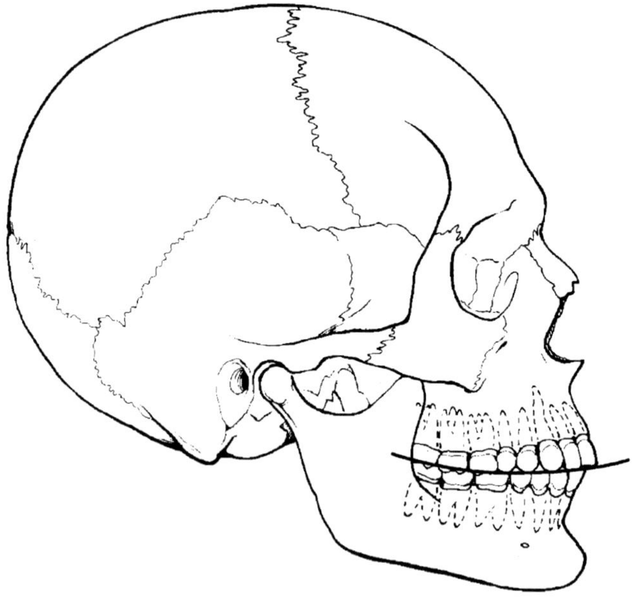

Figure 10 Curve of Spee.

2–3 mm, known as the "freeway space," is present between the upper and lower teeth.

B. Centric Relation and Centric Occlusion

Centric occlusion is a position determined by the way the teeth fit best together with the greatest amount of intercuspation and maximal occlusion. It is related to tooth occlusion and not muscle or bone (Fig. 11). Centric relation or terminal hinge position is the most retruded unstrained position of the mandibular condyle in the glenoid fossa. Thus it does not indicate occlusion or interdigitation of teeth. It is considered a stable, reproducible position that relates bone to bone. Ideally, centric occlusion and centric relation should coincide combining bilateral symmetrical occlusal contact with a balanced and unstrained relationship of the condyle in the glenoid fossa. If this does not exist as a consequence of premature cuspal contacts, it can distract the condyle either anteriorly or too far posteriorly within the glenoid fossa and thus strain the temporomandibular joint complex. The loss of centric relation can in turn lead to muscle imbalance with increased muscle tonus, muscle overactivity, spasm, and pain due to a change of the condylar position in the fossa. Occlusal adjustment, orthodontics, or even orthognathic surgery may be necessary to reestablish a harmonious occlusion, normal jaw

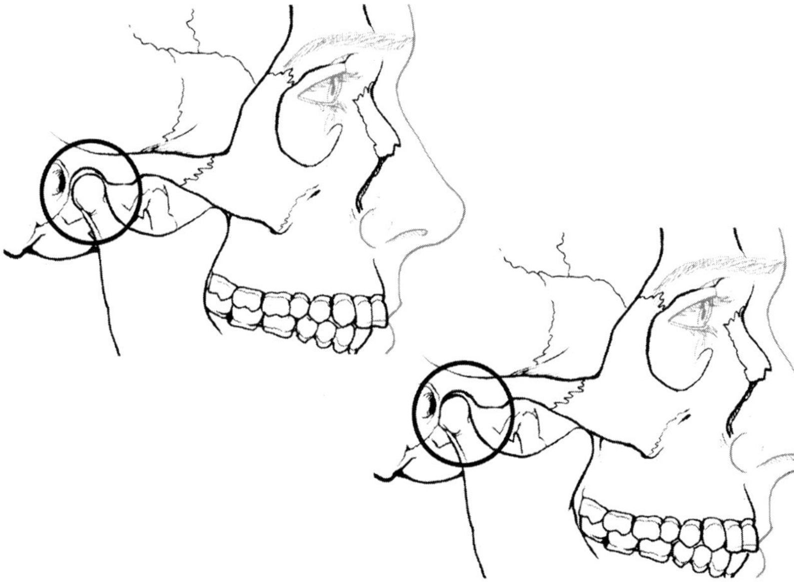

Figure 11 Centric occlusion and centric relation.

relationship, and apposition where centric occlusion coincides with centric relation. When we are reducing facial fractures, patients are being placed in maxillary mandibular fixation in centric occlusion.

C. Overbite, Overjet, Crossbite

The relationship between the upper and lower arches can be described in terms of horizontal or vertical overlap of the anterior teeth. Overbite is the amount of vertical overlap measured between the upper and lower incisal edges when the teeth are in centric occlusion. Overjet is the horizontal overlap measured from the labial surface of the lower incisors to the labial incisal edge of the upper incisors, parallel to the occlusal plane (Fig. 12). A deep bite will have an increased overbite whereas an edge-to-edge bite will have no overbite at all. Some patients may even have an anterior open bite where a distinct gap exists between the incisal edges when the molars are in centric occlusion. When lower incisors are labial to the upper incisors, the condition is referred to as an anterior crossbite. Normally the buccal maxillary molar buccal cusps also overlap the mandibular molar buccal cusps when viewed anteriorly. This is the most common, or "normal," relationship (Fig. 13a). A posterior open bite exists when there is a gap between the

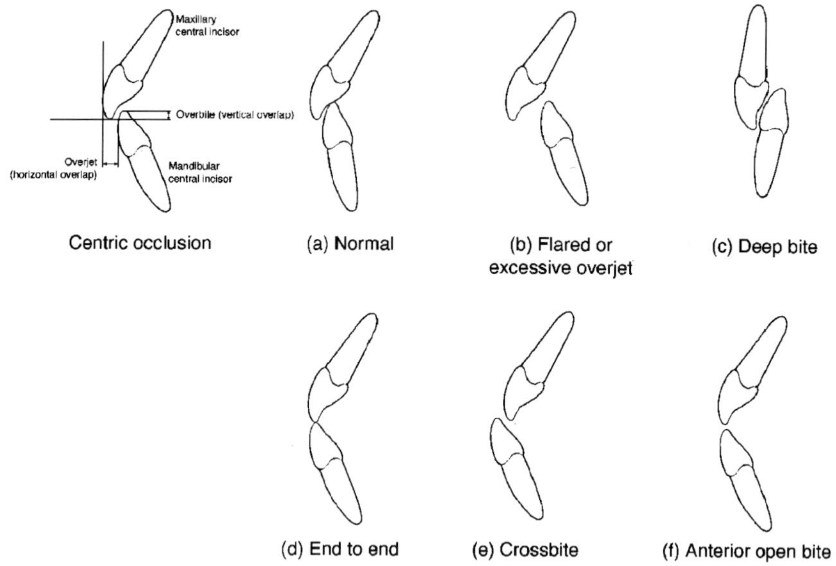

Figure 12 (a) Normal relationship, overjet, and overbite of maxillary and mandibular central incisors. (b–f). Abnormal relationships or malocclusion.

maxillary and mandibular posterior occlusion (Fig. 13b). A buccal crossbite results from tilting of the maxillary teeth toward the cheek (Fig. 13c). A lingual crossbite results from lingual displacement of the upper posterior teeth in relation to the lower teeth (Fig. 13d). Therefore, the buccal cusps of the upper teeth no longer overlap those of the lower teeth. These malocclusions may be either unilateral or bilateral.

D. Wear Facets

As maxillary and mandibular teeth continue to contact one another they start to wear flat planes in each other. These are referred to as wear facets (Fig. 14). These are excellent clues regarding how teeth relate to one another when placing a patient into maxillomandibular fixation to establish preinjury occlusion. Some anatomical variations can tell us there has been no functional contact between teeth. This is true if mamelons (small bumps on the occlusal surface central incisors) are found on teeth. When central incisors erupt, mamelons are seen (Fig. 15). As teeth function and maxillary and mandibular teeth are in contact, mamelons are worn off, creating a smooth occlusal plane. If mamelons are seen in an adult, it is evident that

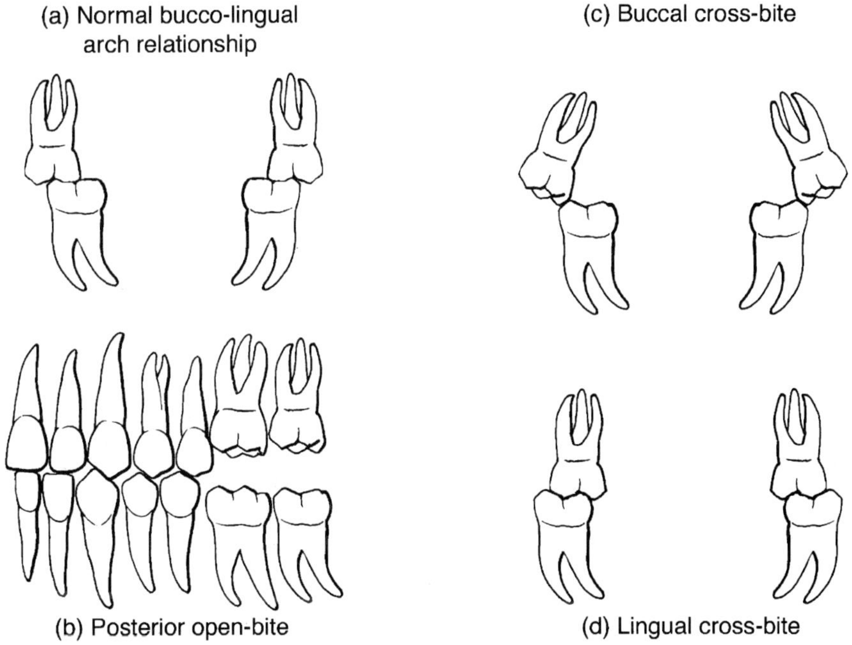

Figure 13 (a) Normal molar buccolingual arch relationship. (b) Posterior open bite. (c) Posterior buccal crossbite. (d) Posterior lingual crossbite.

these teeth have not been functioning against the opposing dentition as may be seen in an anterior open bite.

E. Classification of Occlusion

In 1890, Edward Angle (1) devised a classification of occlusion based on the anterior-posterior relationship between the maxillary and first mandibular molars. It describes only the first maxillary-molar to mandibular-molar relationship. Angle divided occlusions into three broad classes: class I, neutro-occlusion; class II, disto-occlusion; and class III, mesio-occlusion. In class I occlusion, or "normal occlusion," the most commonly found in the population, the mesiobuccal cusp of the maxillary first molar occludes with the mesiobuccal groove of the mandibular first molar (Fig. 16).

In class II occlusion, the lower first molar is distal to the upper first molar, usually one-half to one full cusp distance. Class II malocclusion is subdivided into two divisions. In class II, division 1, the upper anterior teeth are flared forward, leading to a significant overjet. In class II, division

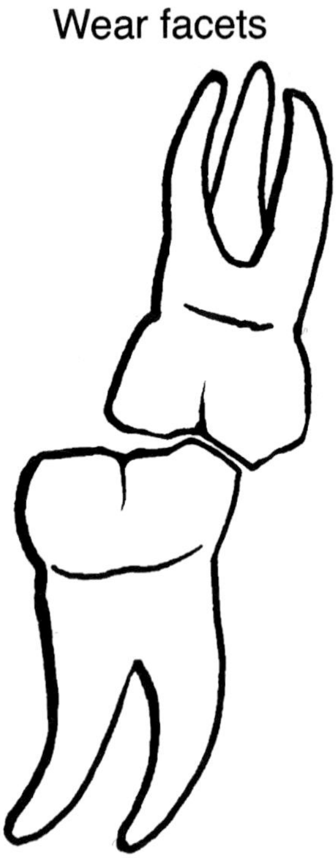

Figure 14 Wear facets on posterior teeth.

2, the anterior teeth of both the maxilla and mandible are retruded with a deep overbite (Fig. 17a and b). This is commonly seen in mandibular hypoplasia.

In class III malocclusion, the lower first molar is mesial to the upper first molar, usually one-half to one full cusp (Fig. 18).

III. DENTAL INJURIES

Orofacial trauma is involved in approximately 15% of all emergency room visits. These injuries can be isolated or in conjunction with multisystem injuries. Dentoalveolar trauma usually results from falls, playground accidents, bicycle accidents, athletic injuries, motor vehicle accidents, abuse and domestic violence, assaults, and altercations. A substantial increase in the frequency of injuries to the dentoalveolar structures occurs as a toddler

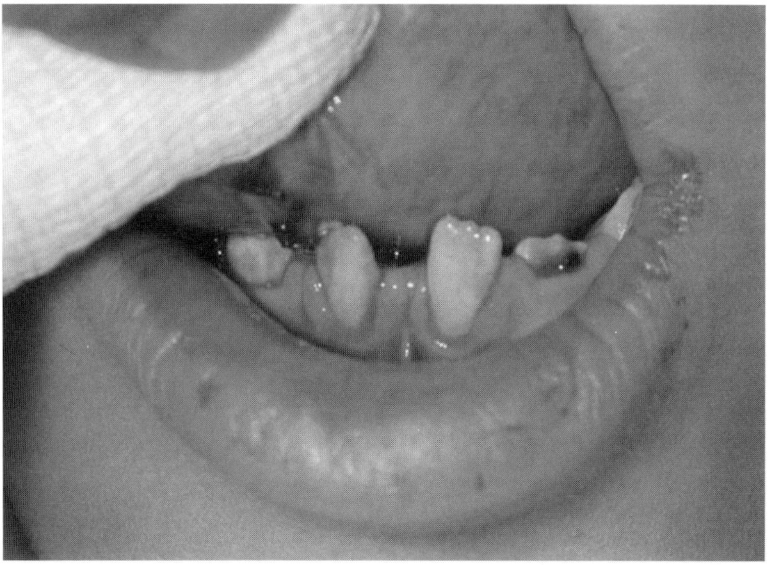

Figure 15 Mamelons (small elevations of the occlusal edge of incisor teeth).

begins to walk and run. The incidence of these injuries is reported to be around 5% in school-aged children with lacerations to the chin and vermilion border of the lip.

Certain predisposing factors can increase the chance of dentoalveolar injuries. These may include abnormal occlusion, labially inclined incisors, overjet in excess of 4 mm, lip incompetence, mouth breathing, and a short upper lip. Some of these conditions may be present in individuals with class II, division I malocclusion or oral habits such as thumb sucking.

A. History and Evaluation

A thorough history can provide valuable information regarding the nature of the injury and any alterations in the normal occlusion, such as crossbites or open bites that were present before the injury. Insight into the type of suspected injury can be provided by the nature of the accident.

Alterations in normal occlusion should be noted. All teeth should be accounted for: Missing teeth or pieces of teeth that have not been left at the scene of the accident must be considered to have been aspirated, swallowed, or displaced into soft tissues of the lip, cheek, floor of the mouth, neck, nasal cavity, or maxillary sinus. Radiological evaluation of the chest,

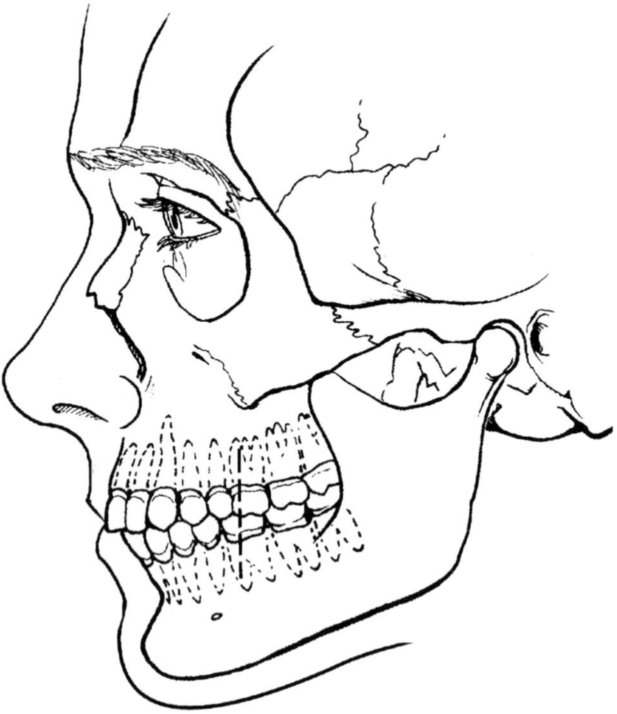

Figure 16 Class I occlusion and soft-tissue profile.

abdomen, and head and neck may be necessary to rule out the presence of teeth or fragments within these tissues or organs.

The length of time that a tooth had been avulsed and the storage media in which it was transported should be determined. Surrounding vital structures, such as the parotid duct, submandibular duct, nerves, blood vessels, and maxillofacial skeleton, should be evaluated carefully.

All teeth should be tested for abnormal mobility, both horizontally and axially, which would suggest displacement of teeth or an alveolar fracture. A bony fracture may present as an uneven contour of the alveolar process. En bloc movement of several teeth may suggest fracture of the alveolar process. Radiographic evaluation of dentoalveolar injuries should include a Panorex and/or periapical dental radiographs. These may provide the following information:

Degree of extrusion or intrusion
Presence of root fractures

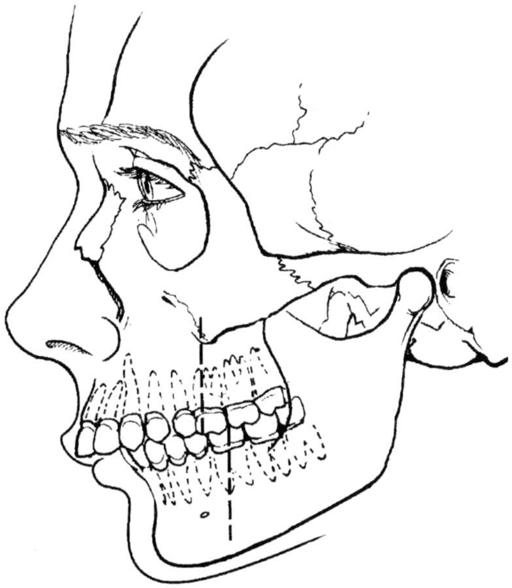

(a)

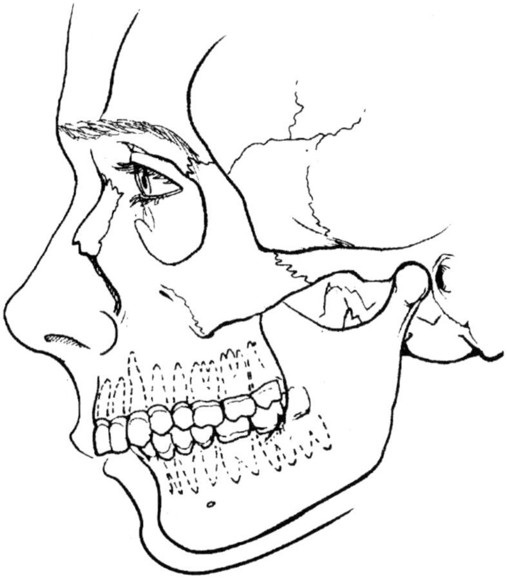

(b)

Figure 17 (a) Class II, division 1. (b) Class II, division 2.

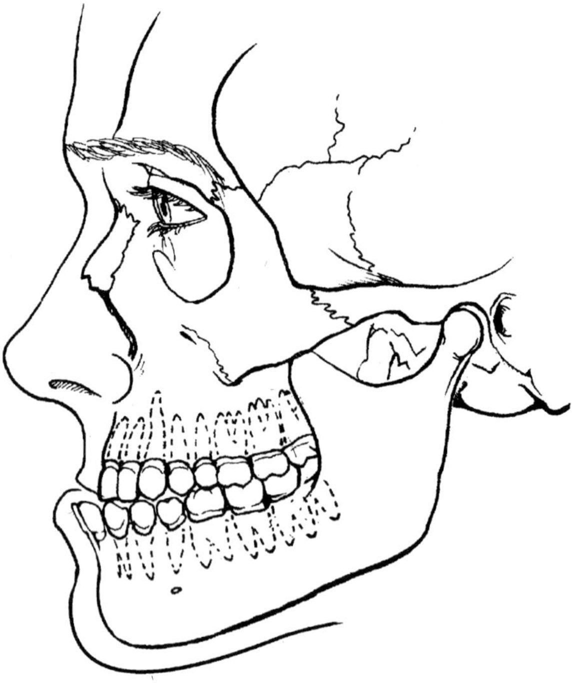

Figure 18 Class III occlusion and profile.

Extent of root development
Presence of pre-existing periodontal disease
Size of the pulp chamber and root canal
Presence of bone fractures
Tooth fragments and foreign bodies lodged in soft tissues

The most reliable clue to an abnormal occlusion from dental injury, bone fracture, or a combination is the patient's perception that his teeth "don't contact normally."

B. Injuries to Dental Tissues and Pulp

A classification of dental injuries has been presented by the World Health Organization (WHO) (Fig. 19a–g).

Figure 19a depicts a crown infraction that is an incomplete fracture of the enamel without loss of tooth structure. This does not usually require any treatment.

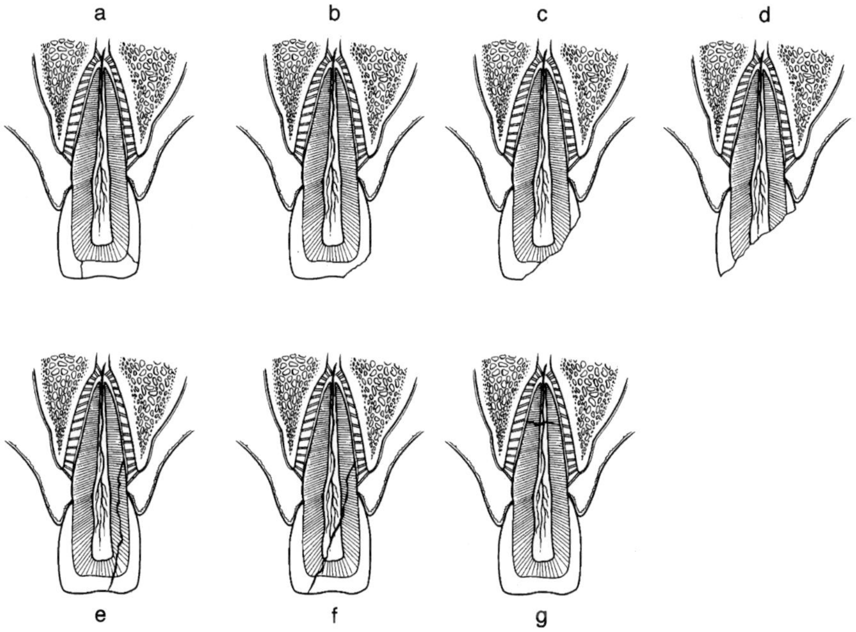

Figure 19 (a–g) WHO classification for injuries to dental tissues and pulp.

Figure 19b depicts an uncomplicated crown fracture confined to the enamel that may be treated with smoothing of sharp edges or restoration with composite resin fillings.

Figure 19c depicts an uncomplicated crown fracture involving the enamel and dentin. This tooth may be sensitive to thermal changes and mastication since the dentinal microtubules carrying the nerve endings from the pulp to the dentinal enamel junction are exposed to bacteria and noxious stimuli. A calcium hydroxide liner is used to seal these dentinal tubules prior to restoration with a tooth-colored composite resin filling.

Figure 19d depicts a complicated crown fracture involving enamel and dentin with exposure of the pulp. A spot of blood may be noted at the area of pulp exposure that would need emergent referral to a dentist. The treatment may range from sealing of the pulp with calcium hydroxide to complete pulp extirpation and endodontic therapy (i.e., root canal therapy) followed by restoration of the remaining tooth with a composite resin filling or a porcelain crown coverage (i.e., cap) if a substantial amount of tooth is missing.

Figure 19e depicts an uncomplicated crown-root fracture involving enamel and dentin and extending into the root structure. The treatment options are dependent on the amount of root remaining. In permanent dentition, if the fracture line is above or slightly below the alveolar bone level, the tooth can be restored with a crown. Primary teeth with any type of crown-root fracture should be extracted, and a dentist should fabricate a space maintainer. Without a space maintainer the adjacent teeth can tip into this space and hinder the proper eruption of the underlying permanent teeth and therefore lead to significant malocclusion.

Figure 19f depicts a complicated crown-root fracture similar to that shown in Fig. 19 with addition of a pulp exposure. Endodontic therapy (i.e., root canal) would be needed prior to crowning of the tooth.

Figure 19g depicts a root fracture involving dentin, cementum, and the pulp. Factures in the apical third, either vertical or horizontal, are an indication for extraction.

C. Injuries to the Periodontal Tissues

These injuries include contusion, luxation, intrusion, or avulsion (Fig. 20). In contusion injuries the tooth would be tender to touch owing to inflammation of the tooth-supporting structures. No treatment is indicated other than palliative therapy.

Of all dental trauma, luxation injuries are the most common in the permanent and primary dentition. This is most commonly seen in the

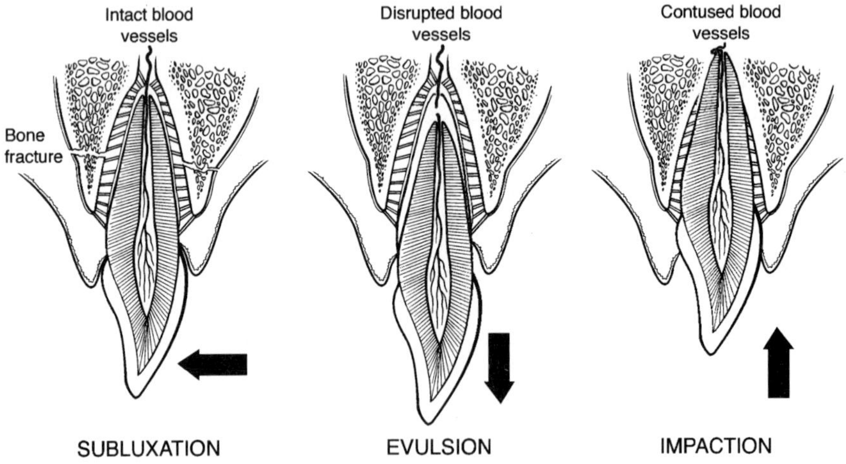

Figure 20 Injuries to the periodontal tissues.

maxillary central incisor region. The type of force and the direction of impact dictate the type of luxation injury. Intrusion injuries involve impaction of the tooth into the alveolar socket. This displacement could be as superior as the nasal cavity leading to bleeding from the nares. An intruded primary or an immature permanent tooth should be allowed to erupt on its own. If the intruded primary tooth impinges on the permanent tooth bud, it should be extracted. An intruded mature permanent tooth requires low-force orthodontic repositioning over 3–4 weeks to minimize the risk of root resorption. Attempts to reposition it immediately at the time of injury must be avoided since this can result in extraction of the tooth. An extruded primary tooth should be extracted to prevent damage to the underlying permanent tooth. An extruded permanent should be repositioned in the socket with gentle pressure and splinted with a thin (28-gauge) wire and/or a segmental arch bar for 1–2 weeks. This tooth should be followed by a dentist periodically since it is common for the pulp to lose vitality owing to the trauma and require endodontic therapy owing to the loss of vitality.

Luxation of a tooth is usually accompanied by comminution or fracture of the alveolar socket. The tooth and alveolar bone can be manipulated digitally into proper position, with concurrent compression forces on both the palatal and labial bone plates. They are then splinted to adjacent stable teeth with a segmental arch bar for 2–8 weeks and covered with appropriate antibiotics. Endodontic therapy may be required since pulp necrosis is prevalent as with extrusive injuries. The patient should therefore be referred to a dentist shortly after treatment of the acute injury. Complete avulsion of a permanent tooth represents a true dental emergency. Avulsed primary teeth should not be reimplanted. These injuries make up to 15% of all traumatic injuries to permanent dentition and 7–13% in the primary dentition. The maxillary central incisor is the most common avulsed tooth. The success of reimplantation is inversely related to the length of time the tooth is out of the socket.

Ideally a tooth should be reimplanted within the first 30 min. This may help maintain the viability of the cells of the pulp and periodontal ligament, which would assist reattachment and avoid posttraumatic complications of root resorption. The stage of root development and the type of extra-alveolar storage medium are also significant factors determining tooth survival. The avulsed tooth should be gently rinsed with saline or milk (hypotonic water is the least desirable storage medium) and placed back into the socket with light pressure and then splinted with an acrylic splint for 7–10 days. If a significant alveolar fracture has occurred, a rigid splint such as an Erich arch bar or a lingual splint should be used for 3–4 weeks. The traumatized tooth should be removed from occlusion and the patient placed on a soft diet for 2–3 weeks. Tetanus prophylaxis should be updated if needed. Antibiotic coverage and 0.12% chlorhexidine rinse are indicated to minimize bacterial activity.

In the case of dentoalveolar injuries the ideal fixation should provide stabilization of traumatized teeth and prevent further damage to the pulp and periodontal tissues during the healing period, allowing the attachment apparatus (periodontal membrane) to regenerate. Arch bar fixation, acrylic splints, or both can be used for stabilization of alveolar process fractures if the teeth within the segment are stable. If the teeth are mobile, apical positioning of the supporting wires to the cervical prominence may have a tendency to elevate the tooth slowly. Therefore, in these situations the ideal splint would be a composite resin in conjunction with a 24- or 28-gauge wire. This splinting technique provides a relatively easy, versatile, aesthetic method for stabilization of teeth without impingement on gingival and periodontal tissues (Fig. 21).

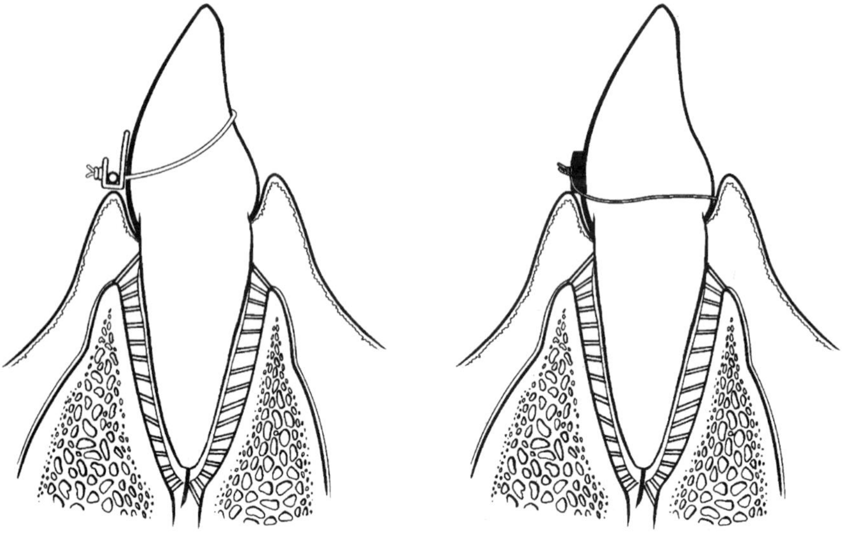

a b

Figure 21 Wire relative to the tooth cingulum for stabilization of avulsed tooth versus fractured alveolar bone. (a) Treatment of evulsed tooth. The wire over the cingulum holds the tooth into the alveolar bone. (b) The wire under the cingulum of the tooth (under the height of contours) that would hold the arch bar to the tooth.

IV. DENTAL SPLINTS

Dental splints are designed to reduce and stabilize fractured tooth-bearing segments to their pretraumatic relationship and to aid in the restoration and occlusion of skeletal relationships. The use of dental splints has diminished with the advent of rigid fixation and application of craniofacial techniques to treat facial fractures. However, in certain situations they can be effectively used for ultimate management of complex maxillofacial fractures. Acrylic dental splints can be very helpful in the anatomical reduction of bony segments. They can help maintain the reduction during the application of rigid fixation and stabilize fractured segments during periods of healing and rehabilitation. Splints can be invaluable in establishing occlusal relationships in patients with comminuted maxillary (palatal) or mandibular fractures. They can also be very useful to obtain maxillomandibular

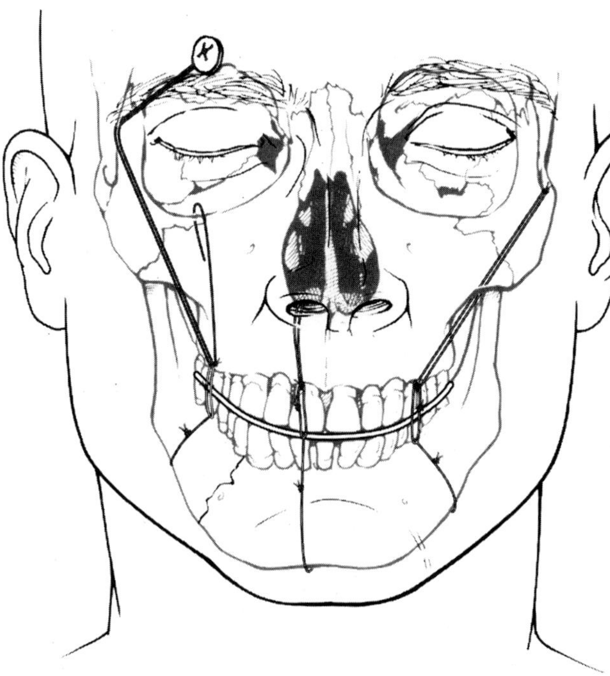

Figure 22 Options for skeletal fixation of a splint: cranial suspension wire, infraorbital rim, piriform rim, circumzygomatic, and circumandibular.

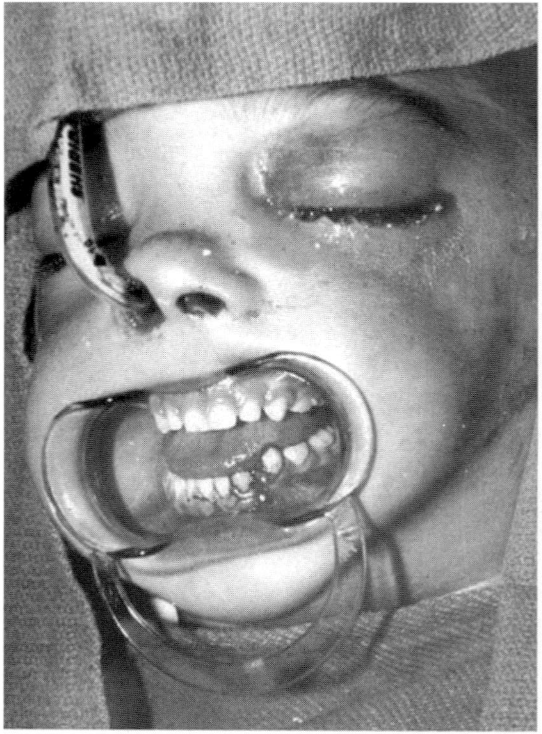

(a)

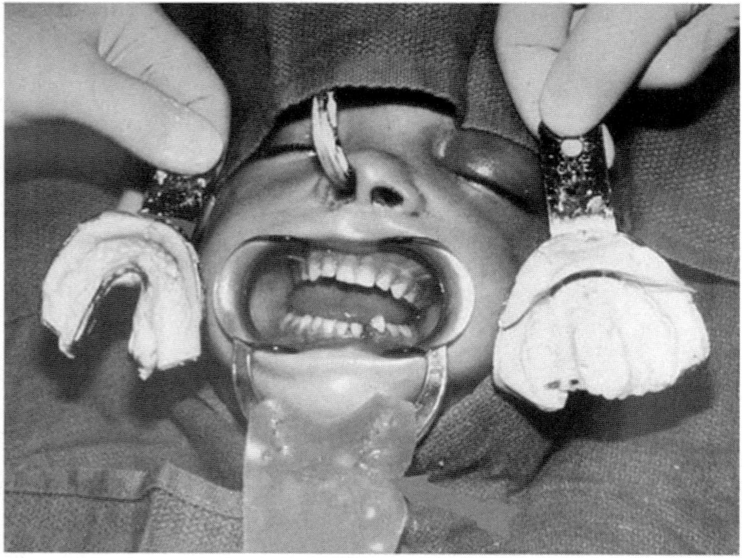

(b)

Figure 23 (Courtesy of W.B. Saunders, from *Plastic Surgery, Indications, Operations, and Outcomes*, Vol. 2, *Craniomaxillofacial, Cleft, and Pediatric Surgery*, Vander Kolk, p. 947, Chap. 63, "Pediatric Facial Trauma," K.J. Kelly.)

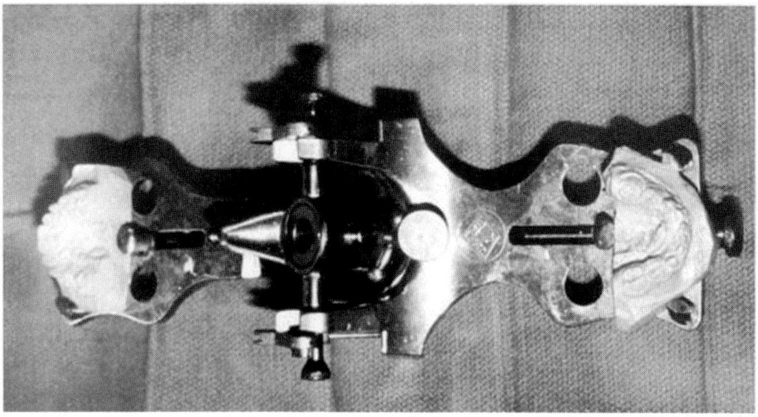

(c)

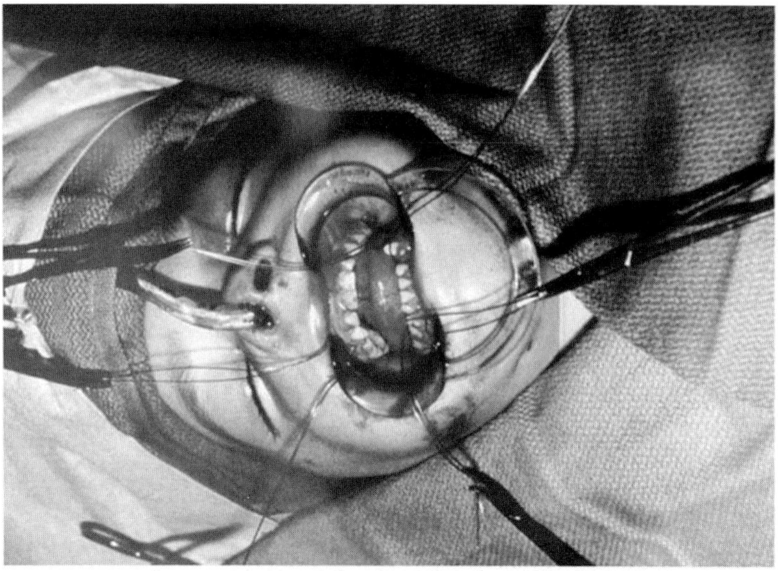

(d)

Figure 23 *(continued)*

fixation in the mixed dentition stage, from age 6 to 12, when children's teeth may not be able to support arch bars.

Dental splints can also have a crucial role in the treatment of multiple dentoalveolar segment fractures in both adults and children. In patients who are partially or fully edentulous, a splint may be used to reestablish the patient's vertical dimension and pretraumatic skeletal relationship as well as stabilize the fractured segments during the healing period. Preexisting partial or complete dentures may be used as intermaxillary splints. This enables one to establish the normal maxillary-to-mandibular relationship for fracture reduction in the absence of teeth. Arch bars are secured to the dentures. A mandibular denture or splint is stabilized with skeletal fixation via circumandibular or circumdental fixation depending on the nature of the fracture. The maxillary denture may be secured by circumdental, circumzygomatic, orbital rim, piriform aperture, or anterior nasal spine suspension wires (Fig. 22). In the endentulous patient, a splint or denture can screwed to the mandibular or maxillary bone to secure the bone to the prostheses. The arch bars are then used to secure maxillomandibular fixation. Once this is done, the buttresses of the fractured bones are exposed and slated.

If open reduction is indicated in an endutulous patient, it may be possible to do anatomical reduction and fixation of fractured bone segments without any splint fixation allowing the patient to remain out of maxillomandibular fixation. This does, however, require perfect reduction of all fractured buttresses to restore preinjury anatomical relationships. It is also necessary in this case to rigidly fixate *all* fractured buttresses.

Once a decision is made to use a dental splint, accurate alginate impression of the patient's maxillary and mandibular out arches should be obtained. This step can be performed under local anesthesia in the adult population, but is best carried out under general anesthesia in the pediatric patient (Fig. 23). It should be emphasized that an impression of the opposing dental arch to the fracture is always required to help reestablish the pretraumatic occlusion. A thorough knowledge of occlusion and dental anatomy is crucial. Information should be obtained about any prior malocclusions from the patient or family members. Pretraumatic photographs or dental orthodontic models may also assist in the reestablishment of the occlusion. Dental cast models are fabricated by pouring dental stone or plaster into the impressions. Cuts are made in the cast model corresponding to the fracture lines.

The segments of the cast models are reassembled against the opposing arch cast, reattached together with wax, and then mounted onto an articulator. The wear facets can be very helpful in reestablishing the normal preinjury occlusion. The quick-cure acrylic resin methyl

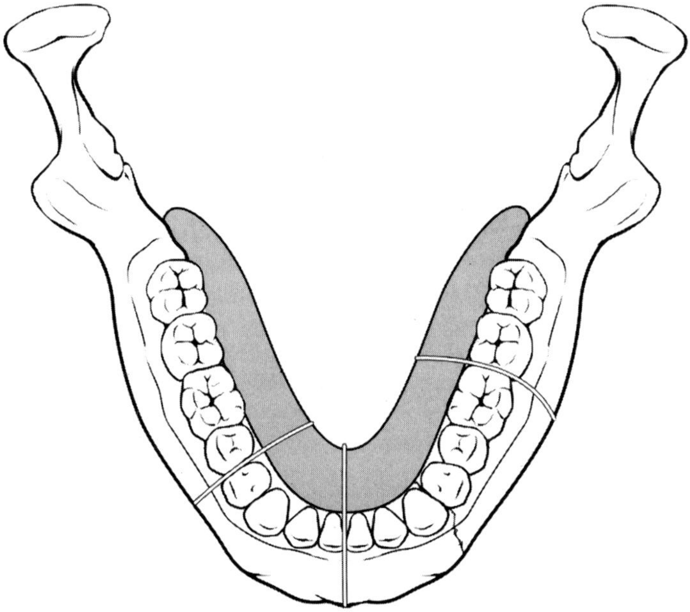

Figure 24 Diagram of a lingual splint realigning fractured segments and stabilizing the reduction. Note that there is no interference with the occlusal surface of the teeth.

methacrylate is the most commonly used material for the fabrication of dental splints. This gives us a guide to know where the normal occlusion should be set.

This splint is then taken to the operating room where the patient is placed in occlusion using the splint as a guide to determine the proper preinjury occlusion. Lingual splints are recommended for the treatment of unstable, complex, bilateral mandibular fractures or fractures of the symphysis or alveolar ridge of both arches. They help prevent lingual tilting of the bony segments and prevent the inferior border of the mandible from being distracted at the fracture site. They should be used in conjunction with a buccolabial arch bar to provide additional support (Fig. 24). Dental splints can be extremely useful for the reduction of splint palatal fractures. Splint fabrication can be very useful in treating facial fractures or in elective orthognathic surgery.

A thorough understanding of dental anatomy and occlusion is critical to anyone treating craniofacial deformities or fractures involving dental-bearing bone segments or dental injuries.

REFERENCES

1. Angle EH. Classification of malocclusion. Dent Cosmos 1899; 41:248.
2. Sicher MD, Harry DSC. Oral Anatomy. St. Louis: CV Mosby Co. 1980.
3. Spee FG. Prosthetic Dentistry. Medico-Dental Publishing Co. 1928.
4. Ferraro JW. Fundamentals of Maxillofacial Surgery. New York: Springer-Verlag Inc. 1997.
5. Kelly KJ. Pediatric facial trauma. Achauer BM, Eriksson E, Guyuron B, Coleman JJ III, Russel RC, Vander Kolk CA. Plastic Surgery Indications, Operations, and Outcomes. St. Louis: CV Mosby Co., 2000:941–969.
6. Eppley BL. Dental and maxillofacial considerations. Achauer BM, Eriksson E, Guyuron B, Coleman JJ III, Russel RC, Vander Kolk CA. Plastic Surgery Indications, Operations, and Outcomes. St. Louis: CV Mosby Co., 2000:1093–1106.
7. Manson PN. Facial fractures. Aston SJ, Beasley RW, Thorne CHM. Grabb and Smith's Plastic Surgery. 5 Philadelphia: Lippincott-Raven1997:383–412.
8. Powers MP. Diagnosis and management of dentoalveolar injuries. Fonseca, Walker. Maxillofacial Trauma.
9. Trope M. Clinical management of the avulsed tooth: present strategies and future directions. Dent Traumatol 2002; 18:1–11.
10. Flores MT, Andreasen JO, Bakland LK. Guidelines for the evaluation and management of traumatic dental injuries. Dent Traumatol 2001; 17:1–4.

4

The Biology of Trauma on Facial Growth

Effects and Noneffects of Personal Surgical Experimentation

Bernard G. Sarnat
University of California and Cedars-Sinai Medical Center, Los Angeles, California, U.S.A.

I. BONE GROWTH

A. General Bone Growth

Growth and development of the skeletal system play an important role in determining body form. The dynamics of growth of bone(s) is a complex process. Although significant articles in regard to bone growth appeared in the literature more than 225 years ago (1), many basis questions are still unanswered. What are some of the problems in need of study? What are the inherent difficulties? Any determination of bone growth must concern itself with one or more of the following questions: What are the sites? The centers? The amounts? The rates? Do they vary? When? What are the directions? What are the changes in size? In shape? What are the changes in proportion? What is the pattern? What are the mechanisms? What factors are influential? Not influential? This chapter addresses the last two questions in particular.

The purposes of this limited chapter are to present several significant basic science methods used for evaluating the effects and noneffects of several surgical factors upon facial growth. Some principles of the biology of bone(s) are central to this presentation. The basic blueprint of a bone is inherent. Postnatal bone growth is but a continuation of prenatal bone growth interrupted by the event of birth. In utero, the fetus with its genetic beginning is subjected to the vicissitudes of the maternal environment. After birth, the individual is subjected to the effects of the general environment. Various factors may affect skeletal growth sites or centers, thereby causing faulty growth of bone(s). The degree of the subsequent deformity will depend not only on the type, intensity, extent, and chronology of the noxious agent but also on the site and its particular susceptibility and growth activity. A growth deformity of bone may be readily produced by interfering with a cartilaginous but not a sutural growth site.

Development of body form is related to the synchronous coordination of three-dimensional, multiple, differential, skeletal growth sites and centers and associated structure activities. The physiological stability of the bony components is the result of many interrelated factors, normal functional use being a prominent one. Well recognized are the effects of either excessive use, with hypertrophy (i.e., an increase in the mass of bone), or disuse, with atrophy (i.e., a decrease in the mass of bone). Thus modifications in the functions of a part are reflected in alterations in the form of the part.

One definition of growth is change over time. A basic physiologial concept is that throughout life, *bone, the tissue*, is in a continuous state of apposition and resorption (Table 1). Consequently, skeletal size and shape are always subject to change. The following generalizations can be made. When skeletal mass increases, as in children, apposition is more active than resorption. Cartilaginous and sutural growth representing *bones as organs* are both active (i.e., *positive growth*). When skeletal mass is constant, as in the adult, apposition and resorption, although active, are in equilibrium (i.e., *neutral growth*). Cartilaginous and sutural growth have ceased. When the skeletal mass decreases, as in old age, resorption is more active than apposition (i.e., *negative growth*). This concept of growth change is not new (2), and is also evidenced in the lay literature by the following passage from *Alice in Wonderland* by Lewis Carroll: "... said Alice, and if it makes me grow *larger*, I can reach the key; and if it makes me grow *smaller*[italics added], I can creep under the door."

B. Craniofacial Bone Growth

The craniofacial skeleton changes, in both size and shape, in all three planes: height, width and depth. However, it grows in these three dimensions of space differentially in both time, amount, and rate (Figs. 1–3). Many sites contribute to the multidirectional growth. The dynamics and details of

Table 1 Bone: Growth, Remodeling, and Repair

	Growth					
	Cartilaginous (bones)	Sulural (bones)	Remodeling (bone)	Skeletal mass	Repair	Clinical considerations
Infancy and childhood	Active	Active (apposition, no resorption)	Apposition greater than resorption	Increasing (positive growth)	Active	Giantism and other growth deformities
Adulthood	Long or tubular bone, skull base, etc. (epiphysis) Inactive Mandibular condyle (epiphyseal-like) Latent (potentially active)	Inactive	Apposition equal to resorption	In equilibrium (neutral growth)	Active	Acromegaly
Old age	Long or tubular bone, skull base, etc. (epiphysis) Inactive	Inactive Mandibular condyle (epiphyseal-like) Latent (potentially active)	Apposition less than resorption	Decreasing (negative growth)	Active	Senile osteoporosis
Clinical considerations	Conditions affecting cartilage: achondroplasia, rickets, etc.	Conditions affecting sutural growth: synostosis, etc.	Skeletal adjustments to various conditions	Changes in size and shape	Fracture, osteotomy, ostectomy, distraction osteogenesis, bone graft	

Source: Adapted from Ref. 24.

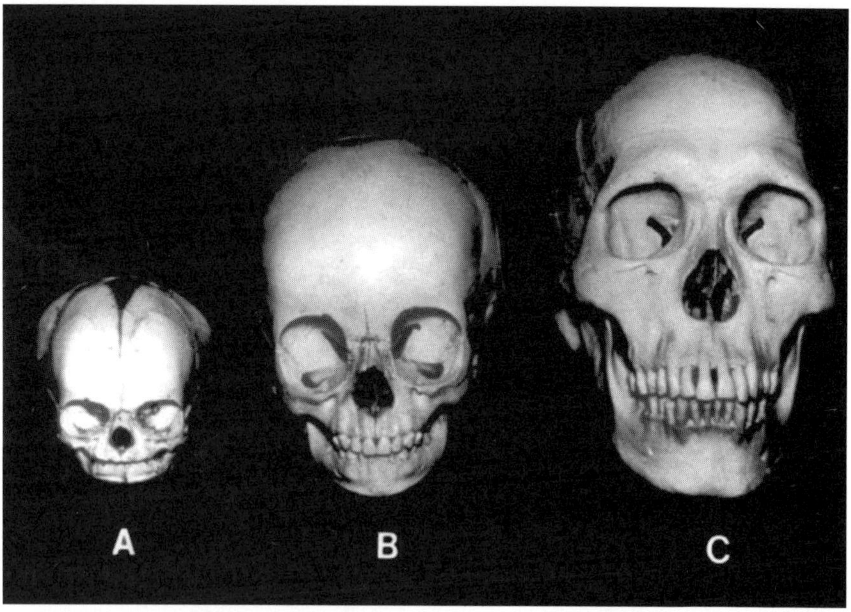

Figure 1 Normal growth of the human skull (A) Clinically edentulous skull at about birth; (B) the skull of a child with completely erupted deciduous primary dentition; (C) the skull of an adult with completely erupted permanent secondary dentition. Note that in the infant the cranium is prominent, and the face is much less so, representing a lesser amount of the total skull size. Also note that the orbit makes up a large part of the face. In the adult, the face is prominent and represents a large part of the total skull size. The orbit makes up a considerably smaller part of the total face in the adult than in the infant. Differential growth takes place at different times and rates in various parts of the skull. (From Ref. 25.)

normal postnatal growth, simultaneity, coordination, and change and nonchange of the craniofacial skeletal system in both the young and the adult are fascinating, complex, and incompletely understood problems in the field of biology.

For the purpose of this chapter the following generalizations apply. Craniofacial bones grow in three principal ways. One is cartilaginous at the nasal septum and as *endochondral growth* (i.e., the replacement of cartilage by bone) at the base of the skull at the spheno-occipital and sphenoethmoidal junctions. These bones are joined by cartilage (synchondroses). In addition, endochondral growth of bones occurs at the septopresphenoid joint and at the mandibular condyle. A second way is by *sutural growth*

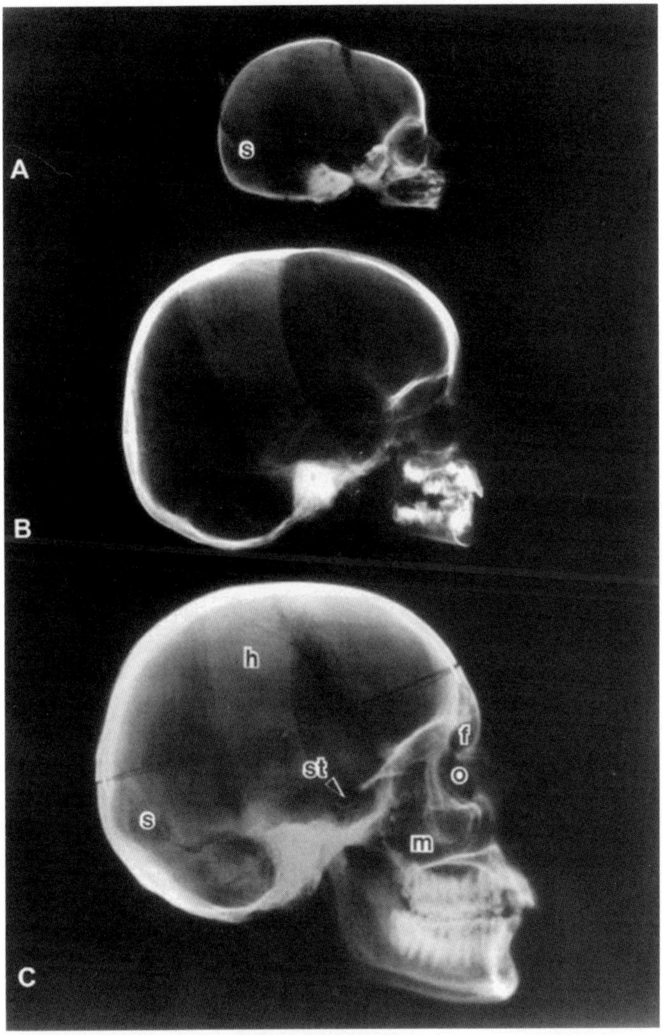

Figure 2 Lateral cephalometric radiographs of skulls shown in Figure 1. (A) Note in the infant skull the presence of unerupted teeth in the jaws. (B) In the child skull, the primary dentition is fully erupted, and the permanent teeth are forming within the jaws. (C) In the adult skull, the permanent teeth are fully erupted and in occlusion. The maxillary (m) and frontal (f) sinuses are not evident in the infant skull, are in early development in the child skull, and are fully developed in the adult skull. Note the open actively growing suture (S) in the infant cranium, in contrast to the closed inactive suture (S) in the adult cranium. st, sella turcica; o, orbit; h, head holder apparatus. (From Ref. 26.)

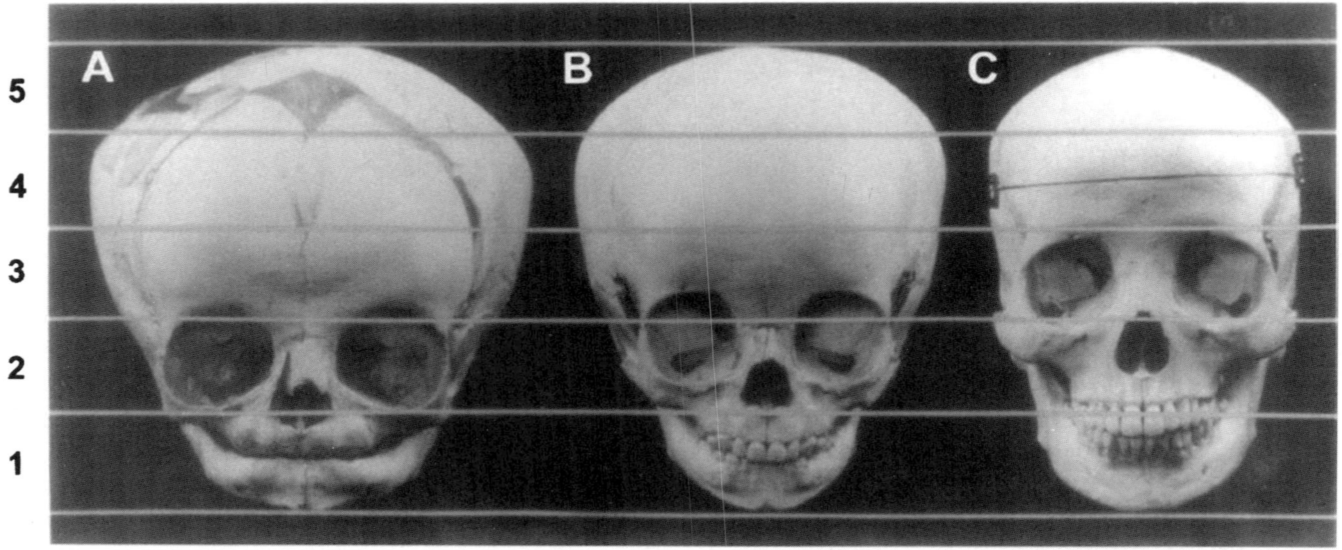

Figure 3 Frontal view of skulls shown in Figures 1 and 2 enlarged to about the same skull height and oriented in the Frankfurt horizontal plane. Note the differences in forms and proportions of the total skulls and their components. The distance between the lower border of the mandible to the superior border of the orbit represents about 40% of the skull height in the infant and 60% in the adult. Orbital height is nearly the same in all three skulls. Cranial height represents about 60% of the skull height in the infant and 40% in the adult. Skull height is divided into fifths. (From Ref. 25.)

where bones are united by connective tissue (synarthroses). This is found only in the skull. Sutures grow differentially by apposition without resorption. The amount of growth may vary on either side of a suture, the rate varies for different sutures at a particular time, and the same suture grows differentially at different times These sites, as well as the endochondral, are of limited growth and usually cease activity as an individual reaches adulthood. A third type is *appositional and resorptive growth* (i.e., remodeling), which occurs on the outer surfaces (periosteal) or inner surfaces (endosteal) of bone throughout life. The differential responses and interrelationships of these processes are important.

The size and shape of the skull are determined not only by the growth of bone(s) but also by its cavities (Table 2). Increases in the size of the contents of the cranial and orbital cavities of the skull influence the growth of adjoining bones and sutures. This occurs by a combination of resorption and deposition of bone on the surfaces and adjustments at the sutures. The cranium and the masticatory facial skeleton are integrated into an anatomical

Table 2 Craniofaciodental Growth

I. Bone(s)
    A. Cartilaginous—bone(s) as organs
        1. Endochondral
        2. Nasal septal
    B. Sutural (appositional)—bone(s) as organs
    C. Remodeling (appositional and resorptive) bone as a tissue
II. Cavities
    A. Matrix
        1. Brain and cranium
        2. Orbital contents and orbit
    B. Matrix and air
        1. Septum and nasal cavity
        2. Tongue and oral cavity
    C. Air
        1. Maxillary sinus
        2. Frontal sinus
        3. Ethmoid sinus
        4. Sphenoid sinus
III. Teeth

Source: Ref. 6.

and biological unit. However, the masticatory skeleton is in part dependent on muscular influences, growth of the tongue, and the dentition. These two parts of the skull follow different paths of development, and the timing of their growth rates is entirely divergent. Nevertheless growth of any one part of the skull is coordinated to the growth of the whole. The air-containing maxillary, frontal, ethmoid, and sphenoid sinuses also increase in size and contribute to growth of the skull.

Growth of the upper facial skeleton is closely correlated with that of the mandible. However, the mode of mandibular growth is entirely different from that of the maxillary part of the face. In the latter, the growth is primarily sutural. In the mandible, an important site of growth is the hyaline cartilage in its condyle. These differences explain a certain independence yet dependence of the growth of these two parts of the facial skeleton.

The growth of the mandible is indispensable for the normal vertical growth of the upper face. Upward and backward growth at the condyle. which rests against the articular fossa of the temporal bone, results in movement of the entire mandible downward and forward. Another concept is that the mandible is distracted and there is secondary growth at the condyle. Thus the upper and lower teeth and alveolar processes become more distant from each other. Since the teeth maintain occlusion by continued vertical eruption, the alveolar processes grow at their free borders. Disorders of mandibular growth, therefore, lead secondarily to changes in the upper face. They generally involve only the subnasal part of the maxilla.

The skull, a complex of bone(s), has proved to be both a rich and challenging source of study, particularly since the combination of different types of bone growth and increase in size of various cavities and growth, calcification, and eruption of teeth is not found elsewhere in the body. Cranial and orbital growth occur predominantly early in life, while facial growth occurs predominantly somewhat later in life, mostly during the periods of growth and eruption of the primary and secondary dentitions and the development of the paranasal sinuses. A number of excellent references are available that describe the anatomical structures and the details of craniofacial growth and movement. Every student of growth will delight in becoming acquainted with the varied seminal works of Hunter (1), Thompson (2), Weinmann and Sicher (3), and Brash et al. (4). Four (5)–(8), relatively recent review and summary retrospective articles plus the original reports offer additional details as well as clinical correlations and are suggested for further reference.

What follows serves as a brief general introduction for consideration of some of the various factors, and their subtleties and nuances that may or may not affect facial growth. In planning experiments to determine either change or nonchange in size and shape with time, as accurately as possible, various approaches were considered and used, both direct and indirect. Although the design of the experiments was such as to obtain either a "yes" or "no" answer, at times a "maybe" answer was the result. Invariably, after completion of the experiments, more questions were raised than answers. The findings were unequivocal but the explanations sometimes left some doubt.

This chapter will be limited to a few selected examples of both extensive gross morphological change and nonchange: (1) resection of the mandibular condyle in both the young and adult with severe changes not only of the mandible but also as a consequence of the ventral skull and midface; (2) resection of the nasal septum with extreme changes in the midface in the young but not the adult; (3) either decrease or increase in orbital contents volume with a resulting either less large or larger-than-normal orbit in the young but not the adult; and (4) resection of the frontonasal, median, and transverse palatine sutures in the young. Thus these models are representative of the lower face, the midface, the upper face, the lateral face, and the ventral skull. Other experiments with either alteration or nonalteration of bone growth are mentioned in Tables 3 and 4.

> . . . find out the cause of this effect,
> Or rather say, the cause of this defect,
> For this effect defective come by cause.
>
> *Hamlet*, Act II, Scene II

II. EFFECTS AND NONEFFECTS OF SURGICAL EXPERIMENTATION ON FACIAL GROWTH: A PERSONAL RETROSPECTIVE

A. Changes After Mandibular Condylectomy in Young and Adult Monkeys

What might be the effects of trauma to the condyle? To find some answers to these and other questions, unilateral mandibular condylectomies were performed on both young (9) and adult (10) monkeys.

After unilateral mandibular condylectomy in young monkeys, the operated-on side showed a lesser total facial, mandibular, and maxillary height and length, a shorter and a less laterally positioned ramus (Figs. 4,5), a coronoid process extending above the zygomatic arch, and an occlusal plane about level with (instead of considerably lower than) the zygomatic arch (Fig. 5A). Contrast this with an unoperated-on animal in Figure 5B. In addition, observation of the ventral side (Figs. 5E, F) of the skull on the operated-on

Table 3 Craniofacial Surgical Experiments That Produced Gross Bony Changes

Site	Animal	Procedure	Findings
Temporomandibular joint (9,10)	Young monkey Adult monkey	Unilateral resection of mandibular condyle and lateral pterygoid myotomy (Figs. 4 and 5)	Severe upper and lower facial and ventral cranial asymmetry
Cartilaginous nasal septum (11)	Young rabbit	Extensive resection of cartilaginous nasal septum (Figs. 6, 7, 8, and 9)	Severe upper and lower facial deformity
Maxillary sinus (12)	Adult dog	Extraction of adjacent teeth	Increase in volume of maxillary sinus
Orbit (13)	Young rabbit	a. Evisceration of eye	Deceleration of orbital growth directly related to volume of tissue removed
		b. Enucleation of eye	
		c. Exenteration of orbit	
		d. Increase in volume of eye (Figs. 11 and 12)	Increase in volume of orbit

Source: Modified from Ref. 6.

Table 4 Craniofacial Surgical Experiments That Produced No Gross Bony Changes

Site	Animal	Procedure	Findings
Temporalis muscle coronoid process (15)	Adult monkey	Unilateral intracranial resection of motor root V nerve	Atrophy of temporalis muscle No change of coronoid process
Cartilaginous nasal septum (16)	Adult rabbit	Extensive resection of cartilaginous nasal septum (Fig. 7B)	Local defect as a result of surgical procedure No gross deformity
Frontonasal suture (17)	Young rabbit	Unilateral and bilateral wide resection of suture not including mucoperiosteum	Regrowth of suture No gross deformity
Midpalatine and transpalatine sutures (18)	Young monkey	Complete resection of sutures including periosteum producing a complete cleft palate (Fig. 10)	Regrowth of sutures and scar tissue No gross deformity
Orbit (19)	Adult rabbit	Enucleation of eye	No change in volume of orbit
Eye, orbit (20)	Adult rabbit	Unable to increase volume of eye as in young	No change in volume of either eye or orbit
Upper and lower jaws (21)	Young human	Experiment of nature, complete absence of both primary and secondary dentitions	Growth of jaws and face within normal limits except for alveolar bone

Source: Modified from Ref. 6.

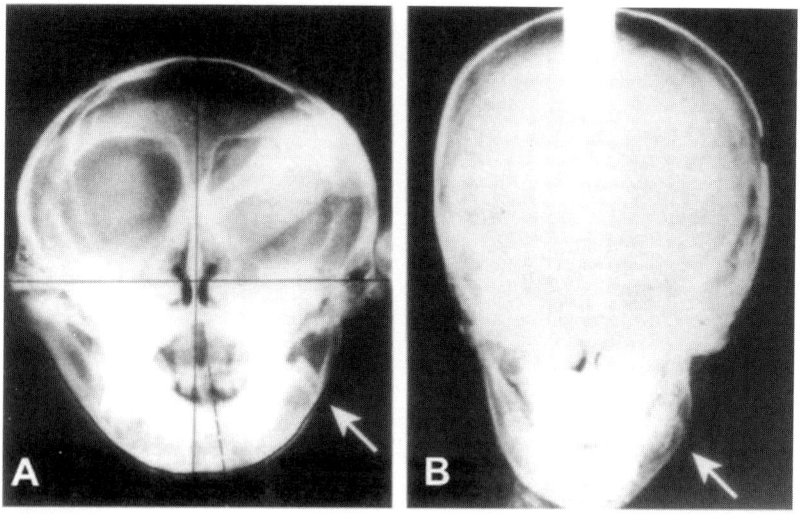

Figure 4 (A) Posteroanterior cephalometric radiograph 15 months after right condylectomy in a monkey. The horizontal plane of reference no longer passes symmetrically through the zygomatic arches. The mandibular asymmetry is especially prominent. The broken line, which corresponds to the midline of the mandibular dentition, emphasizes the considerable shift toward the operated-on side. Note that the right ramus (arrow) is in a more vertical rather than oblique direction and is less lateral than on the unoperated-on side. See B. (B) Posteroanterior radiograph of patient with mandibular condylar fracture dislocation. Note the vertical direction of the ramus on the side of the injury (arrow) compared with the oblique inclination of the ramus on the uninjured side. Compare with A, showing the monkey after condylectomy. (From Ref. 25.)

side revealed a number of differences, some of which were a lesser development of the temporal bone, a less long and rounder zygomatic arch, and a more anteriorly positioned external auditory canal and articular fossa.

Since the craniofacial skeletal changes were quite similar to but not the same as following condylectomy in adult monkeys (10), it seems that removal of the condylar growth site in the young monkey is not the principal factor responsible for the extreme changes. Rather, the alterations are probably secondary to disruption of normal temporomandibular joint function, muscular imbalance, and modification of sensory receptors. The direction and amount of muscle pull with altered position and motion of the mandible were modified by loss of the anatomical and physiological integrity of the temporomandibular joint. These include loss of function

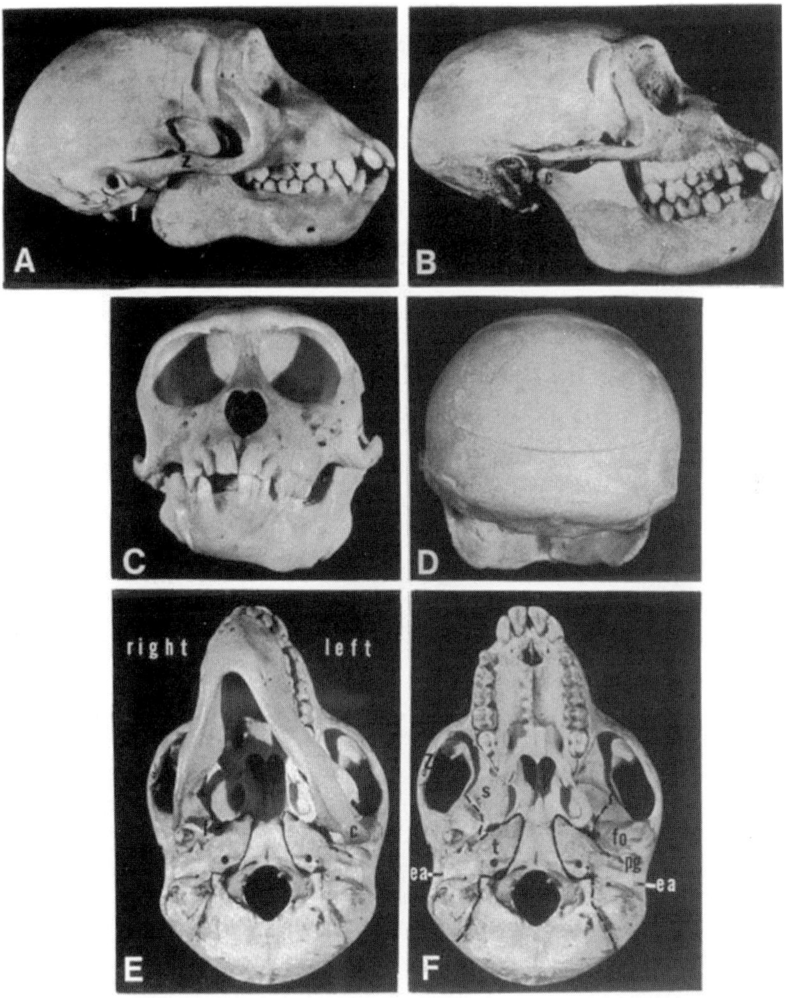

Figure 5 Skulls of young rhesus monkeys. Right mandibular condyle was resected at about 8 months of age (A, C, D, E, and F) with postoperative survival of 29 months. (E, F) Ventral views of skulls, with and without mandible in occlusion. Note, on operated-on right side, that the postglenoid process is less prominent, mandible articluates with temporal bone anterior to fossa, and the body is less long than the unoperated-on left side so that entire mandible is directed toward operated-on side (ea, external auditory canal; f, false articulation). (B) Unoperated-on animal. (From Ref. 9. Copyright 1957 from Excerpta Medica, Inc.)

of the lateral pterygoid muscle, altered function of the medial pterygoid, masseter, temporalis, and suprahyoid muscles, and establishment of a false joint. The remodeling of the ramus and adjacent bony structures, with changes in the bony trabecular pattern, followed these functional alterations (22). Is the mandibular condyle either a primary or a secondary site of growth? Condylectomy experiments in both the young and adult monkeys have demonstrated extreme lack of and/or loss of bone. However, these experiments do not prove that the condyle is not a site of growth.

B. Effects of Extirpation of the Cartilaginous Nasal Septum in Young and Adult Rabbits

Major amounts of the septovomeral regions and/or the cartilaginous nasal septum were resected in both young (11) and adult (16) rabbits (Figs. 6, 7, 8 and 9).

1. *Antemortem Observations*

As early as 4 days after resection of the cartilaginous nasal septum in young rabbits, there was a reversal of the relationship of the incisors, with the upper ones now being lingual to the lower ones (Figs. 6 and 9). As a result, the sharp incisal edge on the labial surface was not maintained. Consequently, considerable overeruption and fractures were frequent of the incisors, which continually erupt throughout life as a logarithmic spiral with a lateral shear. The long, smoothly curved, tapered face seen in unoperated-on control animals was in considerable contrast to the face of the experimental rabbit (Figs. 6 and 7). The snout became progressively stubby with postoperative survival, and a pronounced indentation appeared above the tip of the nose. This was suggestive of the face of a bulldog and certainly not that of a rabbit and was prominent within 3 weeks postoperatively.

2. *Postmortem Observations*

Changes noted in the dissected skulls of the experimental animals were limited to the snout in the region anterior to the orbits, zygomas, and molars (Fig. 7). Although the findings were not always consistent, generally the degree of change varied directly with the amount of septum resected and the postoperative survival period.

The snout, when seen from the side, was tapered and less long than that of the unoperated-on control. Whereas the snout in the control animal was the prominent part of the anterior face, this was not so in the

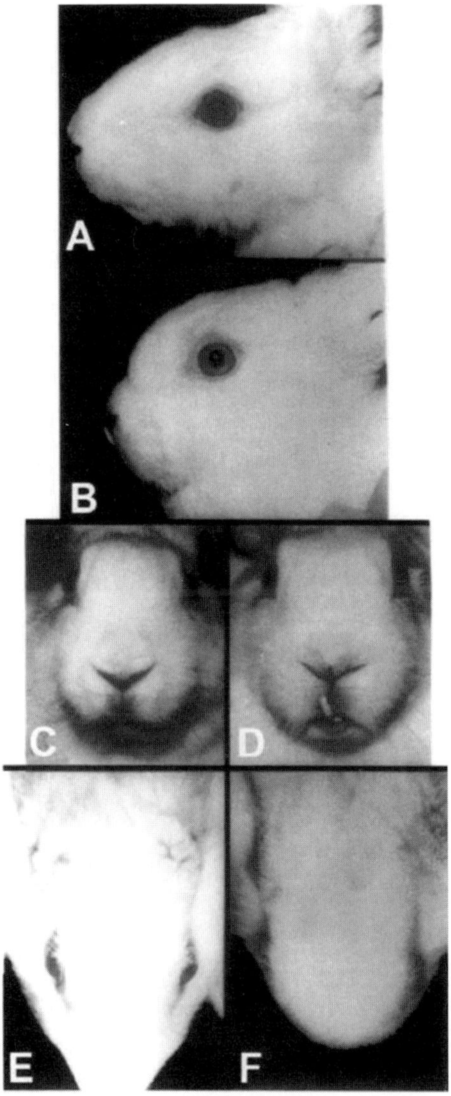

Figure 6 Antemortem photographs of a rabbit (A, C, and E) that had a minor amount of the nasal septum removed and a rabbit (B, D, and F) that had a major amount of the nasal septum removed at 21 days of age. Note the contrast in facial appearance. Also note the short, stubby, rounded face with an indentation above the nostrils and an overerupted lower incisor (B and D). (From Ref. 11a. Copyright 1966, Am J Anat. Wiley-Liss, a division of John Wiley & Sons, Inc.)

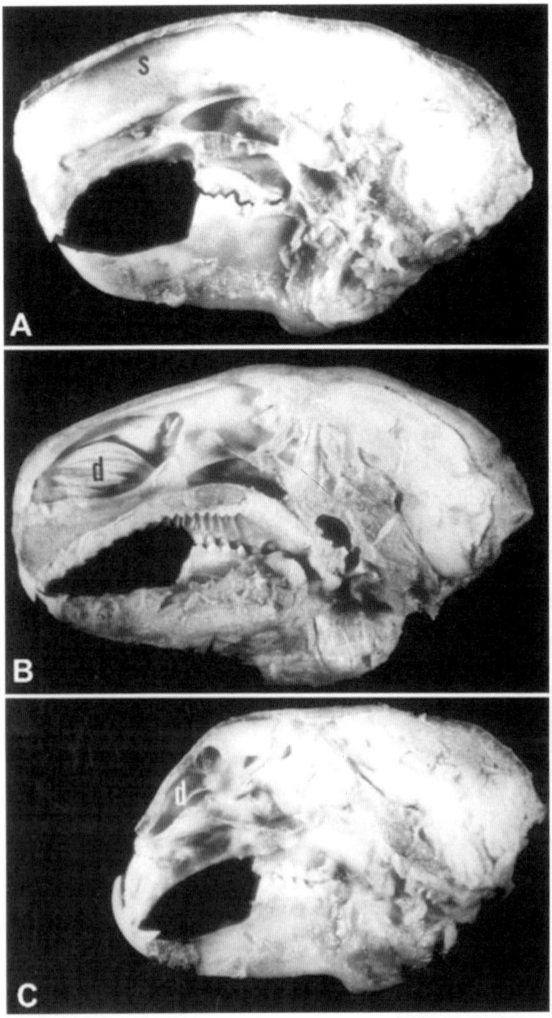

Figure 7 Postmortem photographs of right halves of parasagittally sectioned rabbit skulls. (A) Unoperated-on control animal. No cartilaginous nasal septum was resected. (B) Cartilaginous nasal septum was resected in this experimental animal when is was an adult. Compare with A and note similarities of size, shape, regularity, and relationship of incisors. Also note regularity of dorsal curvature uninfluenced by underlying septal defect (d). (C) Cartilaginous nasal septum was resected in this experimental animal at 3 weeks of age and it was euthanized about 4 months of age. Note short snout in an anterior direction beginning in the region of septal defect. (d). (From Ref. 16. Copyright 1967, American Medical Association.)

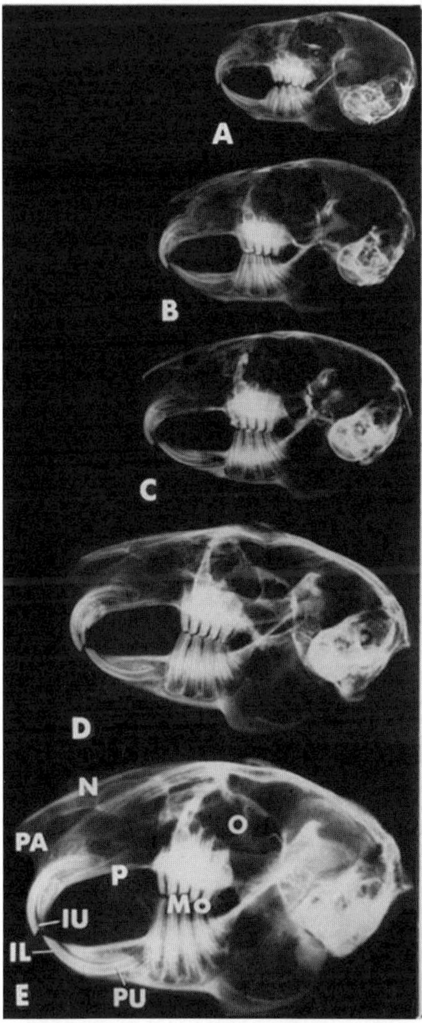

NO.	AGE IN DAYS AT DEATH
6-11	19
6-15	37
3-4	52
1-12	95
3-13	131

Figure 8 Reproduction of lateral radiographs, arranged according to age from 19 to 131 days at death (A–E), of parasagittally sectioned skulls of rabbits with cartilaginous nasal septum intact. Note downward smooth curve of anterior dorsum; length and anterior extension of nasal bone; size of pyriform aperture; length of palate; and form a position, and relationship of incisors. Contrast these with experimental animals in Figure 9. IL, lower incisors; IU, upper labial and lingual incisors; Mo, premolars and molars; N, nasal bone; O, orbit; P, palate; PA. pyriform aperture; PU, pulpal cavity. (From Ref. 27.)

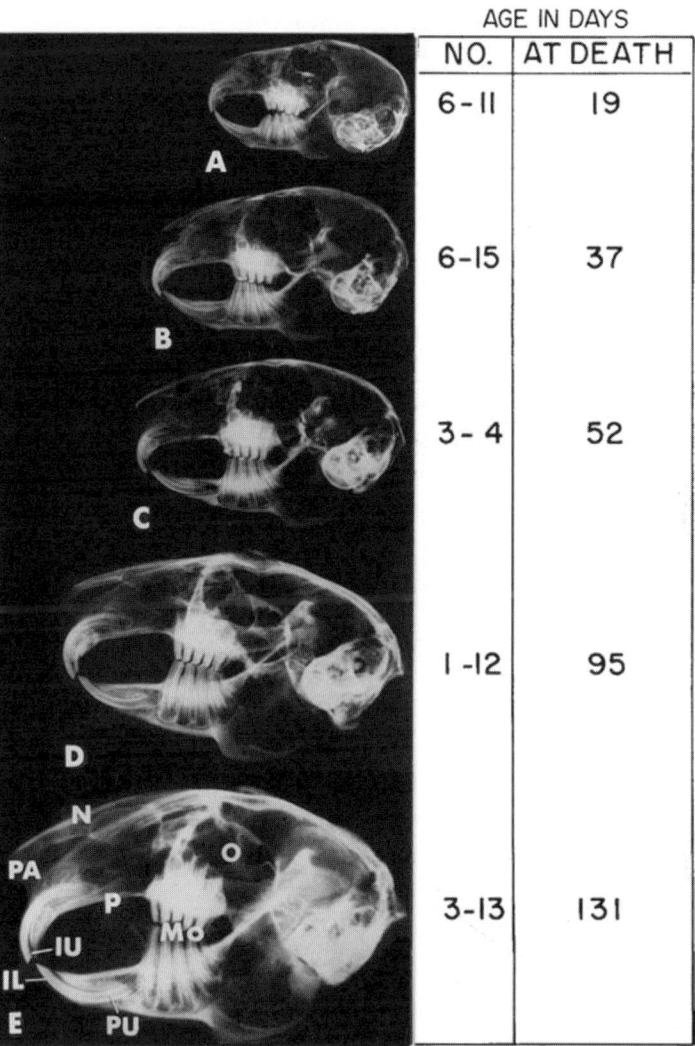

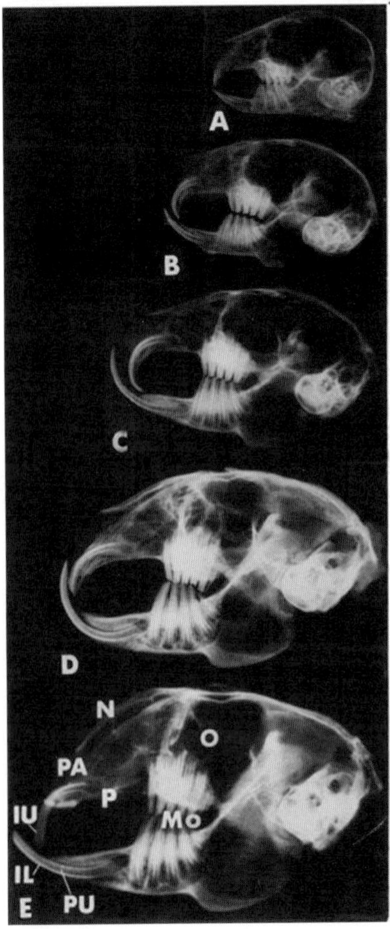

	AGE IN DAYS		
NO	AT OPER.	POSTOP. SURV.	AT DEATH
8-14	14	4	18
8-22	21	14	35
8-25	21	34	55
8-20	21	70	91
3-14	21	110	131

Figure 9 Reproduction of lateral radiographs, arranged according to postoperative survival, of parasagittally sectioned skulls of rabbits that had cartilaginous nasal septum resected at 14 or 21 days of age with postoperative survival of 4–110 days. Note flat anterior dorsum with increasing downward deflection in anterior direction with postoperative survival. Deflection begins at posterior site of resection. Contrast these with control animals in Figures 6, 7 and 8. Note less long snout, nasal bone, and palate and less large pyriform aperture. Also note in A that upper incisal edge is just lingual to lower one. This is more extreme in animals with longer postoperative survival (B–E). Also in contrast with Figure 8, incisors are considerably overerupted and longer and not in occlusion. Abbreviations as in Figure 8. (From Ref. 27.)

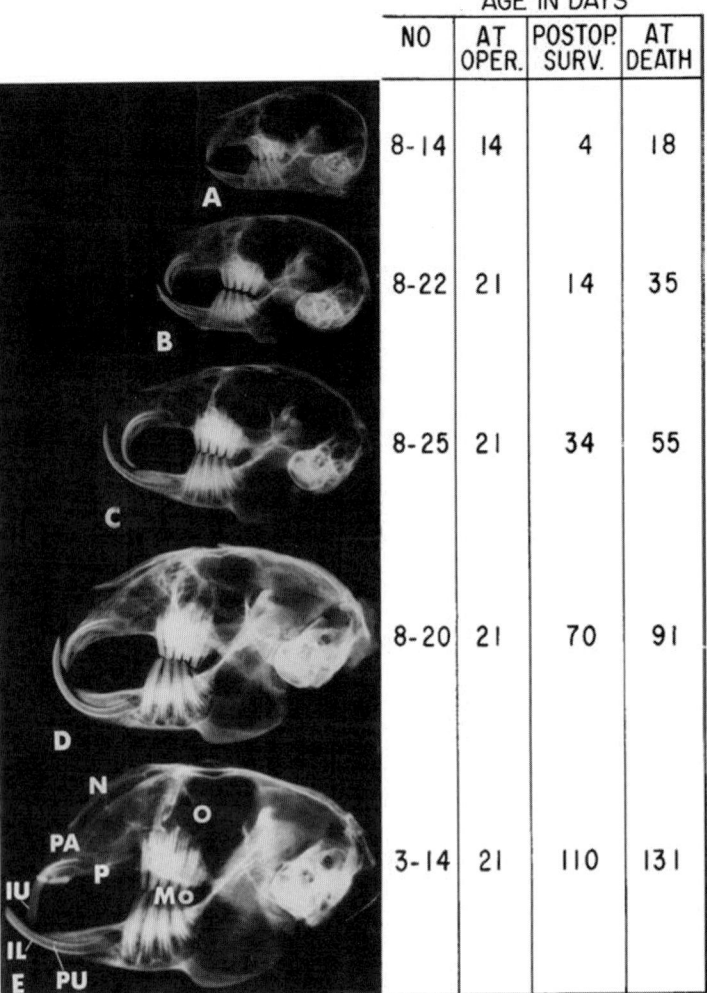

experimental rabbit. There was considerable deflection of the snout in a forward direction, beginning anterior to the frontonasal suture, in contrast to the smoothly curved dorsum of the control animals. From below, the palate and the incisive foramen were less long. From in front, the nasal aperture was less large. The snout from above was considerably less long than that of the littermate control animal. The nasal bones were considerably less long and narrower than those of the control animals and converged toward the premaxilla, with nasal height and volume being considerably less. The premaxilla and its frontal process were also less long. The end of the snout was tapered in the dorsoventral direction.

Examination of the parasagittally sectioned crania revealed in the experimental animals the extent of the septal defect in relation to the remaining septum and deformity of the snout and in the control animals the relation of the extent of the nasal septum to the snout. The site of the beginning of the downward deflection of the nasal bones was correlated with the posterior border of the septal defect, which was anterior to the frontonasal suture (Fig. 7C). Whereas in the control animal the nasal bones and hard palate were about parallel, in the experimental animal anterior projections of straight lines from the surfaces of these bones would soon intersect. Nasal septal resection in adult rabbits (16) did not result in these changes (Fig. 7B).

C. Extirpation of the Frontonasal Suture in Young Rabbits

The purpose of this experiment was to study the effects of trauma on the frontonasal suture (17). The maximal injury, that of extirpation of the suture, was imposed. Growing female New Zealand albino rabbits, 42–48 days of age at the time of the surgical procedure, were used. A dental *bur* mounted in a handpiece was used to extirpate the frontonasal suture either unilaterally of bilaterally. About a 1.0-cm channel was cut equally from the frontal and nasal bones. The nasomucoperiosteum was preserved wherever possible.

Dental amalgam was placed into 0.1-cm prepared cavities as radiographic markers 0.5–1.0 cm from the channel edge. The distance between each pair of implants was recorded. This distance between each implant and its adjacent channel border, and the width of the extirpated area, was measured on a line between the corresponding frontal and nasal bone implants. Immediately on completion of the surgical procedure, a cephalometric radiograph was taken. This was repeated at 14-day intervals. The 14-day increments and total amount of increased separation between implants in the frontal and nasal bones after bilateral or unilateral extirpation of the frontonasal suture were studied. Postoperative survival ranged from 14 to 84 days. The distances between the implants and extirpation borders were determined directly at the beginning of the experiment as well as at death.

The gross size and shape of the snout in the rabbits in which the frontonasal suture had been either bilaterally or unilaterally extirpated were similar to those of the unoperated-on control rabbits. No lateral deviation of the snout was observed in the rabbits with a unilateral extirpation. A less long snout was not seen in the rabbits after bilateral extirpation of the frontonasal suture. Rather, it was found that total longitudinal growth was esentially the same in both the control animals and those animals in which the suture was either bilaterally or unilaterally extirpated. With respect to the increased separation of the implants, the nasal part of the frontonasal suture contributed about half, the extirpation site a fourth, and the frontal part a fourth. The channel width increased as longitudinal growth proceeded. Thus, a wedging or expansive force between the frontal and nasal bones by the frontonasal suture apparently was not necessary for growth in that region. Separation of the nasal and frontal bones, in the absence of the normal suture, continued at all times in an amount not significantly different from normal.

These studies indicate the maximal injury as severe as extirpation of a facial suture failed to produce a growth arrest. Thus, although the frontonasal suture is a site of active growth, it is secondary rather than primary growth. What might be the primary site? Nasal septum?

D. Extirpation of the Median and Transverse Palatine Sutures in Young Monkeys

The purposes of this experiment were to determine (1) the gross effects of complete unilateral removal of the hard palate, including the median and transverse palatine sutures, upon palatal and facial growth and (2) the fate of the sutures after total resection in the otherwise normal monkey (18). Because the growth activity of the face is greatest during early life, the youngest *Macaca mulatta* obtainable were used. Their dental age at the beginning of the experiment was estimated to be about 8 months. The oral mucoperiosteum was first removed from the left half of the hard palate; then the exposed left bony palate was resected, including the median and left transverse palatine sutures, the major palatine foramen, and the nasal mucoperiosteum. Thus, open communication was established between the oral and nasal cavities by the complete surgical cleft. Care was taken not to disturb either the alveolar processes or the teeth. The postoperative survival period ranged from 1 to 34 months.

The surgically produced clefts of the hard palates, with complete communication between the oral and nasal cavities, persisted in varying degrees (Fig. 10). The postmortem examination of the soft tissue revealed the absence of rugae on the operated-on side in contrast to the regular and bilaterally symmetrical rugal pattern in the unoperated-on animals. The size of the clefts ranged from a narrow slit with overlapping of epithelial-covered scar tissue to an extensive cleft, including the boundaries of the surgical procedure (Fig. 10). In every animal the extensiveness of the bony palatal defect was masked by the overlying soft tissues. Where the palatal defect had been bridged by bone, an eccentrically placed suture was found, not in the midline, but rather on the operated-on side. No definite correlation could be made between the length of postoperative survival and either the size of the soft tissue or the bony cleft at postmortem.

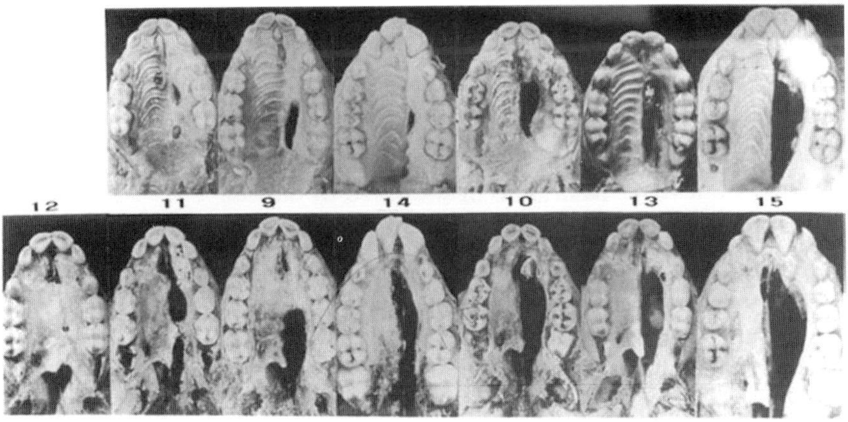

Figure 10 Postmortem photographs of oral palatal regions of monkeys arranged in approximate order of increasing unilateral defect in bony palate. The animals had both the median and transverse palatine sutures and both the oral and nasal palatal mucoperiosteum resected producing a complete cleft. The postoperative survival ranged from 1 to 34 months. There was no correlation between the postoperative survival and the palatal defect. The upper row of photographs was taken before the removal of the soft tissues. The lower row of photographs is of the corresponding animals after removal of the soft tissues. Note how the soft tissues mask the underlying bony defect. The rugal pattern is absent in the epithelial scarred surface of the healed operated-on side. Note, in the lower-row, animals 12, 11, and 9, that there is partial bony healing of the palatal defect and that the reformed suture line is eccentric toward the operated-side. (From Ref. 18.)

Both the operated-on and unoperated-on sides of the skulls were compared. In addition, skulls of operated-on monkeys were compared with unoperated-on controls. No significant gross difference was noted in growth and development of the hard palate, maxillary arch, mandibular arch, maxillomandibular relationship (arch form, occlusion, and tooth relationships), or total face. Within the limits of this experiment, it was concluded that extirpation of the median and transverse palatine sutures did not produce a grossly apparent growth arrest in either the palate or the face. Thus, it might be assumed either that these sutures do not make an important primary contribution to maxillary growth, or that other growth sites adjusted to the altered conditions. Since the jaws were in occlusion at the beginning of the experiment, the mandible may have guided maxillary growth.

After resection of the frontonasal suture with preservation of as much as possible of the nasomucoperiosteum, the suture reformed. And of course, after resection of cranial sutures with the dura and brain intact, the sutures reformed. The midpalatine suture was next selected because it could be completely resected without any underlying tissue remaining — no dura, no brain, no oral nasomucoperiosteum. Since a complete cleft could be produced, this seemed to be the ideal model to test the issue of sutural regrowth.

E. Findings After Decrease or Increase of Orbital Contents Volume in Young and Adult Rabbits

Facial growth is related to orbital growth (13). The shape and size of the orbit result from the balance of a number of genetic and epigenetic factors that may function on a systemic, regional, and local basis. Is there a key factor or are there many factors that influence orbital growth? Is there a correlation between orbital size and intraorbital mass? If so, what role do the vitreous and the aqueous humors, the lens, the globe, the muscles, and other extraocular structures play?

The relative capacity of the orbit and the size of the eye diminish with increase in body weight and size. In the human fetus and the newborn, the eyeball is so large in relation to the socket that it projects beyond the orbital rim so that a normal fetal exorbitism exists. In infants, the eyes are larger not only in proportion to body weight than in the adult but also in proportion to the size of the orbit. The growth of the zvgoma is related to the growth of both the orbit and the eyeball. In humans at birth, the orbital height is about 55% of the adult size and 79% at 3 years of age. At 7 years of age, orbital height is about 94% of the adult size, while facial height is still only 80%.

A series of experiments was carried out to evaluate the effects of either decrease or increase of volume of the orbital contents on orbital growth in both young (Figs. 11 and 12) and adult rabbits. These studies suggest that orbital volume in the young rabbit is dependent, at least in part, on the volume of the contents.

In three groups of young rabbits, varying amounts of intraorbital tissue were removed unilaterally (13). In one group, the intraocular contents, but neither the cornea nor the sclera. were extracted (evisceration) In a second group, the eye was removed (enucleation), and in a third group, the contents of the orbit were removed (exenteration). The postoperative survival was as long as 283 days. A removal permanent elastic rubber base imprint was made of the clean orbit. Orbital volume was calculated from the weight and specific gravity of the orbital imprint. A comparison of the orbital volume data after evisceration, enucleation, and exenteration showed a direct relationship between the lack of orbital mass and the subsequent lack of growth and development of the orbit. The orbit of the operated-on side did increase in volume but did not increase as much as on the unoperated-on side. Examination of orbits after enucleation of the eye in adult rabbits did not show such results (19).

After periodic intrabulbar injection of silicone to increase ocular mass in young rabbits, the orbital volume was grossly increased over the noninjected side (14) (Figs. 11 and 12). Repetition of this experiment in adult rabbits (20) did not produce such gross results (Table 4). Since the eye did not increase in size, another experiment should be done wherein bulbar expansion occurs.

III. THE FRACTURED RAT MANDIBLE: DIFFERENTIAL HEALING OF BONE, CEMENTUM, DENTIN, AND ENAMEL

A gross, radiographic, and histological study was based on 38 rats, ranging in age from 15 to 550 days, 29 of which were subjected to unilateral and nine to bilateral fractures to both the mandible and incisor (23). Since the rodent (and lagamorph) incisor constitutes a large part of the mandible, alveolar rather than body (as in most mammals) bone is fractured (Fig. 13B). The animals were anesthetized with diethyl ether, and the mandible and incisor were fractured with a pair of cutting pliers. The fracture was confined to the embedded portion of the incisor just anterior to the molars and was usually at 90° to the long axis of the body of the mandible and the incisor (Fig. 13). The fractured jaws were not immobilized. The diet of the experimental animals was adequate and balanced. Records of weight, general health, and

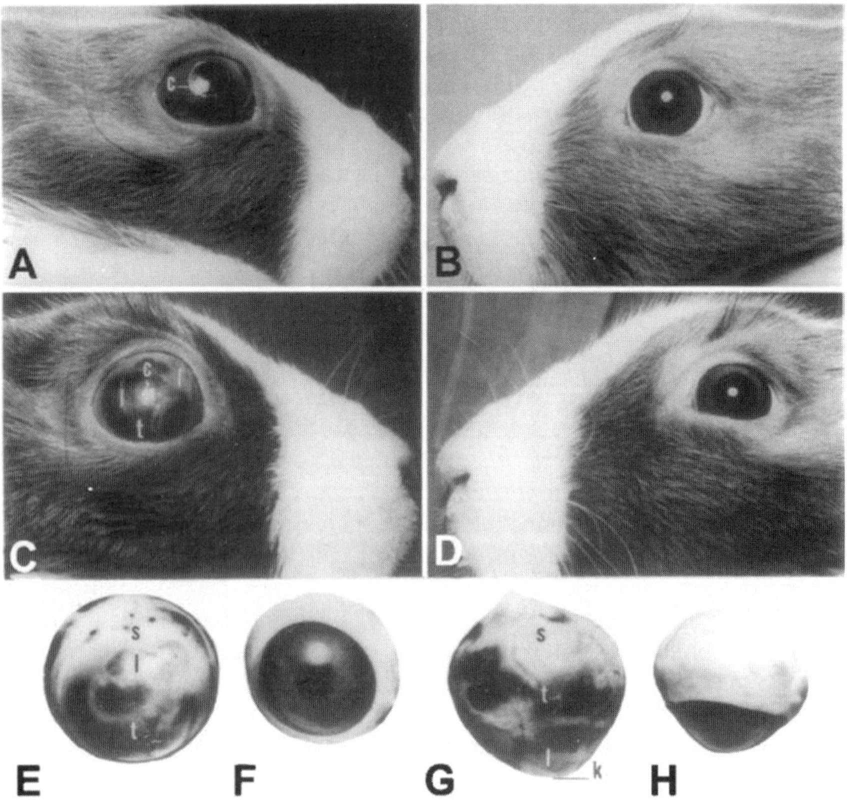

Figure 11 (A) Dutch rabbit, 6 weeks of age. After two injections, 2 weeks apart, a total of 0.2 mL of silicone had been instilled into the anterior chamber of the right eye. Note bulging of eye compared with B, left noninjected eye. (C) Same rabbit at 15 weeks of age after 10 injections at weekly intervals for a total of 1.6 mL of silicone. Note megalocornea with widening of interpalpebral fissure and distortion of corneal light reflex (c) as a result of corneal aberration and presence of globule of silicone in anterior chamber of the right eye. Note increased bulging of eye in C compared with A 9 weeks earlier, and D, left noninjected eye; 1, distortion of corneal light reflex, c; scleral thinning; t, with choroidal pigment visible as dark area. (D) Left noninjected eye. (E) Anterior enucleated injected eye in C. Note enlarged bulbus; megalocornea; corneal leukoma, 1. (F) anterior view of enucleated noninjected eye in D. Compare with E. (G) Superior view of enucleated injected eye in C. Note keratoconus, k, with megalocornea; corneal leukoma, l; sclera, s; and equatorial scleral thinning, t, with dark diffusely distributed choroidal pigment visible. (H) Superior view of enucleated noninjected eye in D. Compare with G. (From Ref. 14. Copyright 1974, Am J Anat, Wiley-Liss, a division of John Wiley & Sons, Inc.)

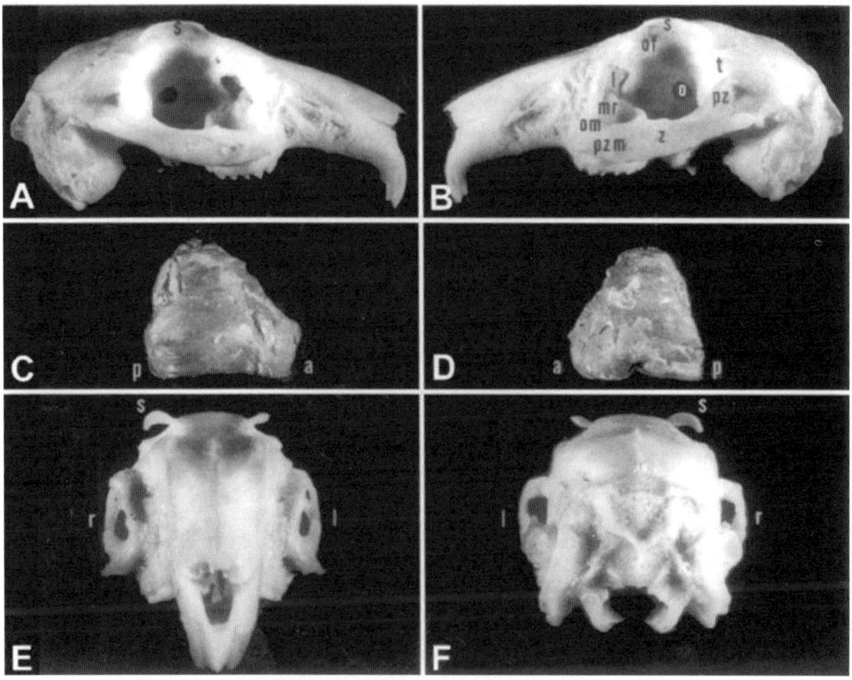

Figure 12 Photographs of skull of Dutch rabbit at 15 weeks of age and superior view of elastic rubber base orbital imprints (C and D). After 10 injections at about weekly intervals, a total of 1.6 mL of silicone had been instilled into the anterior chamber of the right eye. (A) Right orbit (volume 3.9 mL) of injected eye. It is 8.3% larger than the left orbit. (B) Left orbit (volume 3.6 mL) of noninjected eye. l, lacrimal bone; mr, molar root region; o, optic foramen; of, orbital part of frontal bone; om, orbital process of maxilla; pz, zygomatic process of squamosal; pzm, zygomatic process of maxilla; s, supraorbital process of frontal bone; t, temporal fossa; z, zygomatic arch. (C) Imprint of right orbit. Note that it is larger than imprint in d, of left orbit (a, anterior, p, posterior). (E) Anterior view of skull. Note that the supraorbital process (s) is larger and higher on the right injected eye side (r). (F) Posterior view of skull. (From Ref. 14. Copyright 1974, Am J Anat. Wiley-Liss, a division of John Wiley & Sons, Inc.)

gross appearance of the mandible and incisors were kept after the surgical procedure.

The animals were killed from $6\frac{1}{2}$ h to 158 days after the surgical procedure. A midsagittal section was made to facilitate radiography of the mandible. Additional dissection consisted of separating the mandible and preparing it for histological study.

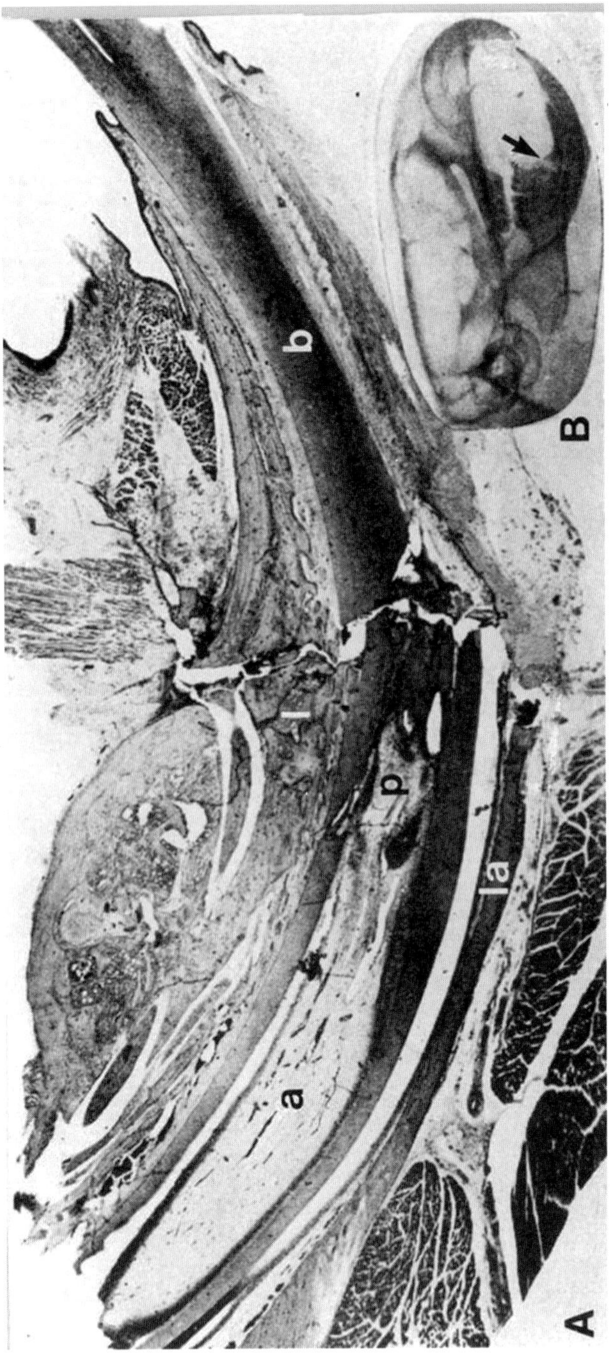

Figure 13 (A) Photomicrograph of demineralized midsagittal section of lower right incisor and madible of a rat that was killed 6 1/2 h after mandibular fracture that divided the incisor into posterior (a) and anterior (b) fragments. The fracture is complete and extends from the lingual bone (l), which is fragmented across the tooth to the labial bones (la). The pulp (p) shows hemorrhage and acute inflammation. (B) Radiograph of the right half of the head of the same animal. The arrow indicates the site of the fracture just anterior to the molars. (From Ref. 23. Copyright 1944, American Medical Association).

A. Bone Healing

Bone healing was active, with rich tissue reactivity. The stages of histological repair of the fractured rat mandible may be summarized in the following chronological order: (1) procallus: (a) hemorrhage and initial blood clot (first few hours); and (b) organization of blood clot and invasion by granulation tissue (first few days); (2) fibrous and/or fibrocartilaginous callus (first few weeks); and (3) bony callus (first and second month) and reorganization of bone (first year). These events were in complete agreement with those occurring in the healing of other bones. Formation of bone was demonstrated histologically during the second month but not radiographically until about the fourth month.

B. Dental Changes

By contrast, the fractured tooth differed from bone by the absence of callus formation and by its limited cellular reaction. Dental changes were chiefly passive and nonregrenerative and were as follows: (1) adult enamel reacted only mechanically and was incapable of response by either inflammation or repair; occasionally, it lost its epithelial covering, which was replaced by connective tissue or cementum; (2) dentin showed no direct reaction, but the region between fragments became infiltrated by cells of either the pulp or periodontal membrane; larger fragments were joined by fibrous union; odontoblasts were injured, and an atypical secondary dentin was formed in the pulp; (3) the pulp showed a rich and varied response, ranging from necrosis to complete recovery, and included bone formation and hematopoiesis (Table 5).

C. Healing of Mineralized Tissues

Experimental complete transverse fractures of the mandible in the rat offered a unique opportunity to both study and compare the effects of simultaneous fractures on the growing bone and the growing tooth (Table 5). While the enamel, dentin, cementum, and bone are all hard, mineralized structures, they differ significantly in their response to injury and their capacity for repair. The dental issues that were capable only of apposition were generally nonreactive, while bone and cementum, which were capable of both apposition and resorption, were highly reactive and able to recover from the trauma. The fractured rat tooth changed from an actively functioning organ to one of deformity and dysfunction, while the repair of bone was frequently effective in restoration of normal function.

Table 5 Differential Reactions of Bone and Teeth to Injury

Formative cells	Bone osteoblasts	Cementum oementoblasts	Dentin odontoblasts	Enamel ameloblasts
Location of formative cells	Periosteum, endosteum, lining of Haversian canals, bone marrow	Single layer, lining the periodontal ligament adjacent to the cementum	Single layer lining pulp adjacent to most recently formed dentin	On surface of enamel in formative stage absent in adult enamel
Cellular contents	Osteocytes	Cementocytes	Acellular	Acellular
Channels	Canaliculi, Haversian canals, Volkmann's canals	Canaliculi in cellular cementum	Dentinal tubules, avascular	None
Contents of channels	Processes of osteoblasts, osteocytes, vessels and nerves, and osteoclasts	Processes of cementocytes	Processes of odontoblasts	None
Response to injury in young	Sensitive to metabolic changes leaving semipermanent record	Sensitive to metabolic changes leaving semipermanent record	Very sensitive to metabolic changes leaving permanent record	Very sensitive to metabolic changes leaving permanent record

Response to injury in adult	Continuous apposition and resorption; rich regenerative power through osteogenic properties of periosteum, endosteum, and bone marrow	Limited regenerative capacity through cementoblastic properties of periodontal cells	Can transmit stimuli through its tubules from dentinoenamel junction to pulp and limited response through odontoblasts (reparative dentin)	Entirely physical, passive, incapable of response by inflammation or regeneration, nonvital
Response to fracture	Very active through rich cellular activity along internal and external surfaces of bone	Partial through periodontal ligament cellular response	Passive or partial through secondary pulpal or cemental reaction	None
Degree of mineralization	70%±	50%±	70%±	96%±

Source: Modified from Ref. 23.

ACKNOWLEDGMENT

I am greatly indebted and thankful to Moira Stovall of the Media Center, School of Dentistry, UCLA, for her unstinting efforts and utter devotion in the development of this chapter.

REFERENCES

1. Hunter J. The Natural History of the Human Teeth. London: J Johnson, 1771.
2. Thompson D. On Growth and Form. Cambridge, England: Cambridge University Press, 1958.
3. Weinmann JP, Sicher H. Bone and Bones. 2d. ed. St Louis, MO: Mosby, 1955.
4. Brash JC, McKeag H, Scott, JH. Aetiology of Irregularity and Malocclusion of the Teeth. 2d. ed. London: Dental Board of the United Kingdom, 1956.
5. Sarnat BG. Some methods of assessing postnatal craniofaciodental growth: a retrospective of personal research. Cl Pal Craniof J 1997; 34:159–172.
6. Sarnat BG. A Retrospective of personal craniofaciodental research and clinical practice. Plast Reconstr Surg 1997; 100:132–153.
7. Sarnat BG. Basic science and clinical experimental primate studies in craniofaciodental biology: a personal historical review. J Oral Maxillofacial Surg 1999; 57:714–724.
8. Sarnat BG. Effects and noneffects of personal environmental experimentation on postnatal craniofacial growth. J Craniof Surg 2001; 12:205–217.
9. Sarnat BG. Facial and neurocranial growth after removal of mandibular condyle in *Macaca* rhesus monkey. Am J Surg 1957; 94:19–30.
10. Sarnat BG, Muchnic H. Facial skeletal changes after mandiublar condylectomy in the adult monkey. J Anat 1971; 108:323–338.

11a. Sarnat BG, Wexler MR. Growth of the face and jaws after resection of the septal cartilage in the rabbit. Am J Anat 1966; 118:755–767.

11b. Sarnat BG. The face and jaws after surgical experimentation with the septovomeral region in growing and adult rabbits. Acta Otolaryngol 1970; 268 (Suppl):1–30.

12. Rosen MD, Sarnat BG. Change of volume of the maxillary sinus of the dog after extraction of adjacent teeth. Oral Surg Oral Med Oral Pathol 1955; 8:420–429.

13a. Sarnat BG, Shanedling PD. Orbital volume following evisceration, enucleation and exenteration in rabbits. Am J Ophthalmol 1970; 70:787–799

13b. Sarnat BG. The orbit and eye: experiments on volume in young and adult rabbits. Acta Ophthalmol 1981; 147 (Suppl):1–44.

14. Sarnat BG, Shanedling PD. Increased orbital volume after periodic intrabulbar injections of silicone in growing rabbits. Am J Anat 1974; 140:523–532.
15. Sarnat BG, Feigenbaum A, Krogman WM. Adult monkey coronoid process after resection of trigeminal motor nerve root. Am J Anat 1977; 150:129–138.
16. Sarnat BG, Wexler MR. The snout after resection of nasal septum in adult rabbits. Arch Otolaryngol 1967; 86:463–466.

17. Selman AJ, Sarnat BG. Growth of the rabbit snout after extirpation of the frontonasal suture: a gross and serial roentgenographic study by means of metallic implants. Am J Anat 1957; 101:273–293.
18. Sarnat BG. Palatal and facial growth in *Macaca* rhesus monkeys with surgically produced palatal clefts. Plast Reconstr Surg 1958; 22:29–41.
19. Sarnat BG. Orbital volume after enucleation and eye volume in the adult rabbit. Graefes Arch Clin Exp Ophthalmol 1978; 208:241–245.
20. Sarnat BG. Adult rabbit eye and orbital volumes after periodic intrabulbar injections of silicone. Ophthalmologica 1979; 178:43–48.
21. Sarnat BG, Brodie AG, Kubacki WH. Fourteen year report of facial growth in case of complete anodontia with ectodermal dysplasia. Am J Dis Child 1953; 86:162–169.
22. Herzberg F, Sarnat BG. Radiographic changes in the bony trabecular pattern in the mandible of growing *Macaca* rhesus monkey following condylar resection. Anat Rec 1962; 144:129–134.
23. Sarnat BG, Schour I. Effect of experimental fracture on bone, dentin and enamel: study of the mandible and incisor in the rat. Arch Surg 1944; 49:29–38.
24. Sarnat BG. Clinical and experimental considerations in facial bone biology: growth, remodeling and repair. J Am Dent Assoc 1971; 82:876–889.
25. Sarnat BG. Normal and abnormal craniofacial growth: some experimental and clinical considerations. Angle Orthodont 1983; 53:263.
26. Sarnat BG: Craniofacial growth, postnatal. In: Delbucco R, ed, Encyclopedia of Human Biology. 2nd ed. San Diego, CA: Academic Press, 1997.
27. Sarnat BG, Wexler MR. Br J Plast Surg 1969; 22:313–323.

5

Maxillofacial and Craniofacial Surgery: Our Family Tree

S. Anthony Wolfe
University of Miami, Miami, Florida, U.S.A.

I. INTRODUCTION

A generation of man—the time from birth to adulthood, and production of the next generation—is generally taken to be 25 years.

The formation of a plastic surgeon takes longer. If one finishes medical school at 25 and takes eight additional years of training, the generation for a plastic surgeon would be 33 years, or three generations per century.

II. EARLY DEVELOPMENTS

Maxillofacial surgery in 1900 did not differ greatly from what surgeons were doing during the American Civil War, except that anesthesia was now available, although it had to be administered by open-drop-ether masks. This limited drastically what surgeons were able to do. Some improved dental splints were available for the treatment of jaw fractures, and one notable individual, Edward H. Angle, M.D., D.D.S., in his publication that was the seminal work in the development of the field of orthodontics, stated bluntly that interosseous wiring of a mandibular fracture should never be done (1). Some pioneering work in the treatment of facial malignancy was performed by David Cheever (2) in the United States and Bernhard von Langenbeck (3) in Germany, who performed a variety of access osteotomies to permit tumor removal. Aside from the precocious and unappreciated mandibular osteotomy performed by Simon P. Hullihen in 1848 in Wheeling, West Virginia, orthognathic surgery was not considered possible (4).

The first generation of the twentieth century, who were active between 1900 and 1933, were responsible for a tremendous flowering in the field of maxillofacial surgery. George Crile (5) developed the radical neck dissection for cervical cancer, Edward Angle and Vilray Blair (6) took pioneering steps in orthognathic surgery with first a body osteotome and then a ramus osteotomy for manibular deformities. Harvery Cushing (7) and Walter Dandy (8) were creating the new subspecialty of neurosurgery. Medical education underwent restructuring after the Flexner report (9), and the Board system for examination and certification of surgeons began.

In England, Sir Harold Gillies made enormous advances in facial reconstruction with soft-tissue flaps, tube pedicles, and autogenous bone grafting (10,11). The use of these methods in the treatment of those with facial injuries sustained in the trench warfare of World War I is considered to be the beginning of the specialty of reconstructive plastic surgery.

In France, Victor Veau (12) focused on the problems of cleft lip and palate, and the Curies investigated radioactivity (13). In Germany, Roentgen (14) developed the x-ray, and Axhausen (15), Joseph (16), Cohn-Stock (17), and Esser (18) made major contributions to maxillofacial surgery.

III. THE MID-TWENTIETH CENTURY

The generation that came after this one spanned the period from 1933 to 1966. The injured of World War II received better treatment than those of the previous war owing to advances in blood transfusion and anesthesia. However, surgical methods had changed little, with head caps and tube pedicles similar to those of the previous generations being widely used. In 1942, Milton Adams (19) brought forward the principle of fixation of facial fractures to the nearest higher intact structure, but facial fractures were still treated by interosseous wires placed through small incisions directly over the fractures. Ralph Millard (20) began his seminal contributions to cleft lip and palate in the late 1950s, and Paul Tessier (21–28) about the same time began his work with the Le Fort 3 type osteotomy, although he did not present the work for another decade [1967, Rome].

IV. THE LATE TWENTIETH CENTURY

From the mid 1960s to the end of the twentieth century—our generation—a number of elements coalesced to make this a period of extraordinary productivity. Some of these areas of progress include:

1. Anesthesia. Endotracheal anesthesia became safe and commonplace, respirators became reliable, monitoring devices much more sophisticated, and intensive care units developed that were run by full-time, on-the-spot intensivists. Storage and testing of transfused blood became better.
2. Imaging devices. CT and MRI have allowed us to see with precision and in fine detail in three dimensions, with much better understanding of the anatomy of the face, making planning and the ability to evaluate our results much better.
3. Surgical equipment. Collaboration between surgeons and manufacturers of medical equipment became closer, with the development of plating systems specifically developed for use on the facial bones, including biodegradable systems, better electrocauteries, and suture material with swagged-on needles.
4. Surgery itself. Development of new surgical principles, tactics, and techniques—in short, how surgeons conceptualize and go about their craft—have taken of all of the above.

Building on the contributions of the prior generation of German-speaking maxillofacial surgeons, Hugo Obwegeser (29) showed the versatility of the sagittal split, and Jacques Dautrey (30) and Bernd Speissl (31) made further improvements in technique and instrumentation. Obwegeser and Karl Hogeman (32) of Sweden made the Le Fort 1 osteotomy commonplace, and Obwegeser was the first to do a simultaneous two-jaw movement (33). With collaboration in preoperative planning and preparation by a new generation of orthodontists accustomed to working with surgeons, orthognathic surgery now could move the tooth-bearing structures predictably and with stability in all directions. Besides his contributions to maxillofacial surgery, Hugo Obwegeser also became a leader in educating a new generation of maxillofacial surgeons, both at the Zahnartliches Institut in Zurich and through his involvement with the European Society of Maxillofacial Surgeons.

Obwegeser added substantially to the existing specialty of maxillofacial surgery; Paul Tessier created an entirely new specialty de novo. After showing the success of the subcranial Le Fort 3–type osteotomy (a subcranial craniofacial procedure that was a higher facial advancement than had been previously performed, but still nevertheless a maxillofacial procedure),

Tessier went on with Gerard Guiot and other neurosurgeons at Hôpital Foch in Paris to show the safety and many possibilities of the transcranial approach to the face. The entire face could be dissected subperiosteally through coronal, intraoral, and lower-eyelid incisions. Segments of facial bones could be displaced and rigidly fixed in any new position desired, and the success of all of the procedures rested on the liberal use of autogenous bone grafts. The demonstrated success of these procedures used for congenital anomalies led to the same methods being used for simultaneous tumor removal and reconstruction, and primary bone grafting in major facial fractures. At the end of the twentieth century, experienced craniofacial teams in a number of centers around the world regularly applied Tessier's methods with rates of morbidity and mortality that became lower and lower.

Other contributions were made in plastic surgery that could be applied to maxillofacial and craniofacial surgery. These included myocutaneous flaps, microsurgical free-tissue transfer, and tissue expanders. Joe McCarthy (34) and Fernando Molina (35) showed how to make small mandibles larger by applying Ilizarov's method of distraction osteogenesis (36), and John Polley (37) and others developed equipment that could distract the maxilla. However, contrary to some initial predictions, distraction osteogenesis does not seem to have supplanted orthognathic surgery in most cases. Rather, it has made it possible to provide earlier treatment for conditions that were not well suited to traditional orthognathic techniques.

Although numerous new antibiotics have been developed, the tremendous ability of microorganisms to reprogram their biochemical structure and rapidly develop resistant strains has been a great disappointment and relative failure. Hopes are high that newer types of antibiotics can be developed, based on having the complete DNA map of the human being available from the Human Genome Project.

Endoscopic surgery, originally developed by gynecologists and then adopted by general surgeons, was tried by plastic surgeons on a number of conditions. The most common use by far is for the endoscopic forehead lift. The technology has been applied to the harvest of certain types of free flaps, and less often in breast augmentation and abdominoplasty. In maxillofacial surgery, the best application so far seems to be in the fixation of condylar fractures and the visualization of hard-to-see areas such as the medial orbital wall through the lower eyelid, where it is in reality not being used for much more than a convenient light source. Each new technology needs to have its proper applications established, and discussion still continues as to whether, for instance, it is better to approach an orbital floor fracture through a Caldwell Luc approach with an endoscope or through a more direct and simpler conjunctival incision. Similarly, it may seem convoluted to some to perform an endoscopic release of a unilateral coronal synostosis simply to avoid a slightly longer incision in the scalp when the tradeoff requires wearing a cranial-molding band for a year after the surgery. New technology will eventually find its appropriate applications.

V. THE FUTURE

What will come for the generation that will extend to 2033? We can expect that biochemical and genetic advances will be made that will help with spontaneous tissue generation, so that instead of a bone graft we will be able to add a material that will lead to bone formation where it is added. Mundane but frustrating problems, such as keloid formation, will hopefully find a cure, as will more and more forms of cancer.

The greatest advances may come, perhaps, if we develop systems of providing medical care that will simply make it possible to apply what we are able to do at the highest level in a regular basis to all comers. Just as designated burn centers have greatly improved the outlook for burn patients, facial fractures, cancer, and congenital anomalies should be treated in designated centers by surgeons with the highest level of expertise. The hideous, convoluted, grotesque, and nightmarish system of medical care currently operating in the United States, wherein bureaucrats who call themselves "medical directors," but have no real expertise in medicine, are rewarded financially for denying as much care as possible, must be dismantled and replaced with a viable system. A certain basic level of care could best be provided by a national health service, but a nightmare in the other direction should be avoided by allowing patients considerable choice in their own medical decisions, and perhaps expecting them to pay for some of it out of their own pocket.

REFERENCES

1. Angle EH. Treatment of Malocclusion of the teeth and Fractures of the Maxilla, Angle's System. Philadelphia: SS White, 1898.
2. Cheever DW. Displacement of the upper jaw. Med Surg Rep Boston City Hosp 1870; 1:156.
3. von Langenbeck B. Dtsch Klin 1861, p. 281.
4. Hillihen SP. Case of elongation of the under jaw and distortion of the face and neck, caused by a burn, successfully treated. Am J Dent Sci (1st Series) 1849; 9:157.
5. Crile GW. Excision of cancer of the head and neck. JAMA 1906; 47:1780–1786.
6. Blair VP. Surgery and Diseases of the Mouth and Jaws. St Louis: Mosby, 1912.
7. Cushing HC. Disorders of the pituitary gland. JAMA 1921; 75:25.

8. Dandy WE, Blackfan KD. An experimental and clinical study of internal hydrocephalus. JAMA 1913; 61:2216.
9. Flexner, AbrahamMedical Education in the United States and Canada. Boston: Merrymount Press, 1910.
10. Gillies H. Plastic Surgery of the Face. London: Henry Frowde, Hodder & Stoughton, 1920.
11. Gillies H, Millard DR Jr. The Principles and Art of Plastic Surgery. Boston: Little, Brown, 1955.
12. Veau V. Bec-de-lievre. Hy othese sur la malformation initiale. Ann Anat Pathol 1935; 12:329.
13. Quin S. Marie Curie: A Life. New York: Simon & Shuster, 1995.
14. Roentgen WK. On a new kind of ray. Proc Wurzburg Phys-Med Soc. December 28, 1895.
15. Axhausen G. Histologische Studien üüber die Ursachen und den Ablauf des Knochenbaus im osteoplastischen Karzinom. Virchows Archi Pathol Anat Physiol 1909; 195:358–462.
16. Joseph J. Ungewohnlich grosse Gesichtsplastik. Dtsch Med Wochenschr 1918; 44:465.
17. Wolfe SA, Gunther Cohn-Stock MS, DDS. father of maxillary orthognathic surgery. J Craniofacial Surg 17:331.
18. Haeseker B. Esser (1877–1946) and the dawn of maxillofacial prosthetics in the Netherlands. Ned Tijdschr Tandheelkd 1991; 98(7):283–286.
19. Adams WM. Internal wiring fixation of facial fractures. Surgery 1942; 12:253.
20. Millard DR Jr. Cleft craft, I. Boston: Little, Brown & Co, 1986.
21. Tessier P. Reflections on cranio-facial surgery in children today and in the future. Ann Chir Plast 1979; 24(2):109–119.
22. Tessier P. Experiences in the treatment of orbital hypertelorism. Plast Reconstr Surg 1974; 53(1):1–18.
23. Tessier P. Orbital hypertelorism. Fortschr Kiefer Gesichtschir 1974; 18:14–27.
24. Tessier P. Orbital hypertelorism. I. Successive surgical attempts. Material and methods. Causes and mechanisms. Scand J Plast Reconstr Surg 1972; 6(2): 135–55.
25. Tessier P. Total osteotomy of the middle third of the face for faciostenosis or for sequelae of Le Fort 3 fractures. Plast Reconstr Surg 1971; 48(6):533–541.
26. Tessier P. The definitive plastic surgical treatment of the severe facial deformities of craniofacial dysostosis. Crouzon's and Apert's diseases. Plast Reconstr Surg 1971; 48(5):419–442.
27. Tessier P. [Orbito-cranial surgery]. Minerva Chir 1971; 26(16):878–904.
28. Tessier P. Treatment of facial dysmorphisms in craniofacial dysostosis (DCF). Crouzon and Apert diseases. Total osteotomy of the facial massif. [Sagittal displacement of the facial massif]. Neurochirurgie 1971; 17(4):295–322.
29. Obwegeser H, Professor Hugo L. Obwegeser on the occasion of his 60th birthday. J Maxillofac Surg 1980; 8:332.
30. Dautrey J. Advantages and difficulties of the sagittal osteotomy of the ascending remus in surgery of the mandible. Rev Stomatol Chir Maxillofac 1970; 71(1):82–87.

31. Speissl B. New concepts in Maxillofacial Bone Surgery. Chapter 6, 1st ed. New York: Springer, 1976.
32. Hogeman KE, Omnell KA, Sarnas KV, Willmar K. Surgical and dental-orthopaedic correction of horizontal and vertical malocclusions. Scand J Plast Reconstr Surg 1967; 1(1):45–50.
33. Trauner R, Obwegeser H. The surgical correction of mandibular prognathism and retrognathia with consideration of genioplasty. Part I. Surgical procedures to correct mandibular prognathism and reshaping of the chin. Oral Surg Oral Med Oral Pathol 1957; 10(7):677–689.
34. McCarthy JG, Stelnicki EJ, Grayson BH. Distraction ostegenesis of the mandible: a ten-year experience. Semin Orthodont 1999; 5(1):3–8.
35. Molina F, Ortiz Monasterio F. Mandibular elongation and remodeling by distraction: a farewell to major osteotomies. Plast Reconstr Surg 1995; 96(4):825–840.
36. Ilizarov GA, Deviatov AA. Surgical lengthening of the shin with simultaneous correction of deformities. Ortop Travmatol Protez 1969; 30(3):32–37.
37. Polley JW, Figueroa AA. Rigid external distraction: its application in cleft maxillary deformities. Plast Reconstr Surg 1998; 102(5):1360–1372.

6

Fracture Healing and Bone Graft Repair

Samuel T. Rhee, Lawrence Tong, and Steven R. Buchman
Mott Children's Hospital, Ann Arbor, Michigan, U.S.A.

I. INTRODUCTION

Fracture healing is a dynamic affair that coordinates a host of complex interacting mechanisms. These remarkable repair processes highlight the powerful regenerative abilities of fractured bone, which can culminate in restoration of the damaged part to a near-anatomical state.

The sequence of events leading to regeneration of bone after fracture healing parallels embryogenic development processes of bone formation. During adult life, continuous remodeling normally occurs as resorption of bone and new bone formation proceeds. The nearly perpetually active state of bone allows significant physiological adaptation in response to a variety of external and internal stimuli.

Although many factors regulating fracture healing and bone remodeling long have been studied, the recent explosive advance of techniques in molecular biology has generated a sudden wealth of information regarding cellular interactions and genetic expression during new bone formation. This advanced understanding is already driving a new generation of enhanced bone regeneration therapies that will transform clinical management of bone repair and grafting.

II. BONE COMPOSITION AND TERMINOLOGY

Bone is a specialized form of connective tissue where the extracellular component is partly mineralized. The inorganic extracellular matrix, which makes up two-thirds of the dry weight of bone, is composed primarily of calcium salts such as hydroxyapatite, which provides the tissue significant rigidity and strength. The organic extracellular matrix ix comprised primarily of collagen (90–95% type I), glycoproteins, and proteoglycans (1).

Three types of cells have been characterized in bone: osteoblasts, osteocytes, and osteoclasts. Osteoblasts, and osteocytes are derived from mesenchymal-type cells termed osteoprogenitor cells (or preosteoblasts or osteogenic cells), while osteoclasts originate from macropage-monocytic cell lines. *Osteoblasts* are immature osteocytes that synthesize organic extracellular matrix called *osteoid*, which subsequently undergoes mineralization to form bone. As osteoblasts become encased in bone, they further differentiate into *osteocytes*, residing in spaces in the calcified extracellular matrix called *lacunae*. Lacunae are interconnected by numerous narrow canals called canaliculi, which contain thin cytoplasmic extensions of osteocytes. *Osteoclasts* are multinucleated cells characteristically found lining bone surfaces in small depressions called Howship's lacunae, where they act to resorb bone tissue. *Osteoprogenitor cells* line several areas, including endosteal surfaces of cortices such as marrow cavities and haversian canals, as well as the inner lining (cambium layer) of the periosteum, which is the surface covering of condensed fibrous tissue investing most bones.

New bone is initially created in a form known as *woven bone*, an immature type that is characterized by coarse, irregular collagen organization. Woven bone is produced during early bone development and fracture healing, and it is subsequently remodeled and organized to form lamellar bone, which constitutes the majority of the mature skeleton. *Lamellar bone* has a characteristic multilayered structure, which results from continuous deposition on existing bone surfaces. This process results in concentrically stratified units termed *osteons* (previously called Haversian systems).

Lamellar bone is divided into two types, cortical (or compact) bone and cancellous (or spongy) bone. *Cortical bone* is comprised of multiple osteons arranged around central neurovascular channels known as haversian canals. Continuing cycles of resorption and deposition of bone result in secondary osteons replacing the initially produced primary osteons. The structure of *cancellous bone* is trabeculated and less dense than cortical bone, which open spaces, spicules, and increased vascular tissue.

A. Osteogenesis and Bone Growth

Osteogenesis during fracture healing recapitulates many of the earliest processes found in bone development and formation. While the most basic cellular processes remain the same for all osteogenesis, two variant methods: initial bone formation occur by intramembranous ossification and endochondral ossification.

Intramembranous (or membranous) *ossification* occurs when bone is deposited directly into embryonic condensations of mesenchymal tissue. Many craniofacial bones, including the cranial vault, the maxilla, and most of the mandible, are formed in this manner. In addition, the iliac crest, scapula, and clavicle also develop in an intramembranous fashion. *Endochondral ossification* occurs by formation of an initial cartilaginous precursor, which is progressively replaced by bone. Cartilaginous epiphyses or epiphyseal grown plates are responsible for continued longitudinal growth. The long bones, vertebrae, pelvis, and the skull base develop via endochondral ossification.

III. FRACTURE REPAIR

A. Macroscopic Aspects of Fracture Repair

When a bone sustains impact, kinetic energy is transferred and the resultant force is dissipated through the tissue. The magnitude and direction of force, the load rate, and the stress duration will determine whether the affected bone will fail. Fracture occurs when the maximum limit of strain or force is surpassed.

In addition to fracture of the bone, additional trauma is sustained at the fracture site aside from the loss of structural integrity. The soft-tissue envelope surrounding the fracture is disrupted, often with associated damage to muscle, tendon, and ligamentous tissue. The vascular supply is compromised as blood vessels rupture. Bleeding ensues with resultant hematoma formation at the site of injury.

Clinical signs of fracture may consist of pain, tenderness, deformity, and decreased range of motion. Functional deficits can be elicited as well as associated neurovascular injuries.

The resultant fracture site immediately after injury is a milieu of devitalized soft tissues, clot, and dead bone. As the healing process commences, the nonviable elements are degraded and the hematoma resorbs. The region of bone bordering the affected area undergoes revascularization, which can be seen grossly as the formation of granulation tissue. This tissue bridges the fracture site and incorporates the interfragmentary gaps.

The clinical signs associated with revascularization are inflammation with swelling and edema.

After 3–4 days, a collar of soft tissue begins to form around the bone in the region of the fracture, which is referred to as *soft callus.* The soft callus may take up to a month to form, binding the fracture fragments. It provides internal support for the injured bone and helps achieve fibrocartilaginous union of the fracture site. The callus forms externally along the marrow cavity and limits motion at the injured area. This immobilization helps prevent reinjury and avoids disruption of newly formed blood vessels and granulation tissue. Clinically, the end of pain and inflammation corresponds with soft-callus formation.

Hard callus is formed by mineralization of the soft callus and conversion to bone. The formation of hard callus may take up to 2 months and upon completion represents bony union. Stability at the fracture site increases with the formation of hard callus since the bone fragments are no longer mobile. The union is substantial enough to allow weight bearing. Once the hard callus is formed and union is achieved, the fracture site will appear healed radiographically. Often excess bone may be visible externally and may fill the marrow cavity internally.

A process of modeling and remodeling beings to replace the initial hard callus with dense compact bone. These changes may take years and serve to recontour the bone and restore the integrity of the marrow cavity. Over time the orientation of bone reflects the strains and loads of use. Modeling ensures that the forces transmitted through the bone are supported by its architecture. In the case of a displaced fracture, these forces work to elicit the best possible conjunction of form and biomechanical function. At the end stages of healing, some residual thickening may be seen radiographically; however, the fracture site can be indistinguishable from normal bone.

In addition to the processes of intramembranous bone repair where mesenchymal tissues condense directly into bone tissue, and endochondral fracture healing in which a cartilaginous intermediate develops, in some instances bone may undergo another fracture healing process known as *primary*, or *osteonal, healing* after a fracture without a cartilaginous intermediate. There is minimal evidence of either soft or hard callus formation, and bone is formed directly at the edges of the fracture. The new bone bridges the fracture site and remodeling begins immediately. Lack of motion, close apposition, and compression at the fracture site foster this process. This is the method of bone healing most commonly seen with compression plates.

Local conditions influence fracture healing. Severe trauma with associated extensive injury to adjacent soft tissues may retard bone healing, and an indadequate reduction or undue distraction at the fracture site can also compromise fracture repair. Indaequate immobilization or tissue interposition between fracture bones may lead to delayed union or nonunion. Concurrent malignancy, poor nutrition, infection, or previous irradiation at the fracture site can impede the healing process.

B. Histological Aspects of Fracture Repair

The disruption of the blood supply to a bone when a fracture takes place leads to ischemia and necrosis (2). The amount of dead bone correlates with ischemic areas created by interruption of the intracortical blood supply and the destruction of the medullary and periosteal capillary systems. Greater levels of injury to bone correlate with increased ischemia due to interruption of the vascular supply. Soft-issue and marrow elements are disrupted and the periosteum is split along with bony fragmentation and shearing of blood vessels. Local osteocyte death leads to release of lysosomal enzymes with subsequent destruction of collagenous and noncollagenous organic matrix. Hematoma floods the wound and the acute inflammtory response ensues. Local tissue reaction results in widespread vasodilatation and edema.

Bloodborne elements are contained in the hematoma and provide the initial population of cells at the fracture site. Platelet degranulation results in an initial release of inflammatory cytokines. As clot forms, platelet deposition continues and a fibrin scaffold develops, allowing migration of new cells to the site of injury. Additional early inflammatory cells include macrophages, polymorphonuclear leukocytes (PMN), and mast cells. In addition, osteoclasts derived from syncytial consolidation of monocytes are present (3). Macrophages and giant cells begin to remove necrotic debris and resorb hematoma as osteoclasts assimilate and remove dead bone while digesting and eroding fracture surfaces (4).

As the healing process continues, precursor mesenchymal cells and osteoprogenitor cells proliferate and migrate into the wound from adjacent muscle and marrow as well as from local layers of endosteum and the cambium layer of the periosteum (5). These cells contribute to the earliest formation of bone at the fracture site (6). The blood supply to the fracture is primarily periosteal in origin, but as the clot continues to organize, neovascularization occurs with endothelial cells and smooth-muscle cells migrating along the fibrin scaffold with ingrowth of capillary buds and granulation tissue (7).

The development of capillaries provides the pool needed for ongoing replacement of cells during fracture repair. There is an influx of mononuclear cells from the blood and local differentiation of cells of the cambium layer of the periosteum. These local precursor cells differentiate into osteoblasts, fibroblasts, and chondroblasts, respectively producing osteoid, collagen, and cartilage (8,9). Initially, type I, II, and III collagen is deposited, but with maturation of the soft callus, type I collagen predominates, forming the framework on which mineralization occurs (10). With the onset of hard-callus formation, there is intensive regeneration of new Haversian systems, and remodeling occurs to accommodate physical forces placed on the injured bone.

As osteoclastic degradation of devitalized fracture fragments continues, there is an increase in cellularity and protein synthesis at the fracture site. The periosteum thickens and a collar of tissue grows around the fragmented bone that consists of inflammatory cells, differentiating multipotential cells, and their products. These cells, which differentiate into fibroblasts, chondroblasts, and osteoblasts, soon produce fibrous tissue, cartilage, and woven bone in a structure termed the soft callus. Found at the external portion of the bone and within the medullary cavity, the soft callus binds the fracture site. This cellular and tissue interaction culminates with a state of fibrous union, bridging and stabilizing the broken bone. The larger the diameter of the callus the more mechanical advantage it possesses (11). The main constituent of the soft callus is unmineralized cartilage, especially at the more peripheral areas. Regulation of the composition of cartilage, fibrous tissue, and bone of the soft callus is poorly understood but seems to be controlled by differences in local factors such as degree of bone displacement, vascularity, soft-tissue injury, and fracture contamination.

The cartilage of the soft callus gradually converts to bone by a process of endochondral ossification. The cartilage intermediate, made up of primarily type II collagen, undergoes degradation, and the cells of the soft callus begin to synthesize and secrete new matrix composed chiefly of type I collagen (12). Calcium hydroxyapatite is deposited in the matrix, and the resultant calcified collagen structure forms a slender perforated labyrinth of interconnecting spaces that are invaded by developing blood vessel (13). Osteoprogenitor cells migrate along the new vascular channels and form a layer on the calcified remnants of cartilage matrix. These osteogenic cells differentiate into osteoblasts, which lay down woven bone with disorganized collagen element (14). The woven bone forms a network of fine trabeculae in the interstices of the capillary channels. This immature woven bone results in bony union of the fracture site; weight stress can be placed on the fracture when this stage is complete.

Once bony union is achieved, the fracture site initially does not resemble the architecture of the original bone, nor does it have preinjury strength and stability. Continued modeling and remodeling restore original form and function. Modeling refers to cellular interactions that result in a normalization of bony macrostructure, while remodeling is the cell-mediated breakdown and reformation of bone leading to reorientation of the bony infrastructure in response to physical forces. These processes work concurrently to complete the sequence of events in bone healing (15). Histologically, the hard callus is made up of woven bone, which is patterned after capillary ingrowth rather than the lines of force. A highly organized set of successive layers of lamellar bone replaces woven bone under the influence of functional stresses.

Cellular modules or units of osteoclasts and osteoblasts are activated in sequences of both bone resorption and formation to convert the preliminary contours of the hard callus to the original bony architecture (16). First, osteoclasts resorb the excess irregular woven bone not subjected to strains or loads. Osteoblasts then deposit a new organic matrix of lamellar bone that later mineralizes, resulting in new struts of mature bone laid down along lines of stress. These sequences continue to cycle, re-establishing the marrow cavity as well as restoring the structure of normal, haversian system (15). Once bony strength and structure are re-established, the processes of modeling and remodeling continue on a lesser scale as part of normal homeostatic mechanisms managing physiological demands on the bony skeleton.

Primary bone healing, or osteonal healing, referred to earlier, differs histologically from the sequence of events just described, which is typically termed secondary healing. In the case of primary bone healing, mechanical factors such as lack of motion and close apposition of the fracture site, which typically occurs in the proper application of rigid compression plates, allow direct internal remodeling and intracortical healing to take place. Primary bone healing occurs in fractures treated with open reduction and rigid internal fixation when the fractured bone ends are closely apposed and immobilized. This sequence of fracture repair lacks significant inflammation, a cartilaginous or mesenchymal intermediate (as found in endochondral or intermembranous healing), or callus formation (17). Existent osteoprogenitor cells differentiate into osteoblasts, and locally derived osteoclasts of osteogenic or hematological origin initiate bone healing. Units or cones of osteoclasts move across the fracture line, resorbing dead bone. Another cone of osteoblasts trails behind, depositing woven bone parallel to the axis of the long bone (18). This process parallels the intramembranous ossification that occurs in embryological development of flat bones. Primary bone healing incorporates and connects haversian systems, remodeling bone at the fracture site. New osteons traverse the fragments of broken bone, culminating in direct osteonal union.

C. Biochemical and Molecular Aspects of Bone Healing

The theory of *regional acceleratory phenomenon* (RAP) is an attempt to explain the complex network of regulatory controls initiating and maintaining fracture repair (19). This theory states that as a response to injury, the ultimate healing of a fracture occurs through a series of interrelated cellular events controlled by local and bloodborne proteins. RAP begins with local changes resulting from an injury to bone and relates these changes to perturbations of local cells. Autocrine, paracrine, and endocrine factors produced by these cells initiate biochemical changes leading to a well-coordinated cascade of reactions between cells and their products, resulting in fracture repair. These interactions may contribute to the communication, timing, and influence of specific elements responsible for bone repair, and information regarding this network could potentially lead to pharmacological intervention to enhance bone repair.

Bone repair is initiated by the activation or induction of local and bloodborne cells and their subsequent proliferation and interaction. Examples include the processes of osteoinduction and osteoconduction as outlined by Urist (20). Osteoinduction involves the transformation of mesenchymal pluripotential cells into bone-forming cells by means of chemical, humoral, and/or physical signals. Osteoconduction refers to the ingrowth of capillaries and osteoprogenitor cells into the fracture from the surrounding bone and soft tissues, interconnecting the fragments and leading to gradual formation of new bone. It has also been referred to as "creeping substitution" in the case of bone graft healing (21). These processes, both of which are active and important in fracture repair, appear to be controlled by local proteins produced by cells at the fracture site and influenced by endocrine signaling as well.

1. Growth Factor Release

Many growth factors and regulatory protein complexes have been isolated that have been demonstrated to influence various portions of the bone-healing cascade (22). These substances are thought to be temporally released to fit into the schema of fracture repair and to drive the coordinated cellular interaction needed for an ordered progression toward bone regeneration.

The cells involved in the early stages of bone repair are essentially those present in any early traumatic wound. Bleeding at the fracture site leads to platelet aggregation and clot formation. PMNs, macrophages, and fibroblasts are attracted to the area of the injured bone in the first several hours and days after injury, when multiple chemoattractant factors and mitogens are present. As part of the first response to injury, platelet-derived growth factor (PDGF) and transforming growth factor-beta (TGF-beta) are released by degranulating platelets (23). This is followed immediately by infiltrating macrophages and other inflammatory cells secreting fibroblast growth factor (FGF) as well as additional TGF-beta and PDGF. IL-I and IL-6 are also thought to be released along with a host of other cytokines; however, this has only been indirectly demonstrated, and much of the proinflammatory and immune cytokine expression during the fracture repair process remains imprecisely identified (24,25).

PDGF has been shown to elicit an endothelial response and to promote fibroblast chemotaxis and proliferation. In addition, PDGF enhances cartilage synthesis and production of type II collagen. Concurrent prostaglandin release recruits monocyte precursors than can then differentiate into osteoclasts. Prostaglandins have been shown to increase the size and number of osteoclasts that can cause profound effects on bone resorption. Lymphokines and monokines derived from bloodborne elements in the hematoma act as mitogens, recruiting and directing cells to move into the wound and begin to divide.

Macrophages and other inflammatory cells express fibroblast growth factors 1 and 2 (FGF-l and FGF-2), which are angiogenic and may foster neovascularization of the fracture site and early formation of granulation tissue. Later in the fracture-healing course, FGFs are expressed by masenchymal cells, chondrocytes, and osteoblasts and have been demonstrated to enhance TGF-beta expression in osteoblastic cells via a receptor tyrosine kinase pathway. FGF-1 (or acidic FGF) appears to be primarily mitogenic for chondrocytes, and expression peaks during chondrogenesis. FGF-2 (or basic FGF) is thought to be more potent and is expressed by osteoblasts. It is thought to influence multiple phases of fracture repair ranging from events in early injury to late callus remodeling. Kallikreins also stimulate the release of vasoactive and angiogenic factors that can affect the local blood supply. Local lymphocytes and monocytes release osteoclast-activating factor (OAF), which stimulates osteoclastic bone resorption.

TGF-beta is a pleiotropic growth factor released by degranulation of platelets within the hematoma and by the extracellular matrix at the fracture site (23,25,26). During the initial stages of fracture healing, TGF-beta is immunolocalized to the region of the hard callus where periosteal proliferation and intramembranous bone formation occur (25,26). In this early stage, TGF-beta likely stimulates proliferation of preosteoblasts within the area of injury. Later during the fracture-healing process, TGF-beta levels increase during chondrogenesis and endochondral bone formation, with peak levels temporally coinciding with chondrocyte hypertrophy (25,26). TGF-beta acts to stimulate undifferentiated mesenchymal and chondrocyte proliferation and associated extracellular matrix production. In addition, TGF-beta may be involved in coordinating bone formation with resorption (25).

Many of the endogenous effects of TGF-beta during fracture healing have been most accurately deduced from studies of exogenously applied TGF-beta in animal models. In vitro studies have shown both inhibitory and stimulatory effects of TGF-beta depending on local cell conditions, suggesting that cell culture results may not accurately reflect in vivo effects of TGF-beta (27). Five isoforms of TGF-beta have been identified to data (28). Isoforms TGF-beta 1 and TGF-beta 2 have been studied most extensively in regard to fracture healing. TGF-beta appears to have the ability to stimulate bone healing, as demonstrated by several studies. Continuous infusion with high-dose TGF-beta at the defect sites in midtibial osteotomies in rabbits resulted in dose-dependent increases in callus volume and increased mechanical strength versus untreated osteotomies (25,29). Similarly, TGF-beta was injected at a fracture site every 2 days for 40 days in a rat tibial fracture study, resulting in a dose-dependent increase in callus cross-sectional area and mechanical strength (30). These improved results in fracture healing with TGF-beta administration appear to require high dosages with persistent treatment (25). Other studies utilizing single-treatment doses at the time of osteotomies have failed to show significant improvement in bone healing. Large calvarial defects in adult baboons treated with human TGF-beta 1 did not result in significant new bone formation compared to untreated defects (31).

Insulin-like growth factors (IGFs), also known as somatomedins, are known to stimulate osteoblastic cell proliferation and type I collagen synthesis in vitro (32). Serum concentrations of IGF are regulated by growth hormone and have a wide range of systemic mitogenic effects. IGFs are incorporated into bone matrix during bone formation and are released during resorption (33). As one of the most abundant growth factors stored in bone matrix, IGFs are released during fracture healing and are present in varying concentrations in fracture callus tissue. Although IGF has a variety of anabolic effects on osteoblasts in vitro, in vivo studies have resulted in varied results. A study with bony defects in rabbits did not demonstrate increased healing with systemic IGF application (34). However, in other studies, subcutaneous IGF infusion did improve bone repair in calvarial and zygomatic arch defects in adult rats (35,36). While the osteogenic effects of exogenous application of IGF in fracture healing are still undergoing further study, it has been hypothesized that physiological IGF acts to modulate coupling of bone formation to resorption (37). Many current studies have focused on utilizing IGF to bolster osteogenesis in osteopenia resulting from increased resorption, such as in postmenopausal and skeletal disuse models (38–40). Owing to the small size of IGF peptides, the bioavailability of systemically administered IGFs is short. Associated protein complexes, known as IGF-binding proteins (IGFBPs), increase the half-life of IGFs and potentiate their effects (41).

2. Osteoinductive Factors

One group of cytokines, *bone morphogenetic proteins* (BMPs), has been demonstrated to have true osteoinductive properties. BMPs have been proven to stimulate new bone formation in vitro and in vivo. In addition, they play critical roles in regulating cell growth, differentiation, and apoptosis in a variety of cells during development, particularly in osteoblasts and chondrocytes.

A subfamily of the TGF-beta superfamily of polypeptides, BMPs are distinguished from other peptides in this group by having seven, rather than nine, conserved cysteines in the mature region (42). There are currently 16 identified BMPs, although only a subset have been found to be expressed in fracture healing (42). BMPs were initially characterized by Urist; their identification was based on the capacity of demineralized bone powder to induce de novo bone formation in an intramuscular pouch, demonstrating the ability to directly induce mesenchymal connective tissue to become bone-forming osteoprogenitor cell (43,44).

BMP signal transduction occurs through serine-threonine kinase receptor-mediated pathways in a manner similar to TGF-beta. BMP signaling involves a complex receptor pattern whereby the BMP protein binds BMP receptor type II, which leads to the association of the complex with BMP receptor type I, resulting in an active receptor-ligand complex. This interaction can be blocked by BMP antagonists noggin and chordin, which prevent receptor binding. Activation of the BMP-signaling pathway is transmitted through a family of signal effectors termed SMADs (an acronym derived from the *C. elegans* gene Sma and the *Drosophila* gene Mad, the first identified members of this family) (25).

During fracture repair, BMP-2, BMP-3 (also known as osteogenin), BMP-4, and BMP-7 (OP-1) have been found to be expressed to varying degrees (25). BMPs are initially released in low levels from the extracellular matrix (ECM) of fractured bone. Osteoprogenitor cells in the cambium layer of the periosteum may respond to this initial BMP presence by differentiating into osteoblasts. Immunolocalization demonstrates an increase in detectable BMP-2/4 near the fracture ends in the cambium region of the periosteum (45,46). BMP receptor IA and IB expression is dramatically increased in osteogenic cells of the periosteum near the ends of the fracture in the early postfracture period (47). Staining for BMP-2, BMP-4, and BMP-7 is minimal around the fracture hematoma, but is upregulated in primitive mesenchymal cells as they infiltrate the fracture site and proliferate (45). Approximately 1–2 weeks postfracture, BMP-2/4 expression is maximal in chondroid precursors, while hypertrophic chondrocytes and osteoblasts show moderate levels of expression. It is hypothesized that the role of BMPs in fracture repair is to stimulate differentiation in osteoprogenitor and mesenchymal cells that will result in osteoblasts and chondrocyte (25). As these primitive cells mature, BMP expression decreases rapidly. BMP expression temporarily recurs in chondrocytes and osteoblasts during matrix formation, and eventually decreases during callus remodeling.

Studies of BMPs in animal models have demonstrated their capability to induce union of large segmental critical size defects that otherwise would fail to heal (25). The addition of partly purified canine BMP to carrier implants significantly increased new bone formation in radial segmental defects in dogs (48). Another canine study showed that the addition of recombinant human BMP-7 (rhBMP-7) to collagen carriers in ulnar segmental defects was associated with complete radiographic bony union, while collagen carrier alone failed to show new bone formation (49). rhBMP-2 has also demonstrated new bone formation in other animals. One report found dose-dependent osteogenesis with BMP-2 treatment in critical-size femoral defects in rats (50). Similar dose-dependent osteogenesis with rhBMP-2 was found in a rabbit ulnar defect model. In this study, high-dose BMP-2 resulted in union for all treated animals, while half of the low-dose-treated animals demonstrated union. Untreated animals had no union. Mechanical testing found that the BMP-2-treated healed ulnae achieved strength and stiffness comparable to that of intact control ulnae (51). Critical size defects in adult baboons have been successfully treated with partly purified BMP-3 (52). BMP-induced osteogenesis in another rhesus monkey cranial defect study demonstrate a histological sequence of mesenchymal cell proliferation, cartilage differentiation, woven bone formation, and lamellar bone formation with nearly complete healing at 16 weeks of a 14–20-mm defect (53). Similar findings in sheep and dogs have been reported (54,55).

Clinical studies utilizing partly purified BMPs have been used in combination with autologous and allogeneic bone grafts to successfully repair large segmental defects of the tibia and femur (56–62). In one study, 30 patients were treated with allograft and partly purified human BMP, supplemented with autograft if the defect was greater than 2 cm. Healing was demonstrated in 24 patients at a mean of 6 months after BMP treatment (56). In prospective randomized study, 30 tibial nonunion patients were treated by reamed nailing with either rh-BMP-7 or autograft, with no significant differences in healing found between the two groups (63). No significant adverse effects were noted. A proliferation of animal and clinical studies are underway to evaluate different BMP delivery systems that modulate the concentration, localization, and duration of administration.

D. Biophysical Aspects of Fracture Healing

1. Oxygen Tension

Changes in oxygen tension influence the formation of bone and cartilage at the fracture site. Relatively hypoxic cells in settings of low oxygen tension are more likely to form cartilage intermediates during bone formation (64). Histologically, nests of persistent cartilage are formed in areas of the fracture callus most distant from the capillary buds. Conversely, higher oxygen tensions are related to the promotion of direct bone healing. In fact, the requisite immobilization needed for primary bone healing is thought to be due to the need to maintain higher oxygen tensions at the fracture site. Rigid fixation may accomplish this by preventing reinjury to blood vessels and preserving oxygen delivery to the wound (4,65).

Although higher oxygen tensions may generate bone without a cartilage intermediate, it should be noted that this level of oxygen tension is high only relative to other areas of healing bone. In fact, the overall partial pressure of oxygen found in tissue during bone repair is low when compared to systemic values. In general, low oxygen tension favors bone healing (66). Experimental evidence of in vitro bone growth shows optimal results in a setting of low partial pressure of oxygen (67). Utilizing organ culture of embryonic chick tibia, one study deomonstrated maximum osteogenesis under 35% ambient oxygen and suppression under 5% oxygen. With high oxygen concentrations (95%), the embryonic cartilage in the explant became damaged and badly eroded by chondroclasis (68,69).

Bone and cartilage cells follow a mostly anaerobic metabolic pathway. The fracture hematoma has a lower pH than serum, and lactate production increases and peaks during the metabolically active period of soft-callus formation. This increase in acid production is in keeping with biochemical evidence of glycolytic enzyme patterns during the proliferation of bone and cartilage cells (13). Brighton's studies support the theory that tissue hypoxia may we play a role in endochondral ossification at the fracture callus. Hypertrophic chondrocytes that have sequestered calcium in their mitochondria release their stores when all of the glycogen available for anaerobic metabolism is consumed. The released calcium aids in the nucleation and mineralization of surrounding matrix (13,66,67).

There is increased vascularity and blood flow in fresh fracture site. Blood flow peaks at 10 days and may take up to 2 months to normalize (70). Despite the increase in perfusion, the oxygen tension in the fracture hematoma is low. In fact, research using microelectrodes indicates that oxygen tension is also low in freshly formed fracture cartilage and bone (66). Furthermore, other experiments confirm that partial pressure of oxygen is low in fresh fracture callus and that oxygen consumption during active bone formation is not increased (71).

The coincident states of increased blood flow, steady-state oxygen consumption, and low oxygen tensions at the fracture site appear contradictory. However, if hypoxia and oxygen utilization are thought of as being measured at the cellular level, a more cogent explanation becomes apparent. If the cellular proliferation at the growing fracture callus outstrips the augmented blood supply, then each cell will show low oxygen tension and a lower-than-expected oxygen consumption. Despite increased perfusion to a fracture site, an increase in cell number greater than the concomitant rise in blood supply would lead to a relative state of hypoxia at the cellular level (13). Perhaps it is this oxygen gradient across the fracture callus that drives the formidable stimulus of induction of bone repair. Although not fully substantiated, this theory remains an active area of continued research.

2. *Mechanobiology*

The biomechanical influences on fracture healing consist of the application of mechanical forces and their effects on healing bone. These forces—tension, bending, and torsion—represent the spectrum of mechanical properties that normal bone must accommodate. During physiological homeostasis of intact bone, the tissue responds to short periods of cyclical mechanical deformation to effect adaptive changes that optimize its mass and architecture to adapt to its current mechanical environment (72,73). Similarly, the repair of bone is modulated by mechanical influences. During fracture healing, formation of the fracture callus reduces interfragmentary movement to the extent that both fragments can be united. Bony union is influenced by the strain magnitude, the strain rate, and the tissue stress experienced at the fracture healing site (72,74). Studies have shown that there exists a specific range of mechanical stimulation that optimizes osteogenesis during fracture healing. One research group demonstrated that short periods of cyclical micromotion increase the rate of fracture healing versus unstimulated controls (74,75); however, exceeding the ultimate strain or yield, point of the callus mass can induce additional damage and inhibit the healing process (72). Conversely. insufficient mechanical stimulation can retard bony regeneration (76).

As the repair process continues, the fracture site increases in stiffness and the differentiating tissue becomes mechanically more stable. The forces experienced at the site result in significant mechanotransduction-induced tissue adaptation. Bending stiffness generally returns more rapidly than bending strength (11). Initially, the bone fails throughout the area of the healing fracture, but as the repair process continues the bone gains strength and resists alteration. Ultimately, a completely healed bone should have an equal probability of failure at or outside the site of previous injury (77).

It has long been known that local mechanical conditions influence the process of fracture healing, and consequently studies of these physical factors in skeletal regeneration have been performed from the macroscopic perspective of the organ and tissue level to the most specific levels of cellular and molecular changes (78). Organ level studies, for example, can characterize the relationship between the force and stiffness properties of fracture fixation devices and the resultant rate and quality of fracture healing. Tissue studies evaluate mechanical characteristics of stress and strain and their effects on tissue differentiation. Cellular and molecular studies relate specific cellular changes such as shape deformation and matrix interactions with signaling cascades and cytokine activation.

One researcher, Pawels, derived seminal mechanobiological principles that predict differentiation patterns found in tissue during fracture healing and osteogenesis (79). Based on initial theories formulated by Roux and Benninghoff in the early 1900s (80,81), his concepts detailed the mechanical influences on mesenchymal tissue development by observation of patterns of growth in vivo (78). Pawels hypothesized that (1) direct intramembranous bone formation is more likely lo occur in areas of low stress and strain; (2) hydrostatic compressive stress is a stimulus for chondrogenesis; and (3) high tensile strain is a stimulus for the net production of fibrous tissue (78).

These concepts correlate with finite element analyses of typical tissue force distributions at healing fracture sites (78). Direct bone formation is generally observed on the endosteal and periosteal surfaces near fracture gaps, and intramembranous bone formation is usually greater on the periosteal surface (78). This osseous bridging usually occurs on the peripheral edges of the callus, where hydrostatic pressure is low. After the initial bridge is formed, the softer inner portion of the callus is shielded from hydrostatic compressive forces, facilitating endochondral ossification, which proceeds from the outer portion of the callus inward toward the center (78). If the fracture site is inadequately immobilized, the resultant bending and torsional displacement creates high hydrostatic-compression pressures and tensile strains within the gap. In addition to the direct physical damage to the callus tissue and angiogenesis at the fracture site, the high compression and strain leads to fibrous tissue and fibrocartilage formation, delaying or preventing bony union (78).

3. Bioelectrical Effects

The study of the effects of electromagnetic fields during fracture healing derived from the discovery that dehydrated bone tissue generated an internal electric field when deformed by mechanical force (82–85). This finding was extended to living tissue when Cochran et al. reported biphasic electric potential generation within bone subjected to mechanical loads in vivo (86). These early investigators hypothesized that these electrical signals were part of a negative feedback loop by which bony remodeling adapted to its mechanical environment (82).

This electromechanical transduction is both piezoelectric and electrokinetic in origin. Piezoelectricity is the generation of electric polarity by pressure within the mineralized bone. Electrokinetic energy arises from the entrainment of ions due to fluid motion within the bone. Alterations in these bioelectrical potentials in bone can experimentally influence osteogenesis, and these signals may have a role in controlling physiological bone cell activity and bone structure (82).

Stress-generated potentials act on bone with distinct polarity so that compressive forces show electronegativity while tensile forces produce electropositivity. Additionally, concave surfaces tend to be electronegative and convex surfaces electropositive (83,84). Clinically, bone develops increased callus on an electronegative concave surface following fracture reduction. Studies have also shown that regions of electropositivity are osteoclastic, while regions of electronegativity are osteoblastic (87). Such evidence suggests a role for bioelectrical potentials in bone repair.

Bioelectrical potentials recorded from a fresh fracture callus are strongly negative at the beginning of the healing process and slowly revert to normal as healing progresses (88). This supports the concept that active bone growth and repair are electronegative. The process has also been reproduced experimentally to show that when electricity is applied to bone at specific currents and voltages, the result is osteoblastic new bone formation. These findings have been used clinically in the treatment of fracture nonunion (89).

Experimental studies applying exogenous electromagnetic fields during fracture healing have typically utilized two modalities: application of direct current with implanted electrodes at the fracture healing site and the use of pulsed electromagnetic fields to the fracture healing area. Attempts to apply direct current to fracture sites were reported as early as the mid-1800s (82,90,91). More recently, researchers have demonstrated accelerated fracture healing with direct current stimulation in a rabbit model (92). Although direct-current electrical stimulation appears to initiate mitosis and recruit osteogenic cells (93), the mechanism is thought to be due to an electrochemical reaction at the electrode-tissue interface where oxygen consumption and pH increase (82,94–96). Another alternative hypothesis is that mechanical micromotion of the electrode provides significant impetus itself for osteogenic upregulation during direct-current stimulation (97).

Pulsed electromagnetic fields have been used clinically to treat nonunions and have been approved by the Food and Drug Administration for that use (98,99). Most devices studied send electric current though a wire coil placed over the fracture site, thus noninvasively producing a magnetic field. Some devices alternatively utilize capactive coupling stimulation using electrodes placed on the skin. Developers of clinical devices use induction waveforms with relatively high-frequency (1–10 kHz) pulses and gated at a low frequency (1–1000 Hz) (82). Several double-blind clinical trials have found mixed results regarding the efficacy of pulsed electromagnetic fields (82). One study found electromagnetic field treatment to be no more effective than conservative management in promoting union in fractures that had not healed in 52 weeks (100). Another trial showed a significant benefit in healing delayed unions after 16–32 weeks with pulsed electromagnetic fields, although the result was not as optimal as that of surgical intervention (101). A study after tibial osteotomies demonstrated a twofold increase in the number of patients demonstrating advanced healing with 60 days of pulsed electromagnetic field treatment compared to controls (102). In contrast to the effects of direct current, pulsed electromagnetic fields appear to affect differentiated bone cells instead of precursor cells, reducing osteoclastic resorption, increasing revascularization of the fracture site, and increasing rates of bone formation by osteoblasts (82,93,98). Although a number of genetic transcriptional changes have been documented, their end results are not yet clear. Several studies have demonstrated increases in IGF, TGF-beta, and BMP growth factors in cell culture models; however, the mechanism by which upregulation occurs remains unclear (103). In addition, the complexity of the pulsed electromagnetic waveforms themselves mike it difficult to elucidate the primary stimulus for increased bone healing (82). Further research is underway to identify the mechanism involved in transducing bioelectric stimuli.

4. Low-Intensity Ultrasound

The efficacious effects of low-pulsed-intensity ultrasound treatment in augmenting fracture healing have been well documented. Researchers first reported in 1983 the successful application of low-intensity-pulsed ultrasound in humans to treat fracture nonunions (104). The energy level, 30 mW/cm^2, is well within the range of diagnostic ultrasound devices (1–50 mW/cm^2), and much lower than energies used for surgical interventions (5–300 W/cm^2) such as tissue ablation and calculi dissolution (105). Animal and clinical studies have documented effects including increased callus formation, increased biomechanical strength, and increased new bone formation by radiographic studies (106–108). Molecular studies have demonstrated upregulated aggregan and osteopontin mRNA transcription in rat fracture healing models (109,110). Tissue selectivity to specific characteristics in the ultrasound signal has been demonstrated by several studies. A pulse width of 200 μs and a 1-Hz repetitive frequency has a significantly greater effect on fracture healing than other tested parameter (105,111).

The mechanobiological mechanism by which ultrasound treatment influences the fracture-healing process is not known, owing to the complex nature of the physiological response of tissue to high-frequency acoustic energy (105). The higher-energy absorption rate of bone, owing to its increased density compared to soft tissue, likely plays a significant role in the targeted nature of ultrasonic treatment of bony injuries. As ultrasonic energy is absorbed, the conversion to heat energy results in a small ($< 1°C$), but possibly significant, rise in temperature (105). One hypothesis is that certain enzymes, particularly collagenases, are extremely sensitive to small temperature changes and may be differentially upregulated (105,112). Another hypothesis regarding fracture healing and ultrasonic energy is that stable cavitation may occur in areas of fluid after ultrasonic treatment. As a result, extremely small pockets of air may become trapped within the fracture site, serving as nucleation sites for growth (105,113). An additional hypothesis suggests that a direct increase in blood flow to the fracture site may be the principal factor accelerating healing by ultrasound treatment (105). Studies in an osteotomized dog ulna fracture-healing model demonstrated increased vascularity at the fracture site after 10 days of ultrasonic energy application, with improvement of blood flow distribution around the fracture compared to untreated controls (114).

Studies are continuing to more precisely elucidate the nature of the ultrasonic-induced effects on fracture healing. Given the noninvasive, relatively safe, and inexpensive treatment modality ultrasound offers, if its mechanism is better understood, ultrasonic energy may become part of standardized therapy for a variety of complicated fractures.

IV. BONE GRAFTS

Surgery involving the craniofacial skeleton often requires the use of bone grafts for reconstruction of congenital and acquired deformities and skeletal augmentation in aesthetic surgery. Bone grafts are used to fill bony defects, provide structural support, and buildup the deficient areas in contour restoration. Nonvascularized autogenous bone grafts (i.e., free grafts) are the gold standard for reconstruction in the craniofacial complex.

A. Nonvascularized Bone Graft Physiology

After a bone graft is harvested and transplanted to a new region, multiple biological processes occur as the graft becomes incorporated into its host bed. Healing and incorporation involve the processes of inflammation, revascularization, osteoconduction, osteoinduction, osteogenesis, and remodeling. An important aspect in (nonvascularized) bone graft healing is that a substantial portion of the biological activity originates from the host. Most viable osteocytes within the graft itself die quickly after transplantation, rendering the graft comparatively inert versus the host. Despite this substantial biological interactions occur between the graft and the host, and the graft has a fundamental role in determining its own fate. This biological interplay between graft and host establishes the final result.

In 1907, Axhausen first described systematically that nonvascularized bone grafts heal through a sequence of events, and his work has been cited frequently (115). He noted that bone grafts initially undergo partial necrosis, followed by an inflammatory stage, in which the existing bone is replaced with new bone by osteoblasts that are brought in through the invading blood vessels. Axhausen coined the term "creeping substitution" to describe the slow process of vessel invasion and bony replacement. More recently, these events have been referred to as *osteoconduction,* and both terms are used interchangeably.

Hematoma formation around the bone graft is the first event that occurs after graft transplantation, usually caused by bleeding from the surgical disruption of host soft tissues and the recipient bony bed. During this early stage, only a small minority of the cells within the bone graft are still viable, located at the graft's peripheral surface. These surface cells survive, owing to early revascularization or by plasmatic imbibition (116,117). An inflammatory reaction around the graft ensues and lasts for 5–7 days. The inflammatory tissue becomes reorganized into a dense fibrovascular stroma around the graft, and the onset of vascular invasion occurs at 10–14 days (118), bringing cells with osteogenic potential into the graft (119). These cells (osteoblasts and osteoclasts) begin to replace the graft, while the interstices of the old bone act as a scaffold for the deposition of new bone. As the deposition takes place through osteoblast activity, resorption of necrotic bone occurs through osteoclastic activity, and the bone graft is slowly penetrated by vascular tissue. These processes continue to occur until revascularization and deposition are complete. The ultrastructural character of the bone graft (whether cancellous or cortical) has significance in determining the extent and manner in which the graft is revascularized and incorporated into the host (120).

B. Cancellous Bone Graft Revascularization and Bone Deposition

Cancellous bone grafts are revascularized more rapidly and completely than cortical bone grafts (120–124). This is thought to occur due to the large spaces between the trabeculae that permit unobstructed invasion of vascular tissue. Osteogenic cells, brought in by the invading vessels, differentiate into osteoblasts and deposit a layer of new bone around the dead trabeculae. An osteoclastic phase then ensues, as osteoclasts enter and resorb the entrapped cores of dead bone. The cancellous grafts are completely revascularized and replaced by new bone; these processes may take weeks or months (120,124).

C. Cortical Bone Graft Revascularization and Bone Deposition

In contrast, cortical bone graft revascularization proceeds slowly and incompletely. Vascular invasion of cortical bone graft is thought to be limited, due primarily to its dense lamellar structure that constrains vessels to invading the graft along the preexisting haversian and Volkmann's canals (120). The revascularization may also be hindered by the limited number of endosteal cells that remain viable after transplantation. These cells are thought to contribute to end-to-end vessel anastomoses during bone graft revascularization (125). While cancellous bone grafts proceed with initial osteoblastic activity, revascularization of cortical bone grafts proceeds with initial osteoclastic activity. Osteoclastic enlargement of the haversian and Volkmann's canals must occur before vessels are able to penetrate the graft. The course of revascularization begins at the graft periphery and progresses to the interior of the graft (126). Osteoblasts are brought in and deposit new bone, refilling the enlarged canal spaces. In cancellous grafts, vessel invasion may begin within a few hours posttransplantation, and the process is completed in a few days. In cortical grafts, the earliest vessels enter the graft at 6 days, and the process of revascularization may take months, often resulting in incomplete graft revascularization (120,124). Incompletely revascularized regions of necrotic graft may persist indefinitely, sealed off from the viable regions of the graft. The final appearance of a cortical bone graft is often a patchwork of necrotic bone, interspersed by areas of new bone. This admixture usually remains unaltered, even after a graft has become fully incorporated. Studies have confirmed that cortical grafts in the onlay position show only superficial revascularization occurring in the first 10–21 days and central revascularization by 8–16 weeks (127,128).

D. The Role of Osteoinduction and Osteogenesis in Bone Grafts

Osteogenesis is the process that occurs when surviving osteogenic cells from within the graft produce new bone. This mechanism of graft healing relies on viable posttransplant osteogenic cells to become the source of new bone formation. Although most cells within the graft die soon after transplantation, some surviving cells are believed to take part in osteogenesis. The superior revascularization qualities of cancellous bone grafts are thought to result in a greater proportion of posttransplant osteogenic cell survival and, consequently, a greater degree of osteogenesis than in cortical bone grafts. The local sources of cells partaking in osteogenesis are believed to be the periosteum, endosteum, marrow, and intracortical elements. The role of osteogenesis as a mechanism of new bone formation during nonvascularized bone graft healing is thought to be of lesser significance than that of osteoconduction. Although osteogenesis has a secondary role in the healing of nonvascularized bone graft, it constitutes the primary mechanism of *vascularized* bone graft healing. Cells within these grafts maintain their blood supply and remain viable after transplantation.

Osteoinduction is the process by which active factors released from the graft matrix stimulate cells from the host to form new bone. Osteoinduction has been studied extensively; however, there is significantly less research within the specific context of bone graft healing. Three phases of osteoinduction—chemotaxis, mitosis, and differentiation—have been described. In response to a chemical gradient during chemotaxis, bone induction factors direct the migration of cells to the area in which they are to be utilized. Following chemotaxis, these factors stimulate intense mitogenic.and proliferative activity in these cells; the cells differentiate into cartilage and become revascularized by invading blood vessels to form new bone. Research on osteoinduction during graft healing has demonstrated that chemical and physical alterations to the graft, such as hydrochloric acid decalcification and freezing, will decrease its osteoinductive properties (129,130). These findings suggest that osteoinduction is most significant when freshly harvested bone grafts are utilized. Burwell suggested that osteoinductive factors within a bone graft are released by the necrotic bone and marrow components of the graft (129). The true mechanisms of osteoinduction during bone graft healing are still unknown and may provide a fertile ground for new research endeavors. Osteoinductive factors have been shown to be powerful stimulators de novo bone production in bony defect healing of animal models; their potential applications in bone graft healing and incorporation have yet to be exploited. Although the roles of osteoinduction and osteogenesis are thought to be of lesser significance than osteoconduction in nonvascularized bone graft healing, these three processes are thought to be intimately connected.

E. Remodeling of Bone Grafts

The mechanical environment of a bone graft affects its growth and morphology. Normal skeletal bone has the ability to adapt to the physical stresses that are placed upon it through the process of remodeling. Wolff's law was postulated in 1892 and is often summarized by the phrase "form follows function" (131). Although the actual cellular mechanisms responsible for regulating the remodeling processes are unknown, the macroscopic effects of these processes are indisputable. It is reasonable to assume that bone grafts are also subject to the influences of physical force and are remodeled through their effects. Although Wolff s law was formulated more than a century ago, and is accepted as one of the fundamental constituents of bone physiology, direct data examining the significance of mechanical factors on bone graft behavior are negligible. Rudimentary questions, such as the mechanism, timing, and effect of mechanical stress, remain open.

F. The Current Science of Graft Survival

The ultimate fate of facial bone grafts has been studied extensively in the surgical literature (129,132–138). Clinically, nonvascularized bone grafts have been observed to decrease variably, maintain, or increase bone volume after transplantation. Clinical and basic scientific research has also established the inconsistent and significant resorptive characteristics of facial bone grafts. The unpredictable nature of volume preservation represents one of the main difficulties encountered by surgeons working with bone grafts in the craniofacial skeleton. Parameters relating to volume and projection are important, since loss of either may have adverse functional and aesthetic implications on the outcome of a surgical intervention. Literature on facial bone graft survival reveals that numerous factors are important variables in the survival of the graft. They include the position (inlay versus onlay), embryological origin (membranous versus endochondral), microarchitecture (cancellous versus cortical), mechanical stress, recipient site, method of fixation, graft orientation, presence or absence of periosteum, and rate of revascularization. The majority of these studies have been performed in the context of nonmorselized onlay grafts.

G. Embryological Origin, Microarchitecture, and Graft Position

Clinical practice and literature concur that bone grafts from calvarial and facial sites have a superior volumetric maintenance and survival over the grafts from rib, tibia, or iliac crest (122,132–138). The search for an explanation has been a succession of research, speculation, and controversy. In 1951, Peer found that grafts harvested from vomer, nasal, or ethmoid bones, transplanted in contact with nonbony tissues (i.e., abdominal fat, intramuscular regions, and subcutaneous tissues), retained their normal bony structure for up to 5 years, whereas rib, tibia, and iliac grafts were replaced by fibrous tissue in 6–8 months (139). He postulated that facial bones that lacked regenerative powers were endowed with a tenacious ability to retain their structure, but he did not elaborate on the mechanism for his hypothesis.

Smith and Abramson proposed two possible mechanisms for calvarial bone graft's volumetric superiority over iliac bone graft (140). They compared calvarial bone grafts to iliac bone grafts in a rabbit model. After 1 year, the calvarial grafts had maintained their size and structure, while iliac grafts had lost at least 75% of their original volume. They postulated that mechanical stress was a key factor in graft survival, believing that iliac bone required mechanical stress to maintain its morphology. After transplantation, loss of this stress led to resorption and poor volume maintenance when compared to grafts from non-stress-bearing donor sites, such as the calvarium. They also hypothesized that the microarchitecture of the bone graft could account for these differences. They noted that iliac grafts had more cancellous bone than calvarial grafts, and they hypothesized that the increased cancellous component would lead to increased revascularization, resulting in more resorption than calvarial bone grafts.

In an effort to explain the significant differences in graft survival between cranial and noncranial sources, researchers recognized that the embryological origins of these bones were different. Bones of membranous origin (bones of the cranial vault and most of the facial bones) arise directly from mesenchymal tissue, while bones of endochondral origin (the majority of long bones and bones of the axial skeleton) undergo initial formation of cartilage and then become ossified. Studies have shown repeatedly that volume retention in membranous bone grafts in the onlay position is better than in a similar graft harvested from an endochondral source (133–140).

In 1979, Zins and Whitaker published a study of bone graft survival for a 20-week follow-up period, harvested from endochondral or membranous sites (133). They found that membranous bone grafts had better volume maintenance properties than endochondral bone grafts. From these and other results, they concluded that the membranous origin of a bone bestowed it with superior volume maintenance. Their data were corroborated by previous research results and supported their hypothesis, but a specific mechanism to explain the "embryology hypothesis" was not given, and the concept of an innate ability continued to be a matter of controversy.

In 1990, a study by Hardesty and Marsh found that calvarial grafts preserved better than iliac grafts (137). They broached the concept of architecture having a role in survival by hypothesizing that the thicker cortex and more stout trabeculae in a calvarial graft was more resistant to resorption than the thinner cortex and trabeculae in an endochondral graft. Chen et al. suggested that the embryological origin of the graft was significant only in that it determined the relative proportions of cortical and cancellous bone within the graft (127). They showed that the cancellous components of bone grafts, regardless of the graft's embroyological origin, had increased degrees of revascularization and osteoclastic activity when compared to the cortical components. They theorized that membranous bone grafts have better volume maintenance properties because they have a large cortical and smaller cancellous component than the endochondral grafts.

This "ultrastructural hypothesis" had only circumstantial evidence until 1998, when Buchman and Ozaki demonstrated that the microarchitecture of a graft was the basis for volume maintenance (141). Their experiments isolated the cancellous and cortical components from membranous and endochondral graft sources. They demonstrated that there was a statistically greater resorption rate in the cancellous endochondral bone graft than in either endochondral or membranous cortical bone graft, but that there was no significant difference in the resorption rates between the endochondral and membranous cortical bone grafts. They believed cortical bone to be a superior onlay grafting material, independent of its embroyological origin. It is now generally acknowledged that the microarchitecture of a bone graft is perhaps the most important determinant of graft volume maintenance. The embryological origin of a bone graft affects its behavior only to the extent that it influences the proportions of cortical and cancellous composition within the graft.

While numerous studies have been conducted using onlay bone grafts, few have examined graft survival in the inlays. In 1989, Whitaker noted that interposition (i.e., inlay) grafts maintained volume and persevered significantly better than onlay grafts and introduced the concept of biological boundaries, hypothesizing that the body has genetically predetermined boundaries that are inclined to remain constant (142). He asserted that onlay bone grafts violated these boundaries, leading to resorption, while interpositional grafts did not violate these boundaries, resulting in superior volume maintenance. LaTrenta et al. reported that inlay bone grafts in a dog model maintained greater volume and weight than onlay grafts (143). He cited favorable remodeling forces present within the inlay position as the reason for the inlay graft's greater weight and volume maintenance. Rosenthal and Buchman performed a series of experiments observing the survival patterns of cortical and cancellous bone grafts in the inlay position in a rabbit model (personal communication). These experiments provided significant findings regarding the behavioral differences of inlay versus onlay grafts. Contrary to most previous onlay bone graft studies, this study demonstrated that bone volume *increases* for inlay grafts at all time points. The data also demonstrated that cancellous inlay bone grafts increased their bone content to a significantly greater extent than the cortical inlay bone grafts, regardless of their embryological origins. These results imply the inlay bone grafts are superior in volume maintenance to onlay bone grafts, and that cancellous inlay bone grafts increase bone content to a greater degree than cortical inlay bone grafts.

The current science of bone grafts suggests that onlay and inlay bone grafts behave differently, with inlay grafts showing superior volume maintenance properties. There is evidence to support the notion that a cortical microarchitecture is an important factor for the volume maintenance of onlay grafts, while a cancellous mircroarchitecture may be more significant for increasing bone content of inlay grafts.

H. Mechanical Stress in Bone Graft Incorporation

Several authors have noted the importance of mechanical stress in relation to graft incorporation (128,140,141). Mowlem supported the notion that different recipient sites had favorable and unfavorable mechanical stress that would affect bone graft survival (144). Smith and Abramson argued that lack of stress following transplantation was responsible for the resorption of grafts (140). LaTrenta et al. cited favorable remodeling forces as the mechanism for improved weight and volume maintenance in inlay versus onlay grafts (143). These hypotheses had only empirical support, based on Wolff's law; however, some more direct evidence has been reported. Recent studies have noted that the adaptation of onlay and inlay bone grafts became morphologically similar to the host site (145). Researchers have used micro-computed tomography (micro-CT) to demonstrate that a bone graft's morphological structure recapitulates to its surrounding bony bed over time. Through these studies, forces were implicated by computer-aided mathematical analysis of anisotrophy and connectivity, giving supporting data to the role of mechanical force in graft incorporation. Empirical and indirect evidence has demonstrated the effect of force on bone graft remodeling; research on the direct effects of mechanical stress on graft survival is limited. Mechanical force may have a profound influence on its volumetric maintenance properties during early and late graft incorporation, just as it has profound effects on normal skeletal bone. Further research in this area and the cellular mechanisms of mechanotransduction is required to further investigate the role of mechanical stress in bone graft physiology.

I. Rigid Fixation in Bone Grafts

The use of rigid fixation in fracture repair results in primary bone healing. The benefits of rigid fixation in fracture repair include early ambulation and more rapid and efficient bone healing. The effect of rigid fixation on bone grafts is less definite and less well understood. Some data do indicate that rigid fixation improves onlay graft survival when compared to bone grafts without any fixation or with wire fixation only (135,143,146). These studies found that there was a more rapid and greater extent of bony union between graft and host when rigid, rather than wire, fixation was used. Lin et al. noted that when onlay bone graft to the cranium was compared to the femur, rigid fixation provided superior survival in areas that were subject to high motion, shear, and torsional forces (femur), but provided no benefit in areas of low motion (cranium) (146). They also found that membranous bone survived better than endochondral bone and that rigid fixation could improve endochondral bone survival to approximate nonfixed membranous bone. The reasons believed responsible for improved survival with rigid fixation included increased primary bone healing and more rapid revascularization by virtue of graft immobility. Phillips and Rahn believed that grafts placed in areas of high motion resulted in a process analogous to a fibrous nonunion in fracture healing (135) and led to bone graft resorption. In some clinical circumstances, rigid fixation of onlay bone grafts is thought to prevent resorption, loss of volume, and loss of projection. For example, rigid fixation of a cantilever bone graft used for nasal reconstruction is thought to improve graft survival over nonrigid fixation. These clinical observations, along with previous studies supporting the notion that rigid fixation of bone grafts improves the rate and effectiveness of graft healing, lend credence to the use of rigid fixation in bone grafting. Further research should uncover the specific principles that dictate when rigid fixation is best utilized.

J. Periosteum and Bone Graft Orientation

Preserving the periosteum on a bone graft during transplantation has been shown to improve graft survival in the craniofacial region (132,147,148). Thompson and Cass studied the effects of periosteum preservation in a canine model and found that onlay bone grafts with retained periosteum showed improved volumetric survival over those without periosteum. They stressed the importance of early revascularization for bone graft survival and believed that the periosteum facilitated this process (132). Knize reported similar results with onlay bone grafts in a rabbit model (147). He emphasized the importance of the periosteum for its role in graft revascularization and believed that the deeper level of periosteal cells was significant in contributing to osteogenesis by transforming into osteogenic cells after transplantation. Lozano et al. published a study comparing grafts with and without periosteal preservation, placed either above or below the recipient periosteum (149). They concluded that there was no difference in graft survival or rate of revascularization between the four groups that were examined. Their study was notable because it failed to find improved survival or revascularization with periosteal preservation. Using rib grafts in a canine model, Burstein et al. found that periosteal preservation significantly enhanced new bone formation when compared with grafts without periosteum (148). They described three layers of the periosteum—an outer vascular network, with communications to the internal portions of the bone, a middle layer of osteogenic reserve cells, and the inner cambial layer. They proposed that bone graft revascularization was enhanced by means of the outer periosteal layer and its direct connections to the interior of the graft.

Many of the same studies also investigated the effect of graft orientation. In 1970, researchers used corticocancellous onlay bone grafts without periosteum, and placed the cancellous surface in contact with either the recipient bone or soft tissue (132). They found that bone grafts had better survival when their cancellous surfaces contacted the bone, even though grafts with cancellous surfaces facing the soft tissue revascularized sooner. These results appear to contradict the hypothesized mechanism in periosteal preservation, which asserts that improved revascularization improves graft survival. Similarly, Knize's study in 1974 found that corticocancellous bone grafts (with periosteum) survived best when the cancellous portion was placed in contact with the host bone (147). Zins and Whitaker observed the effect of graft orientation using (periosteum preserved) corticocancellous iliac bone grafts in a rabbit model (133) and corroborated earlier findings by demonstrating that grafts with cancellous surfaces placed in contact with bone had increased volumetric survival. An additional study by Hardesty and Marsh did not support previous findings on bone graft orientation (137). They used onlay bone grafts in a rabbit model and found no relationship with respect to graft orientation and survival, concluding that graft orientation was not a factor in survival.

The literature confirms that the significance of periosteal preservation and graft orientation on craniofacial bone graft survival remains controversial. Preservation of periosteum may be a favorable factor for improved graft survival, although the mechanisms are not completely understood. The role of graft orientation and its mechanism of action are still a matter of debate, and further research of the two variables is warranted to isolate the specific role and mechanism of action for each.

K. Bone Graft Recipient Site Physiology

The recipient site may have a profound effect on the outcome of graft healing and incorporation, and studies have demonstrated that grafts placed in an avascular bed to not survive well (139); other factors at the recipient site include prior irradiation, infection, and tissue scarring. Different sites of transplantation have been shown to affect graft persistence. Although bone grafts are usually placed in contact with bone, some studies have investigated the effects of placing bone grafts in different tissue environments. Ermis and Poole placed endochondral bone grafts in subcutaneous and muscular pockets, and found that bone graft resorption was greater when grafts were covered by muscle (150). They postulated that excessive graft movement and increased revascularization from the muscle resulted in increased graft resorption.

The site of a bone graft may affect its survival. In 1963, Mowlem advanced the concept of orthotopic and heterotopic locations (144). A bone graft placed in a defect normally occupied by bone is known as *orthotopically transplanted*; a graft placed in a site normally not occupied by bone is *heterotopically transplanted*. Mowlem observed that orthotopic conditions favor new bone formation and heterotopic conditions lead to resorption. Enlow advanced another theory that implicated the bone graft recipient site as a significant factor for graft survival (151). Through his theories of transformative and translational growth in the craniofacial skeleton he asserted that certain areas of the face remodel by bony deposition, whereas other areas remodel by bony resorption. He believed that different aspects of bony growth and remodeling in the craniofacial skeleton work together to create the adult form. In an effort to extend Enlow's theories of craniofacial bone growth to craniofacial bone graft applications, Zins et al. performed experiments that placed corticocancellous onlay bone grafts in resorptive and depository fields of rabbits (152). Their results showed significant differences in volume maintenance in accordance with the resorptive or depository nature of the recipient bed.

In 1989, Whitaker introduced the concept of the *biological boundary* (142), which is an extension of Wolff's law and Moss' functional matrix theory. Moss' theory (153) states that as the craniofacial skeleton grows, its soft-tissue environment may have a significant role in shaping its morphology. The deformative effects on craniofacial growth in a child with congenital or acquired torticollis are examples of his theory in clinical practice. Whitaker applied Moss' theory to bone grafts. He believed that the body has predetermined physical boundaries that have a major role in bone graft survival. He hypothesized that onlay grafts, by virtue of their position, generally disturbed these boundaries and would elicit a response from the body's natural tendency to maintain the boundary by resorbing the graft. Whitaker noted that inlay bone grafts did not disturb biological boundaries, while basal bone advancements established new ones. Although his concepts provided a consistent explanation for the behavior of craniofacial bone grafts, Whitaker did not offer a mechanism for his theory, stating only that these boundaries were genetically predetermined.

L. Discussion and Proposal of New Concepts in Bone Grafting

A better understanding of bone graft physiology will result in more intelligent grafting of facial bone. However, the multitude of factors purported to be important for graft survival makes it difficult to obtain a "big picture" view of graft behavior.

Accurate clinical predictors of nonvascularized bone graft survival in the craniofacial skeleton may be related to the mechanical environment in which a bone graft is transplanted and to the extent to which a bone graft is revascularized. Numerous variables deemed important for bone graft survival may be reduced to an association with the recipient site's mechanical environment. They include graft position (inlay versus onlay), the concept of depository/resorptive fields, biological boundaries, and recipient bed environment. Similarly, many variables have a direct effect on bone graft revascularization, including the recipient bed environment, graft position (inlay versus onlay), graft microarchitecture (cancellous versus cortical), presence of rigid fixation, and presence of periosteum. By distilling these factors into the two parameters—mechanical environment and graft revascularization—a simple, logical, and consistent theory of bone graft behavior may be formulated.

M. Mechanical Environment in Graft Survival

The mechanical environment of the graft recipient site is of paramount importance to graft survival and that mechanical force influences bone graft physiology in the same way as does normal skeletal bone. The recipient site affects the mechanical environment of a graft by virtue of the tissue envelope in which the graft sits. Onlay grafts within a tight tissue envelope will experience forces that are different from grafts within a loose soft-tissue envelope.

Onlay grafts that underlie muscle (an example of a tight tissue envelope) may be expected to encounter an increased magnitude of compressional forces when compared to grafts transplanted within the subcutaneous tissues. As a clinical example, onlay grafts placed under the temporalis muscle invariably show significant resorption. The compressional forces in this region may be significant in effecting graft resorption.

The position of the graft with respect to the surrounding bone (inlay or onlay) is another factor that affects the graft's mechanical environment. Onlay bone grafts are placed in positions that are normally occupied by soft tissues and therefore tend to stretch their soft-tissue envelope. Disruption of the soft-tissue envelope generates recoil forces that act directly upon the onlay bone graft. These "recoil" forces may be an essential component of the mechanism that is responsible for the net resorption that occurs with onlay bone grafts. Ozaki et al. noted that the top edges of onlay cortical grafts circumferentially demonstrated preferential resorption (145). This suggested an effect of the skin envelope's recoil forces exerting pressure and causing focal resorption at the points of contact with the graft. In contrast, inlay bone grafts reside in locations where bone is normally present. A bone graft placed in an inlay position, does not result in the creation of recoil forces because it does not affect the soft-tissue envelope. In addition to being "shielded" from the recoil forces of the soft tissues, inlay bone grafts benefit from receiving the physical stresses identical to those received by the surrounding recipient bone bed. The absence of recoil forces and the presence of these "functional" forces may act to bring about the graft survival that occurs with inlay bone grafts.

It is important to note that the forces acting on a graft vary by graft position (inlay versus onlay), as well as the location of the recipient bed. Two grafts placed in the same inlay or onlay position but in different locations in the craniofacial skeleton will not behave in the same fashion owing to the differences in the mechanical environment at each location. The wide variation of mechanical forces and their influence on bone grafts may represent a critical component in graft survival.

N. Revascularization of Bone Grafts

In addition to the concept that location and position may affect the nature of forces a bone graft encounters, the ability of these forces to render changes on the graft may be a second key component in graft behavior. The ability of force to render changes in bone is a function of the effector cells in the bone—the osteoblasts and osteoclasts. Therefore, the effectiveness of force to make changes in a bone graft will be proportional to the degree of osteoclastic and osteoblastic activity that occurs during graft healing. In turn, osteoclastic and osteoblastic activity is determined primarily by the degree of revascularization, which in turn is dependent on the environment of the recipient bed. Conditions that adversely affect revascularization include presence of dead/necrotic bone, prior irradiation, presence of scarring, and presence of infection; the type of soft tissue that overlies the graft may be another factor. The degree of vascularization of a tissue envelope may affect the rate and extent of bone graft revascularization. A study by Ermis and Poole notes that muscle coverage can result in increased revascularization and serves as an example (150).

As stated previously, the microarchitecture of a bone graft has profound implications on the rate and completeness of revascularization. Cancellous bone grafts have been shown to revascularize quickly and completely, while cortical bone grafts revascularize slowly and incompletely. Therefore, the microarchitecture of a bone graft determines the degree of biological bone activity it will have. The position of a bone graft (inlay or onlay) also affects its degree of revascularization. Inlay grafts have their base and sides in contact with the recipient bed; an onlay graft has the base only. Increased bone-to-bone contact provides more area for graft/host interaction. Theoretically, this results in increased potential for posttransplant cell survival and, therefore, increased osteogenesis. An increased area of direct contact also results in increased potential for osteoinduction and osteoconduction. In general, increased contact results in more rapid and complete revascularization, resulting in greater biological activity. Using the unifying concepts of revascularization and the effects of mechanical force, the behavior of bone grafts can be explained and even predicted.

O. Interaction of Mechanical Force and Revascularization in Bone Grafting

The effects of revascularization and mechanical force establish fundamental principles that have their origins in Wolff's law; they may be used to explain the phenomena observed in clinical practice and to unify apparent inconsistencies in previous research. The difference in resorptive behavior of a cancellous onlay bone graft (versus an onlay cortical bone graft) is its greater capacity to remodel, by virtue of its more rapid and extensive revascularization. A cancellous graft, placed in the onlay position, is subject to recoil forces; in the face of the intense bone remodeling climate, resorption of the graft ensues. In contrast, when a cortical graft is placed in the onlay position and is subject to the same recoil forces, its revascularization proceeds more slowly and less completely. The graft has less osteoclastic and osteoblastic activity, making it relatively unresponsive to the recoil stresses. A cortical graft in the onlay position, therefore, maintains its volume better than a cancellous graft.

Inlay grafts have superior volume maintenance characteristics when compared to onlay grafts. As mentioned previously, increased bone-to-bone contact provides more area for graft/host interaction, resulting in greater potential for revascularization, osteogenesis, osteoinduction, and osteoconduction. By virtue of its inlay position, the graft is shielded from the recoil forces that an onlay graft experiences. Additionally, the mechanical forces experienced by an inlay graft are physiologically reinforcing or "functional" in nature. The combination of "functional" mechanical forces and intensified osteogenic activity results in superior volume maintenance of inlay over onlay bone grafts. In the early phases of bone healing, the mechanical effect of the inlay position may be primarily shielding it from soft-tissue recoil forces, while later in healing and incorporation, the functional forces exert their remodeling effects. More investigation is required to corroborate or refute these ideas.

The role of microarchitecture for graft persistence in the inlay circumstance is less well defined than in the onlay position. In a recently presented study of inlay bone, no statistical difference was found in the final volume of inlay cancellous bone graft when compared to inlay cortical bone graft. It was found however, that the change in the amount of bone produced was significantly higher in defects filled with cancellous bone grafts than in those filled with cortical grafts. These changes were manifested in the thickening of the trabeculae and obliteration of the interstices in cancellous grafts. It was also noted that, over time, the cortical grafts became more porous but the cancellous graft less porous in nature. It was suggested that the effects of the surrounding physiological "functional" forces led both types of graft to converge toward one phenotype in an effort to recapitulate the recipient bed.

Although revascularization may be detrimental to graft survival in some cases (e.g., onlay cancellous graft), the converse (i.e., absence of revascularization) may result in graft resorption. Some authors have described a type of graft resorption replaced with fibrous tissue that histologically demonstrates the absence of osteoclastic activity (132,154). Absence of revascularization leading to resorption through these nonosteoclastic mechanisms might be used to explain the resorption of bone grafts placed in the abdominal wall, as seen by Peer (139), since a source of osteoclasts in the abdominal wall region would be difficult to explain. Although cortical bone graft contains regions of nonrevascularized necrotic bone that remain indefinitely after incorporation, these areas are sealed off with viable bone, which may prevent resorption through these nonosteoclastic mechanisms. Lack of revascularization may be the basis for Lin's results in his study that demonstrated the effectiveness of rigid fixation for bone graft survival in areas of high motion (146). High motion may have prevented the invasion of blood vessels resulting in significant resorption through nonosteoclastic mechanisms. Rigid fixation could prevent this disruption and promote revascularization as the mechanism of improving bone graft survival.

These unifying concepts may be used to explain the theories of biological boundaries and resorptive and depository fields, espoused by Whitaker (142) and Enlow (151). Whitaker states that interpositional grafts survived well, as did onlay grafts, when used to correct a disruption of the bony surface by trauma or tumor resection. These results may reflect the fact that these grafts were essentially used in an inlay position. Although his observations regarding the behavior of bone grafts were accurate, his explanation for biological boundaries proposed a genetically predetermined innate ability for the body to maintain "boundary homeostasis." The concepts of functional mechanical force and revascularization offers a mechanism that may help to explain his concepts in terms of mechanical force and remodeling activity.

Enlow's theories of resorptive and depository fields (151) may also be explained through mechanistic concepts. Results from an earlier publication by Zins et al. examining the effect of these fields showed that identical bone grafts, differing only in positions on the face, could have different graft behavior (152). They used a rabbit model and placed grafts at the mandibular ramus, body, and dorsal surface of the snout. It is interesting to note that the (resorptive) region at the mandibular ramus correlates with the area that the masseter muscle overlies, and that the (depository) region of the snout correlates with the absence of compression from overlying soft tissue or muscle. The differing mechanical forces in these regions, caused by the differing overlying soft tissues, may have had a role in their findings. In an earlier study, researchers demonstrated that grafts survived better when placed on the maxilla than on the mandible (132). Again, differences in soft tissue and their forces at the maxillary and mandibular regions may have had a role in these results. Recent findings support the notion that grafts placed submuscularly demonstrate increased local resorptive and remodeling activities compared to grafts placed in a subcutaneous pocket (155).

When the soft-tissue envelope is altered, one might expect that the forces it exerts on an onlay graft may be altered. A study by Goldstein et al. (156) utilized supraperiosteally placed tissue expanders to alter the recipient bed. They placed rigidly fixed membranous bone grafts under the expanded soft tissues and demonstrated increased survival of these grafts when compared to grafts placed in nonexpanded sites. Goldstein et al. postulated that an increase in recipient bed vascularity was a reason for the results. Although this may be true, their results also support our hypothesis that mechanical forces are an important component in bone graft survival. It is possible that the alterations of the soft tissue led to decreases in the soft-tissue tension that resulted in alteration in graft volume.

P. Summary of Bone Grafting

Bone grafts are the building blocks of the craniofacial surgeon. To use bone grafts optimally, a clear understanding of graft physiology and the current scientific research is required. An analysis of the basic science currently available on facial bone grafts has demonstrated that numerous factors may impact on bone graft healing and incorporation. Many of the previously studied factors affecting bone graft healing may be condensed to the bone graft's mechanical environment and degree of revascularization. These concepts are based on the knowledge accumulated from clinical and basic scientific research and must be further critically assessed. Just as bone is a dynamic entity that continually regenerates and redefines itself, the ultimate test of validity for these and other concepts will be continual scientific examination, evaluation, and reexamination.

V. CONCLUSION

The study of fracture healing and bone grafting continues to provide novel insights into every aspect of bone growth and repair. Biochemical and molecular studies have given impetus to pioneering clinical trials that may revolutionize treatment of fractures in the future. In addition, the brugeoning research regarding biophysical aspects of fracture repair is resulting in elucidation of many fundamental mechanobiological mechanisms that allow adaptation to physiological stimuli. Bone regeneration continues to be a challenging field of study that will require continued sustained effort to illuminate many of the most fascinating processes of the human body.

REFERENCES

1. Hobar P. Implantation: bone, cartilage, and allografts. Selected Readings Plast Surg 1992; 7:1–2.
2. Uam A. A histologic study of the early phases of bone repair. J Bone Joint Surg 1930; 12:927–944.
3. Benfu C, Xueming T. Ultrastructural investigation of experimental fracture healing. I. Electron microscopic observation of cellular activity. Chinese Med J 1979; 92(8):530–535.

4. Ashhurst DE. The influence of mechanical conditions on the healing of experimental fractures in the rabbit: a microscopical study. Phil Trans Roy Soci Lond Ser B Biol Sci 1986; 313(1161):271–302.
5. Ashton BA, et al. Formation of bone and cartilage by marrow stromal cells in diffusion chambers in vivo. Clin Orthopaed Rel Res 1980; 151:294–307.
6. Tonna EA, Cronkite EP. The periosteum: autoradiographic studies on cellular proliferation and transformation utilizing tritiated thymidine. Clin Orthop Rel Res 1963; 30:218–233.
7. Trueta J. The role of the vessels in osteogenesis. J Bone Joint Surg 1963; 458:402–418.
8. Nemeth GG, Bolander ME, Martin GR. Growth factors and their role in wound and fracture healing. Prog Clin Biol Res 1988; 266:1–17.
9. Sandberg M, et al. In situ localization of collagen production by chondrocytes and osteoblasts in fracture callus. Bone Joint Surg Am Vol 1989; 71(1):69–77.
10. Lane J, Boskey A, Li W. A temporal study of collagen, proteoglycans, lipids, and mineral constituents in a model of endochondral osseous repair. Metab Bone Dis Rel Dis 1979; 1:319–324.
11. Davy DT, Connolly JF. The biomechanical behavior of healing canine radii and ribs. J Biomech 1982; 15(4):235–247.
12. Lane JM, et al. Immunofluorescent localization of structural collagen types in endochondral fracture repair. J Orthop Res 1986; 4(3):318–329.
13. Brighton C. Principles of fracture healing. In: Murry J, ed. Instructional Course Lectures. St. Louis: CV Mosby, 1984:60–82.
14. Wheater P, Burkill U, Daniels V. Functional Histology. London: Churchill Livingston, 1980.
15. Frost H. Skeletal physiology and bone remodeling. In: Urist M, ed. Fundamental and Clinical Bone Physiology. JB Lippincott: Philadelphia, 1980:208–241.
16. Frost H. Bone Remodeling and Its Relation to Metabolic Bone Disease. Springfield, IL: Charles C. Thomas, 1973.
17. Rahn BA, et al. Primary bone healing. An experimental study in the rabbit. J Bone Joint Surg Am Vol 1971; 53(4):783–786.
18. Perren SM. Physical and biological aspects of fracture healing with special reference to internal fixation. Clin Orthop Rel Res 1979; 138:175–196.
19. Frost HM. The biology of fracture healing: an overview for clinicians. Part I. Clin Orthop Rel Res 1989; 248:283–293.
20. Urist M. Bone Transplantation. In: Urist M, ed. Fundamental and Clinical Bone Physiology. Philadelphia: JB Lippincott, 1980:331–368.
21. Phemister D. The fate of transplanted bone and regenerative power in its various constituents. Surg Gynecol Obstet 1914; 19:303–333.
22. Reddi AH, Ma SS, Cunningham NS. Induction and maintenance of new bone formation by growth and differentiation factors. Ann Chir Gynaecol 1988; 77(5–6):189–192.
23. Bolander ME. Regulation of fracture repair by growth factors. Proc Soci Exp Biol Med 1992; 200(2):165–170.

24. Einhorn TA, et al. The expression of cytokine activity by fracture callus. J Bone Miner Res 1995; 10(8):1272–1281.
25. Barnes GL, et al. Growth factor regulation of fracture repair. J Bone Miner Res 1999; 14(11):1805–1815.
26. Joyce ME, Jingushi S, Bolander ME. Transforming growth factor-beta in the regulation of fracture repair. Orthop Clin North Am 1990; 21(1): 199–209.
27. Centrella M, et al. Transforming growth factor-beta gene family members and bone. Endocr Rev 1994; 15(1):27–39.
28. Kingsley DM. The TGF-beta superfamily: new members, new receptors, and new genetic tests of function in different organisms. Genes Dev 1994; 8(2): 133–146.
29. Lind M, et al. Transforming growth factor-beta enhances fracture healing in rabbit tibiae. Acta Orthop Scand 1993; 64(5):553–556.
30. Nielsen HM, et al. Local injection of TGF-beta increases the strength of tibial fractures in the rat. Acta Orthop Scand 1994; 65(1):37–41.
31. Ripamonti U, et al. Limited chondro-osteogenesis by recombinant human transforming growth factor-beta 1 in calvarial defects of adult baboons (Papio ursinus). J Bone Miner Res 1996; 11(7):938–945.
32. Canalis E. Insulin like growth factors and the local regulation of bone formation. Bone 1993; 14(3):273–276.
33. Sandberg MM, Aro HT, Vuorio EI. Gene expression during bone repair. Clin Orthop Rel Res 1993; 289:292–312.
34. Aspenberg P, Albrektsson T, Thorngren KG. Local application of growth-factor IGF-1 to healing bone: experiments with a titanium chamber in rabbits. Acta Orthop Scand 1989; 60(5):607–610.
35. Thaller SR, Dart A, Tesluk H. The effects of insulin-like growth factor-1 on critical-size calvarial defects in Sprague-Dawley rats. Ann Plast Surg 1993; 31(5):429–433.
36. Thaller SR, et al. Effect of insulin-like growth factor-1 on zygomatic arch bone regeneration: a preliminary histological and histometric study. Ann Plast Surg 1993; 31(5):421–428.
37. Linkhart TA, Mohan S, Baylink DJ. Growth factors for bone growth and repair: IGF, TGF beta and BMP. Bone 1996; 19(1 Suppl):1S–12S.
38. Ammann P, et al. IGF-1 and pamidronate increase bone mineral density in ovariectomized adult rats. Am J Physiol 1993; 265(5 Pt 1):E7770–776.
39. Machwate M, et al. Insulin-like growth factor-1 increases trabecular bone formation and osteoblastic cell proliferation in unloaded rats. Endocrinology 1994; 134(3):1031–1038.
40. Mueller K, et al. Stimulation of trabecular bone formation by insulin-like growth factor 1 in adult ovariectomized rats. Am J Physiol 1994; 267 (1 Pt I):E1–6.
41. Bagi CM, et al. Benefit of systemically administered rh1GF-1 and rh1 GF-1/IGFBP-3 on cancellous bone in ovariectomized rats. J Bone Miner Res 1994; 8(9):1301–1312.

42. Hogan BL. Bone morphogenetic proteins: multifunctional regulators of vertebrate development. Genes Dev 1996; 10(13):1580–1594.
43. Urist M. Bone formation by autoinduction. Science 1965; 150:893–899.
44. Urist MR, DeLange RJ, Finerman GA. Bone cell differentiation and growth factors. Science 1983; 220(4598):680–686.
45. Onishi T, et al. Distinct and overlapping patterns of localization of bone morphogenetic protein (BMP) family members and a BMP type II receptor during fracture healing in rats. Bone 1998; 22(6):605–612.
46. Nakase T, et al. Transient and localized expression of bone morphogenetic protein 4 messenger RNA during fracture healing. Bone Miner Res 1994; 9(5):651–659.
47. Ishidou Y, et al. Enhanced expression of type I receptors for bone morphogenetic proteins during bone formation. J Bone Miner Res 1995; 10(11):1651–1659.
48. Heckman JD, et al. The use of bone morphogenetic protein in the treatment of non-union in a canine model. J Bone Joint Surg Am Vol 1991; 73(5): 750–764.
49. Cook SD, et al. Recombinant human bone morphogenetic protein-7 induces healing in a canine long-bone segmental defect model. Clin Orthop Rel Res 1994; 301:302–312.
50. Yasko AW, et al. The healing of segmental bone defects, induced by recombinant human bone morphogenetic protein (rhBMP-2). A radiographic, histological, and biomechanical study in rats. J Bone Joint Surg Am Vol 1992; 74(5):659–670.
51. Bostrom M, et al. Use of bone morphogenetic protein-2 in the rabbit ulnar nonunion model. Clin Orthop Rel Res 1996; 327:272–282.
52. Ripamonti U, et al. Initiation of bone regeneration in adult baboons by osteogenin, a bone morphogenetic protein. Matrix, 1992; 12(5):369–380.
53. Ferguson D, et al. Bovine bone morphogenetic protein (bBMP) fraction-induced repair of craniotomy defects in the rhesus monkey (Macaca speciosa). Clin Orthop Rel Res 1987; 219:251–258.
54. Lindholm TC, et al. Bovine bone morphogenetic protein (bBMP) induced repair of skull trephine defects in sheep. Clini Orthop Rel Res 1988; 227: 265–268.
55. Sato K, Urist MR. Induced regeneration of calvaria by none morphogenetic protein (BMP) in dogs. Clini Orthop Rel Res 1985; 197:301–311.
56. Johnson EE, Urist MR. Human bone morphogenetic protein allografting for reconstruction of femoral nonunion. Clin Orthop Rel Res 2000; 371:61–74.
57. Johnson EE, Urist MR. One-stage lengthening of femoral nonunion augmented with human bone morphogenetic protein. Clin Orthop Rel Res 1998; 347:105–116.
58. Johnson EE, Urist MR, Finerman GA. Resistant nonunions and partial or complete segmental defects of long bones: treatment with implants of a composite of human bone morphogenetic protein (BMP) and autolyzed, antigen-extracted, allogeneic (AAA) bone. Clin Orthop Rel Res 1992; 277:229–237.

59. Johnson, EE, Urist MR, Finerman GA. Distal metaphyseal tibial nonunion: deformity and bone loss treated by open reduction, internal fixation, and human bone morphogenetic protein (hBMP). Clin Orthop Rel Res 1990; 250:234–240.
60. Johnson EE, Urist MR. Distal metaphyseal tibial nonunion associated with significant bowing deformity and cortical bone loss: treatment with human bone morphogenetic protein (h-BMP) and internal fixation. Nippon Seikeigeka Gakkai Zasshi—J Jpn Orthop Assoc 1989; 63(5):613–620.
61. Johnson EE, Urist MR, Finerman GA. Repair of segmental defects of the tibia with cancellous bone grafts augmented with human bone morphogenetic protein: a preliminary report. Clini Orthop Rela Res 1988; 236:249–257.
62. Johnson EE, Urist MR, Finerman GA. Bone morphogenetic protein augmentation grafting of resistant femoral nonunions: a preliminary report. Clin Orthop Rel Res 1988; 230:257–265.
63. Cook SD. Preclinical and clinical evaluation of osteogenic protein-I (BMP-7) in bony sites. Orthopedics 1999; 22(7):669–671.
64. Bassett C. Current concepts of bone formation. J Bone Joint Surg 1962; 44A:1217–1244.
65. Jargiello DM, Caplan AI. The establishment of vascular-derived microenvironments in the developing chick wing. Dev Biol 1983; 97(2):364–374.
66. Brighton CT, Krebs AG. Oxygen tension of healing fractures in the rabbit. J Bone Joint Surg 1972; 54(2):323–332.
67. Brighton CT, et al. In vitro epiphyseal-plate growth in various oxygen tensions. J Bone Joint Surg 1969; 51(7):1383–1396.
68. Sevitt S. Bone Repair and Fracture Healing in Man. Edinburgh: Churchill Livingstone, 1981.
69. Shaw JL, Basett CA. The effects of varying oxygen concentrations on osteogenesis and embryonic cartilage in vitro. J Bone Joint Surg 1967; 49(1):73–80.
70. Brockes M. The Blood Supply of Bone. New York: Appleton-Century-Crofts, 1971.
71. Heppenstall RB, Grislis G, Hunt TK. Tissue gas tensions and oxygen consumption in healing bone defects. Clin Orthop Rel Res 1975; 106:357–365.
72. Goodship AE, Cunningham JL, Kenwright J. Strain rate and timing of stimulation in mechanical modulation of fracture healing. Clin Orthop Rel Res 1998(355 Suppl):S105–115.
73. Lanyon LE, et al. Mechanically adaptive bone remodelling. J Biomechan 1982; 15(3):141–154.
74. Goodship AE, Kenwright J. The influence of induced micromovement upon the healing of experimental tibial fractures. J Bone Joint Surg Br Vol 1985; 67(4):650–655.
75. Kenwright J. Goodship AE. Controlled mechanical stimulation in the treatment of tribal fractures. Clin Orthop Rel Res 1989; 241:36–47.
76. Goodship AE, et al. The role of fixator frame stiffness in the control of fracture healing: an experimental study. J Biomechan 1993; 26(9):1027–1035.
77. White AA III, Panjabi MM, Southwick WO. The four biomechanical stages of fracture repair. J Bone Joint Surg 1977; 59(2):188–192.

78. Carter DR, et al. Mechanobiology of skeletal regeneration. Clin Orthop Rel Res 1998; (355 Suppl):S41–55.
79. Pawels F. Biomechanics of the Locomotor Apparatus. Berlin: Springer-Verlag, 1980.
80. Benninghoff A. Experimentelle untersuchungen uber den einfluss verschiedenartiger mechanischer beanspruchung auf den knorpel. Verh Anat Ges 1924; 33:194.
81. Roux W. Terminologie der entwicklungsmechanick der tiere und pflansen. Leipzig: Wilhelm Engelmann, 1912.
82. Otter MW, McLeod KJ, Rubin CT. Effects of electromagnetic fields in experimental fracture repair. Clin Orthop Rel Res1998(355 Suppl):S90–104.
83. Bassett CA, Generation of electric potentials by bone in response to mechanical stress.
84. Fukada E, Yasuda I. On the piezoelectric effect of bone. J Phys Soc Jpn 1957; 10:1158–1169.
85. Yasuda I. Fundamental aspects of fracture treatment. J Kyoto Med Assoc 1953; 4:395–406.
86. Cochran GV, Pawluk RJ, Bassett, CA. Electromechanical characteristics of bone under physiologic moisture conditions. Clin Orthop Rel Res 1968; 58:249–270.
87. Simmons D. Fracture healing. In: Urist M, ed. Fundamental and Clinical Bone physiology. Philadelphia: JB Lippincott, 1980:283–330.
88. Friedenberg ZB, Brighton CT. Bioelectric potentials in bone. J Bone Joint Surg 1966; 48(5):915–923.
89. Brighton CT. The semi-invasive method of treating nonunion with direct current. Orthop Clin North Am 1984; 15(1):33–45.
90. Hartshorne E. On the causes and treatment of pseudoarthrosis and especially that form of it sometimes called supernumerary joint. Am J Med 1841; 1: 121–156.
91. Lente F. Cases of ununited fractures treated by electricity. NY J Med 1850; 5:317–319.
92. Friedenberg ZB, et al. Stimulation of fracture healing by direct current in the rabbit fibula. J Bone Joint Surg 1971; 53(7):1400–1408.
93. Luben RA. Effects of low-energy electromagnetic fields (pulsed DC) on membrane signal transduction processes in biological systems. Health Phys 1991; 61(1):15–28.
94. Black J. Tissue response to exogenous electromagnetic signals. Orthop Clin North Am 1984; 15(1):15–31.
95. Brighton CT, Friedenberg ZB. Electrical stimulation and oxygen tension. Ann NY Acad Sci 1974; 238:314–320.
96. Renooij W, et al. Electrode-oxygen consumption and its effects on tissue-oxygen tension: a study by mass spectrometry. Clin Orth Rel Res 1983; 173:239–244.
97. Spadaro JA. Mechanical and electrical interactions in bone remodeling. Bioelectromagnetics 1997; 18(3):193–202.

98. Bassett CA. Biomedical implications of pulsing electromagnetic fields. Surg Rounds 1983.
99. Bassett CA. Fundamental and practical aspects of therapeutic uses of pulsed electromagnetic fields (PEMFs). Crit Rev Biomed Eng 1989; 17(5):451–529.
100. Barker AT, et al. Pulsed magnetic field therapy for tibial non-union. Interim results of a double-blind trial. Lancet 1984; 1(8384):994–996.
101. Sharrard WJ. A double-blind trial of pulsed electromagnetic fields for delayed union of tibial fractures. J Bone Joint Surg Br V 1990; 72(3):347–355.
102. Mammi GI, et al. The electrical stimulation of tibial osteotomies: double-blind study. Clin Orthop Rel Res 1993; 288:246–253.
103. Ryaby JT. Clinical effects of electromagnetic and electric fields on fracture healing. Clin Orthop Rel Res1998(355 Suppl):S205–215.
104. Xavier C. Duarte L. Estimulaci ultra-sonica de callo osseo: applicaca clinica. Rev Brasileira Orthop 1983; 18:73–80.
105. Hadjiargyrou M, et al. Enhancement of fracture healing by low intensity ultrasound. Clin Orthop Rel Res 1998; (355 Suppl):S216–229.
106. Duarte LR. The stimulation of bone growth by ultrasound. Arch Orthop Traum Surg 1983; 101(3):153–159.
107. Heckman JD, et al. Acceleration of tibial fracture-healing by non-invasive, low-intensity pulsed ultrasound. J Bone Joint Surg 1994; 76(1):26–34.
108. Wang SJ, et al. Low intensity ultrasound treatment increases strength in a rat femoral fracture model. J Orthop Res 1994; 12(1):40–47.
109. Yang KH, et al. Exposure to low-intensity ultrasound increases aggrecan gene expression in a rat femur fracture model. J Orthop Res 1996; 14(5):802–809.
110. Wu JJ, et al. Comparison of osteotomy healing under external fixation devices with different stiffness characteristics. J Bone Joint Surg 1984; 66(8):1258–1264.
111. Jinguishi S, Azuma Y, Ito, M. Effects of noninvasive pulsed low-intensity ultrasound on rat femoral fracture in Third World Congress of Biomechanics, Sapporo, Japan, 1988.
112. Welgus HG, Jeffrey JJ, Eisen AZ. Human skin fibroblast collagenase: assessment of activation energy and deuterium isotope effect with collagenous substrates. J Biol Chem 1981; 256(18):9516–9521.
113. Coleman DJ, et al. Therapeutic ultrasound. Ultrasound Med Biol 1986; 12(8):633–638.
114. Rawool D, Goldberg B, Forsberg F. Power doppler assessment of vascular changes during fracture treatment with low intensity ultrasound. Trans 83rd Radiol Soc North Am 1997; 83:421.
115. Chase S, Herndon, C. The fate of autogenous and homogenous bone grafts. J Bone Joint Surg, 1955; 37A:809–841.
116. Mulliken JB, Kaban LB, Glowacki J. Induced osteogenesis—the biological principle and clinical applications. J Surg Res 1984; 37(6):487–496.
117. Heslop B, Zeiss I, Nisbet N. Studies on transference of bone. I. A comparison of autologous and homologous bone implants with reference to osteocyte survival, osteogenesis, and host reaction. Br J Exp Pathol 1960; 41:269–287.

118. Gross TP, et al. The biology of bone grafting. Orthopedics 1991; 14(5):563–568.
119. Schmitz JP, Hollinger JO. The critical size defect as an experimental model for craniomandibulofacial nonunions. Clin Orthop Rel Res 1986; 205:299–308.
120. Burchardt H. Biology of bone transplantation. Orthop Clin North Am 1987; 18(2):187–196.
121. Stevenson S, Emery SE, Goldberg, VM. Factors affecting bone graft incorporation. Clin Orthop Rel Res 1996; 324:66–74.
122. Sullivan WG, Szwajkun, PR. Revascularization of cranial versus iliac crest bone grafts in the rat. Plas Reconstr Surg 1991; 87(6):1105–1109.
123. Pinholt EM, et al. Revascularization of calvarial, mandibular, tibial, and iliac bone grafts in rats. Ann Plas Surg 1994; 33(2):193–197.
124. Burchardt H. The biology of bone graft repair. Clin Orthop Rel Res 1983; 174:28–42.
125. Heiple KG, et al. Biolog of cancellous bone grafts. Orthop Clin North Am 1987; 18(2):179–185.
126. Enneking WF, et al. Physical and biological aspects of repair in dog cortical-bone transplants. J Bone Joint Surg 1975; 57(2):237–252.
127. Chen NT, et al. The roles of revascularization and resorption on endurance of craniofacial onlay bone grafts in the rabbit. Plast Reconstr Surg 1994; 93(4):714–722; discussion 723–724.
128. Ozaki W, Buchman SR. Volume maintenance of onlay bone grafts in the craniofacial skeleton: micro-architecture versus embryologic origin. Plast Reconstr Surg 1998; 102(2):291–299.
129. Burwell RG. Studies in the transplantation of bone. 8. Treated composite homograft-autografts of cancellous bone: an analysis of inductive mechanisms in bone transplantation. J Bone Joint Surg Br Vol 1966; 48(3):532–566.
130. DeBruyn P, Kabisch W. Bone formation by fresh and frozen autogenous and homogeneous transplants of bone, bone narrow and periosteum. Am J Anat 1955; 96:375.
131. Albee F. The fundamental Principles Underlying the Use of Bone Graft in Surgery. Philadelphia: WB Saunders, 1915.
132. Thompson N, Casson JA. Experimental onlay bone grafts to the jaws: a preliminary study in dogs. Plast Reconstr Surg 1970; 46(4):341–349.
133. Zins JE,Whitaker, LA. Membranous vs endochondral bone autografts: implications for craniofacial reconstruction. Surg Forum 1979; 30:521–523.
134. Kusiak JF, Zins JE, Whitaker LA. The early revascularization of membranous bone. Plast Reconstr Surg 1985; 76(4):510–516.
135. Phillips JH, Rahn BA. Fixation effects on membranous and endochondral onlay bone-graft resorption. Plast Reconstr Surg 1988; 82(5):872–877.
136. Phillips JH, Rahn BA. Fixation effects on membranous and endochondral onlay bone graft revascularization and bone deposition. Plast Reconstr Surg 1990; 85(6):891–897.
137. Hardesty RA, Marsh JL, Craniofacial onlay bone grafting: a prespective evaluation of graft morphology, orientation, and embryonic origin Plast Reconstr Surg 1990. 85(1) p. 5–14; disussion 15.

138. Alonso N, et al. Cranial versus iliac onlay bone grafts in the facial skeleton: a macroscopic and histomorphometric study. J Craniofac Surg 1995; 6(2):113–118; discussion 119.
139. Peer L. The fate of autogenous bone grafts. Br J Plast Surg 1951; 3:233–243.
140. Smith J, Abramson M. Membranous vs endochondral bone autografts. Arch Otolaryngol 1974; 99(3):203–205.
141. Buchman SR, Ozaki W. The ultrastructure and resorptive pattern of cancellous onlay bone grafts in the craniofacial skeleton. Ann Plas Surg 1999; 43(1):49–56.
142. Whitaker LA. Biological boundaries: a concept in facial skeletal restructuring. Clin Plast Surg 1989; 16(1):1–10.
143. LaTrenta GS, et al. The role of rigid skeletal fixation in bone-graft augmentation of the craniofacial skeleton. Plast Reconstr Surg 1989; 84(4):578–588.
144. Mowlem R. Bone grafting. Br J Plast Surg 1963; 16:293.
145. Ozaki W, et al. A comparative analysis of the microarchitecture of cortical membranous and cortical endochondral onlay bone grafts in the craniofacial skeleton. Plast Reconstr Surg 1999; 104(1):139–147.
146. Lin KY, et al. The effect of rigid fixation on the survival of onlay bone grafts: an experimental study. Plast Reconstr Surge 1990; 86(3):449–456.
147. Knize DM. The influence of periosteum and calcitonin on onlay bone graft survival: a roentgenographic study. Plast Reconstr Surg 1974; 53(2):190–199.
148. Burstein FD, et al. The effect of periosteal preservation on osteogenesis in a canine rib autograft model: tetracycline fluorescence incident photometry. J Craniofac Surg 1994; 5(3):161–171.
149. Lozano AJ, Cestero HJ Jr, Salyer KE. The early vascularization of onlay bone grafts. Plast Reconstr Surg 1976; 58(3):302–305.
150. Ermis I, Poole M. The effects of soft tissue coverage on bone graft resorption in the craniofacial region. Br J Plast Surg 1992; 45(1):26–29.
151. Enlow D. The Handbook of Facial Growth. Philadelphia: WB Saunders, 1982.
152. Zins JE, et al. The influence of the recipient site on bone grafts to the face. Plast Reconstr Surg 1984; 73(3):371–381.
153. Moss M. Facial growth: the functional matrix concept. In: Grabb W, Rosenstein S, Bzoch K, Cleft Lip and Palate. Boston: Little Brown & Co., 1971:97–107.
154. Ham A. Some histophysiological problems peculiar to calcified tissues. J Bone Joint Surg Am 1952; 34:701–728.
155. Alberius P, et al. Influence of surrounding soft tissues on onlay bone graft incorporation. Oral Surg Oral Med Oral Pathol Oral Radiol Endodont 1996; 82(1):22–33.
156. Goldstein J, Mase C, Newman MH. Fixed membranous bone graft survival after recipient bed alteration. Plast Reconstr Surg 1993; 91(4):589–596.

7

Optimizing Bony Repair

Stephen M. Warren, Tony D. Fang, Kenton D. Fong, HanJoon M. Song, and Michael T. Longaker
Stanford University School of Medicine, Stanford, California, U.S.A.

I. INTRODUCTION

In this chapter, we present the hypotheses and current research that have furthered our knowledge of the molecular and cellular mechanisms that govern fracture healing. Our purpose is to integrate animal and human data to present the biological basis for successful and unsuccessful fracture healing. By developing a dynamic biological blueprint for angiogenic and osteogenic cascades, we hope to begin to anticipate complications, learn to improve patient outcomes, and drive research in new directions.

To date, most of the fracture-healing benchwork has been performed on endochondral bone and we will reference this work as a foundation for current/future studies in the intramembranous craniofacial skeleton. It is important to note that disparities may exist in endochondral and intramembranous fracture-healing cascades, so results from the long bones may not, for example, be directly translated to the craniofacial skeleton. This brings up a critical point: do endochondral and intramembranous fracture healing share ontologically conserved common final pathways? While there the obvious differences in endochondral and intramembranous bone development, evidence suggests that there is astounding conservation in their molecular and cellular repair mechanisms. While this conservation provides the foundation for general endochondral to intramembranous fracture healing extrapolation, more research is still needed to validate this point.

Understanding the molecular and cellular events leading to intramembranous fracture healing has important clinical implications as it is a fundamental step toward the evolution of targeted therapeutic interventions designed to accelerate osseous regeneration. Indeed, the development of novel recombinant proteins, gene and cellular transfer techniques, minimally invasive approaches, and the identification of objective endpoints will propel the field of craniomaxillofacial fracture repair, reducing complications (e.g., infections and nonunions) and optimizing patient outcomes.

II. THE FRACTURE HEALING PROCESS

There are two types of fracture healing: primary (direct) fracture healing and secondary (indirect) fracture healing. Primary fracture healing occurs without intermediate callous formation. Both cancellous and cortical bone will heal primarily when rigid fixation assures minimal interfragmental movement (1,2). Primary fracture healing can be subclassified into *contact healing* and *gap healing* (3–5). Contact healing leads to lamellar bone formation across the fracture line via direct extension of the osteons (6). Gap healing occurs when the intercalary space cannot be bridged directly with lamellar bone; therefore, a provisional woven bone interstage develops until remodeling produces mature bone (6). Unlike secondary healing, primary fracture healing does not have distinct remedial stages.

Secondary fracture healing commonly occurs when severe injury or comminuted high-energy fractures limit fixation; consequently, these resilient fractures heal through a callous intermediate. Secondary fracture healing can be divided into four stages: (1) inflammatory phase with hematoma formation; (2) proliferation phase with soft callous formation; (3) modeling phase with hard callous formation; and (4) remodeling phase with sustained bone turnover (7). Since both primary and secondary healing can result in successful fracture repair, it should be emphasized that primary fracture healing is not equated with early healing and secondary healing is not delayed.

Successful fracture healing is a unique form of wound healing. Unlike soft tissue, successful fracture healing produces scarless regenerate bone that is architecturally, histologically, and mechanically indistinguishable from native bone (6). However, the conditions required for successful fracture repair are not always present; therefore, surgeons must learn to anticipate *delayed unions, malunions,* or *nonunions.* Delayed union, also known as slow union, occurs when the fracture-healing process extends over an abnormally long period of time. Marsh, correlating his material testing data with histological analysis of fracture healing, described a delayed union as a fracture that fails to achieve normal histology and a bending stiffness of $7\,N/m^2$ within 20 weeks (8). While delayed unions eventually heal, the long-term care and rehabilitation of these problematic fractures is a significant bio-medical burden (9,10). Malunion refers to fracture healing with angular and/or translational deformation in one or more planes (including foreshortening). Long-bone malunions commonly cause loss of intra-articular congruity (7). Nonunion is the cessation of the fracture-healing process without bony bridging of the fracture gap. While nonunions are commonly defined as fractures that do not spontaneously heal in the experimental animal's or patient's lifetime, Marsh defined nonunions as fractures that never achieve normal histology or a bending stiffness of $7\,N/m^2$ (8). In practice, nonunions are fractures that do not heal after the first intervention and require a secondary procedure. Finally, nonunions may be described as *hypertrophic, atrophic,* or *fibrous*, and they may cause *pseudarthroses*.

III. TISSUE DIFFERENTIATION THEORY

We have attempted to categorize the cascading events that affect fracture repair into boundary parameters to describe the interrelationship of the convergent molecular and cellular tributaries that nourish the fracture microenvironment. Understanding the parameters that influence successful and unsuccessful fracture healing may help us envisage novel ways to intervene to optimize fracture repair. We use a triangular model based on conventional tissue differentiation theory to unite the components of the fracture microenvironment (Fig. 1). The three main components of the fracture triangle are: (1) *mechanical loading history* (stress and strain); (2) *angiogenesis* (new vessel formation); (3) *osteogenesis* (new bone formation). The complex interactions between each component of this triad guide the fate of the tissues at the fracture site and, ultimately, determine successful or unsuccessful healing.

To discuss the effects of fracture microenvironment biomechanics on tissue differentiation, we first define a few basic engineering terms. Bone is a biphasic (mineral and ground substance) composite material with viscoelastic properties (11). Bone has inherent time-dependent deformational properties that are related to the rate of loading, hysteresis, creep, and stress relaxation (11). Three types of *loads* may act on the fracture microenvironment: *tension forces, compression forces*, and *shear forces*. Since *stress* is defined as load per unit area, these forces when analyzed per unit area become the three principal stresses: *tensile stresses* are generated in response to loads that pull an object apart, *compressive stresses* push objects together,

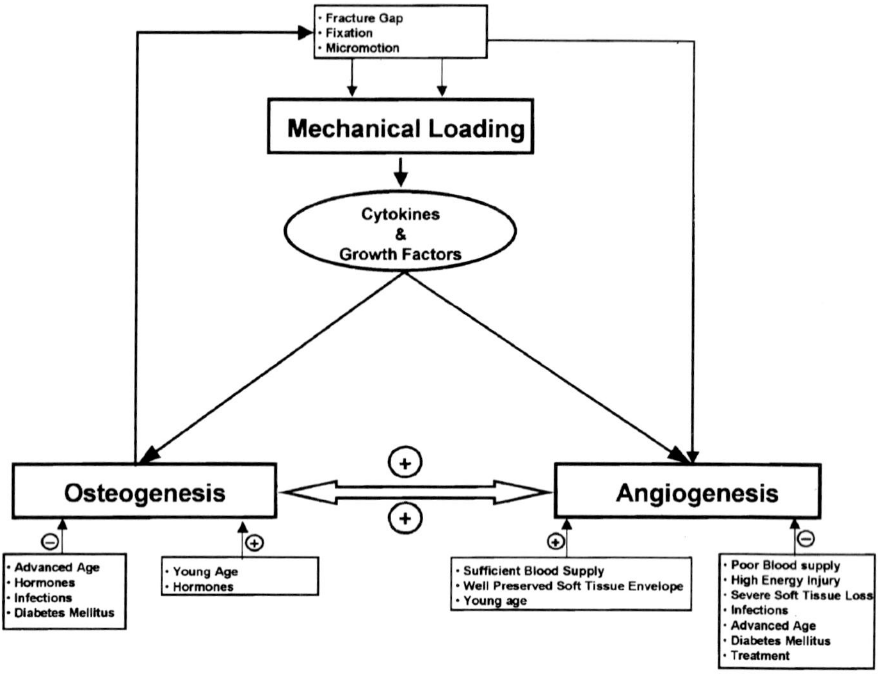

Figure 1 Triangular relationships between mechanical loading, angiogenesis, and osteogenesis during fracture repair. Mechanical loading (stresses or strains) is imposed on the regenerative tissue in the fracture gap. This mechanical loading activates transcription pathways (mechanotransduction) that result in angiogenic and osteogenic cytokine and growth factor production and release. In addition, mechanical loading has direct physical effects on angiogenesis. The relationship between angiogenesis and osteogenesis is mutual. Each affects the other by altering matrix deposition and the mechanical loading environment. There are many individual factors that affect each component of the triangle.

and *shear stresses* deform or separate objects by sliding molecule layers past each other on one or more planes. *Strain* is the deformation of an object in response to an applied load. Using these basic biomechanical engineering terms we can discuss tissue differentiation theory.

Pauwels, based on ideas originated by Roux and Benninghoff, hypothesized that intermittent mechanical stresses guided tissue differentiation (12–14). Since then, many have investigated the relationships between mechanical forces and cellular differentiation. For example, Perren et al., using a long-bone model, demonstrated that intercalary forces influenced the fate of fracture healing (15,16). Then, in a series of pioneering studies,

Dennis Carter's group applied tissue differentiation theory to skeletal tissue regeneration by linking the mechanical loading history with cellular differentiation (Fig. 2) (17–21). Carter highlighted the importance of cyclical mechanical loading history on tissue differentiation and developed a method to calculate the local stress-and-strain history (17–21). Their model predicts: (1) low stress-and-strain environments promote direct intramembranous bone formation; (2) poor blood supply favors chondrogenesis in an otherwise osteogenic environment; (3) hydrostatic compressive stress encourages chondrogenesis; (4) high tensile strain tips the balance in favor of net deposition of fibrous tissue; and (5) hydrostatic compressive stress superimposed on tensile strain produces fibrocartilage. Carter showed that mechanical forces not only determine early tissue differentiation, but also affect the rate of bony remodeling. For example, intermittent compressive stress may slow or stop endochondral ossification, but intermittent octahedral shear stress (or stain) will accelerate ossification (22,23).

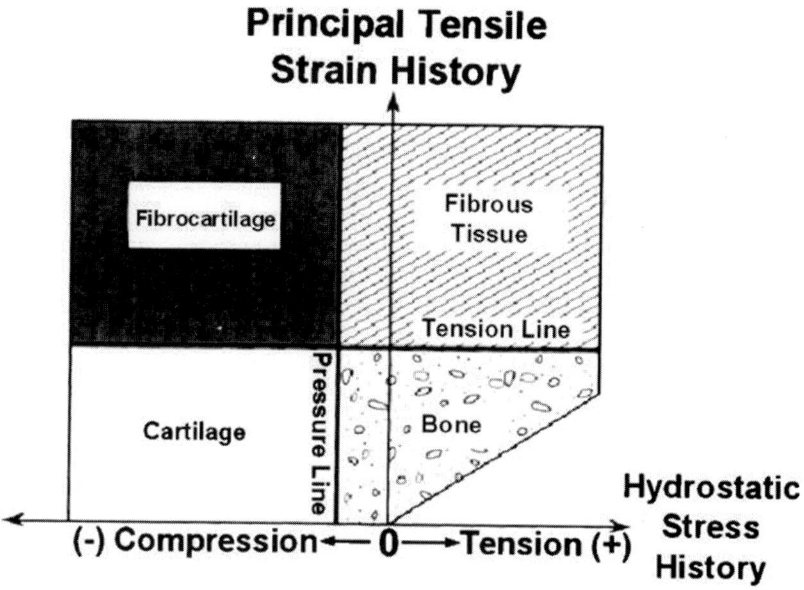

Figure 2 Carter Phase diagram. Loading history has important implications for tissue differentiation. With low strain and low tensile stress, bone will form. If the strain increases beyond a certain level, even with the same tensile stress, fibrous tissue will form. In general, compressive stress will promote chondrogenesis. Low strain levels favor cartilage formation, while a high-strain environment will lead to fibrocartilage formation. (Adapted with permission from Ref. 22)

A. Mechanical Loading and Angiogenesis

Mechanical loading, or mechanotransduction, affects angiogenesis on at least three levels: (1) tissue (e.g., pressure gradients, distortion, energy dissipation); (2) cell (e.g., cell shape changes, cell pressure, local oxygen tension, effects on extracellular matrix (ECM), temperature changes, and electric potential); and (3) subcellular (e.g., cytoskeletal changes, integrin expression, growth/transcriptional factor production, stretch-activated ion channels). We hypothesize that mechanotransductive signaling must act locally on established vasculature (neoangiogenesis) and/or initiate signaling cascades to attract bone-marrow-derived/circulating angioblasts (neovasculogenesis) to mediate successful facture healing (24–30).

Stresses and strains can support or physically disrupt the neovasculature. For example, micromotion stimulates new vessel formation, but excessive motion (gap strain $\geq$15%) prunes budding capillaries (31,32). In our rat distraction osteogenesis (DO) model, successful DO (bony union) experienced average daily strains of 9–12%, while unsuccessful DO (fibrous union) experienced stains level more than 400% initially, which ultimately led to nonunions (E. Loboa, personal communication, 2002) (33). Moreover, since capillary hydrostatic pressure is only 0.0023 MPa, even small amounts of tissue hydrostatic pressure can compress the microvasculature and compromise blood flow (34). In addition to the physical effects on blood vessel formation or blood flow, cells may directly translate mechanical signals into neoangiogenic cascades by producing angiogenic factors (e.g., VEGF) of upregulating angiogenic cell surface proteins (e.g., Flk-1/Flt-1 or $\alpha v\beta 3/\beta 5$) (35–37). Fracture site mechanical stimuli have profound effects on angiogenesis, and angiogenesis temporally and spatially precedes osteogenesis; the direct link between angiogenesis and osteogenesis is described below.

B. Angiogenesis and Osteogenesis

Today, many studies have demonstrated that blood flow increases during fracture healing. In a rat femoral fracture model, Grundes and Reikeras found that there was more than a 10-fold increase in blood flow in the fracture callus 4 weeks after osteotomy (38). Using an iatrogenically manipulated form of fracture healing (i.e., distraction osteogenesis) to illustrate the magnitude of new vessel formation during fracture healing, Aronson demonstrated that there was a peak 8.5–9.5-fold increase in blood flow to the distracted segment (i.e., osteotomized) bone within 2 weeks of osteotomy and bone lengthening. This dramatic hyperemia persisted throughout the consolidation and remodeling period (39). We have found similar results in the craniofacial skeleton. In our rat mandibular distraction osteogenesis mode, Rowe et al. demonstrated intense neovessel formation during the early time points of distraction that was decreased but remained at high levels throughout distraction and consolidation (40).

Although the increase in blood flow during fracture healing and distraction osteogenesis was likely due to new blood vessel formation in the intercalary gap, there was no evidence to support this supposition. Moreover, there was no direct evidence to link angiogenesis to osteogenesis. However, in 2001, using TNP-470, a potent angiogenesis inhibitor, Hausman et al. demonstrated that successful angiogenesis was a prerequisite for successful osteogenesis. The authors used plain film, mechanical testing, and histology to compare control and TNP-470-treated femoral fracture healing over 24 days. Interestingly, all TNP-470 treated animals had roentgenographic evidence of nonunion, which was confirmed by histology to be atrophic nonunion. Furthermore, the TNP-470-treated fractures recovered only 16% of normal strength and 7% of normal stiffness. In contrast, control fractures recovered 56% and 48% strength and stiffness, respectively. The authors concluded that antiangiogenesis therapy inhibited both intramembranous and endochondral osteogenesis and angiogenesis was essential to both bone formation pathways (41).

While the preceding study convincingly demonstrated that new vessel formation is essential for successful fracture healing, the origin of the endothelial cells in the nascent fracture vasculature remains debatable. Traditionally, we have assumed that the fracture microenvironment stimulates the sprouting of new capillaries from pre-existing vessels. Accordingly, local endothelial cell proliferation, migration, and remodeling hypothetically lead to wound revascularization. More recent work suggests that bone-marrow-derived angioblastic cells can traffic to healing wounds (27–30). These startling reports suggest that postnatal neovasculogenesis may be naturally occurring during normal wound healing; however, more evidence is needed to support this idea.

If bone-marrow-derived angioblastic cells traffic to healing wounds, can osteoblastic cells traffic? In 1999, Hou et al. reported that bone-marrow-derived osteoblastic precursors engraft at osseous sites following intravenous administration (42). Taken together, these findings rouse an intriguing way of conceptualizing fracture healing: the fracture microenvironment must contain (or be manipulated to contain) the appropriate molecular and cellular milieu to attract *local* and *systemic* angioblastic, osteoblastic, and mesenchymal cells necessary for successful angiogenesis, osteogenesis, and fracture healing. While further work is still needed, we can look forward to a series of insightful studies that will either prove or disprove this exciting new hypothesis.

IV. SYSTEMIC FACTORS AFFECTING FRACTURE HEALING

A. Age

Children have a greater capacity to heal fractures than adults. For example, a displaced femoral fracture in a 3-year-old often heals within a month, while it takes a 70-year-old more then 5 months to heal the same fracture (6). Age-specific healing is even more dramatic in the craniofacial skeleton. For example, total calvariectomies will completely reossify in children younger than 2 years, but even a cranial burr hole usually will not heal in an adult (43).

Why are there dramatic differences between juvenile and adult fracture healing? Anatomically, children have a thicker, more cellular and vascular periosteum than adults (44–47). While the periosteum may be critical for rapid fracture healing in the young, other factors are certainly involved. Bone marrow cellularity and function decline with age (48–50). This decline may reduce the number/function of marrow-derived osteoblastic and angioblastic precursors and contribute to slower healing in the adult. Furthermore, our laboratory has recently demonstrated marked differences in juvenile and adult osteoblast biology (C. Cowan, personal communication, 2002) (51). For example, we have found that juvenile osteoblasts proliferate more rapidly and produce greater amounts of osteogenic proteins at baseline and when stimulated with osteogenci cytokines, such as fibroblast growth factor-2 (FGF-2). We have learned that as osteoblasts age they express more antiproliferative factors (i.e., Tob and PC3) that may be primarily responsible for impairing their response at the fracture site (51). Furthermore, adult osteoblasts are more differentiated [high fibroblast growth factor receptor-1 (FGFR1)] and less proliferative [low fibroblast growth factor receptor-2 (FGFR2)] than juvenile osteoblasts. Finally, even after treatment with FGF-2, adult osteoblasts cannot increase their expression of genes necessary for bone formation [e.g., osteopontin (OP)] (51).

Why are there more dramatic age-dependent differences in the calvarium than, for example, in the long bones? We feel some answers may relate to the anatomy (and paracrine signaling) of overlying cranium and underlying dura mater. Our laboratory has demonstrated that in addition to effects on osteoblast biology, age dramatically affects underlying dura mater biology (52,53). By comparing juvenile (6-day-old) and adult (60-day-old) Sprague-Dawley rat nonsuture associated dura mater, we demonstrated that not only was the juvenile dura mater producing significantly more osteoinductive growth factors [e.g., transforming growth factor-beta (TGF-β1)] and FGF-2 and primary extracellular matrix scaffolding proteins (e.g., collagen I), but it was also expressing markers of the osteoblast lineage (osteocalcin), suggesting that juvenile dura mater may contain a subpopulation of cells with an osteoblast-like phenotype. This osteoblast-like subpopulation appears to be severely attenuated in adult dura mater. Collectively, these studies suggest that juvenile dura mater expresses critical levels of osteoinductive paracrine factors and may supply sufficient osteoblast-like cells to orchestrate successful calvarial reossification. While we cannot change the age of a patient, we have tried to determine if we can turn back the "biological clock" to improve local fracture healing in the adult (*see "Viral Vectors,"* Sec. IX. A).

B. Nutrition Status

Both preoperative and postoperative nutrition can affect fracture healing (54). Nutrition may have an enormous impact on fracture healing because the complex cascades (i.e., osteoblast, endothelial, and inflammatory cell proliferation, migration, and matrix biosynthesis) that mediate successful healing require tremendous energy. For exampled, simple long-bone-fracture repair increases a patient's metabolic expenditure by 25%, but repair of a comminuted infected fracture, irrespective of other injuries, can increase metabolic demand by 55% (54–56). In addition to supplying fuel for cellular machinery, good nutrition provides trace elements (e.g., calcium, zinc, and phosphorus) that are essential for callous formation, collagen cross-linking, and mineralization (57).

C. Diabetes Mellitus

Diabetes mellitus (DM) impairs wound and fracture healing (58). the effects on fracture healing may be due to inhibition of angiogenesis and, consequently, osteogenesis. While DM compromises tissue perfusion at baseline, untreated and poorly controlled DM compromises callous maturation and fracture healing (58). For example, Gooch et al. demonstrated that, in addition to adversely affecting endothelial biology, elevated blood glucose impairs the conversion of collagen production in chondrocytes from type II to type X (59). This suggests that DM prevents chondrocyte maturation and fracture healing (59). Funk et al. also showed that even if a fracture does heal despite elevated blood glucose, diabetic rats exhibited inferior healing compared to control animals (60). For example, torque failure, stress failure, structural stiffness, and material stiffness of healed DM femur fractures were significantly less ($^{*}p < 0.05$) than healed control femur fractures (60).

Moreover, the healing rate in diabetic animals was significantly delayed (60). When DM animals were treated with insulin to control blood glucose, DM healing rates and mechanical strength returned to near-normal levels, suggesting that tight blood sugar control dramatically improves fracture healing (58). It is important to note, that it is not clear whether the fracture healing augmentation observed with tight glucose control was due to decreasing blood glucose level (and, consequently, improved endothelial, chondrocyte, and osteoblast biology) or the direct pro-osteogenic effects of insulin (see below).

D. Hormonal/Metabolic Factors

Many hormones and metabolic factors are pro-osteogenic. For example, growth hormone (GH), thyroid hormone, vitamin A, vitamin D, androgens, calcitonin, parathyroid hormone (PTH), insulin-like growth factors (IGF), and insulin stimulate new bone formation (61,68). Conversely, some hormonal/metabolic factors (e.g., corticosteroids) can impair fracture healing (69–71). How exactly do hormones affect fracture healing? The answer is unclear, but different hormones, presumably, act through different mechanisms. For example, vitamin D_3 seems to affect fracture healing by regulating mineralization (6), while corticosteroids adversely affect healing by inhibiting osteoblast differentiation and decreasing matrix synthesis (69,71). Clinical observations suggest that hormone levels tend to affect the rate of fracture healing and, therefore, may account for delayed unions; however, hormone levels are rarely responsible for nonunions (6).

E. Smoking

Smoking profoundly impairs fracture healing by causing both delayed unions and nonunions. For example, Schmitz et al. demonstrated that smoking significantly delays tibial fracture healing (62% longer in the smoking patients than the nonsmoking patients) (72). Cobb et al. found that the relative risk of nonunion in the patients who smoke was 3.5–16 times that of the patients who did not smoke (73). In studies of craniofacial fractures, Haug and Schwimmer analyzed 27 nonunions out of 704 mandibular fractures, and found 41% of the nonunions were associated with smoking (74). Furthermore, Brown et al. demonstrated that smokers were 5 times more likely to develop pseudarthrosis than nonsmokers (75). Brown et al. suggested that the elevated pseudarthrosis rate was due to lower peripheral oxygen saturation and, consequently, lower tissue oxygen delivery in smokers (75).

Most research is in agreement with Brown's hypothesis: carbon monoxide displaces oxygen from hemoglobin, reducing oxygen saturation and, in turn, oxygen content (CaO_2). However, in addition to decreasing CaO_2, cigarette smoke compromises local circulation by causing profound vasoconstriction (76,77). Equally important, cigarette smoke may impair fracture healing by directly inhibiting neoangiogenesis (78–80). With our new understanding of the importance of postnatal neovasculogenesis, we would predict that smoking may also impair bone-marrow-derived angioblasts trafficking to sites of fracture healing (81). Finally, cigarette smoke has been shown to directly inhibit osteoblast differentiation and may even increase osteoblast apoptotic rates (82). Collectively, there is strong evidence to conclude that smoking impairs fracture healing by compromising both angiogenesis and osteogenesis.

V. LOCAL FACTORS AFFECTING FRACTURE HEALING

A. Oxygen Tension

Oxygen plays an important role in fracture healing. Normal oxygen tension (pO_2) in bony tissues is about 150 mm Hg. The oxygen-carrying capacity of blood (i.e., CaO_2) is determined by the hemoglobin concentration (Hb), the oxyhemoglobin saturation (SaO_2), and the partial pressure of oxygen dissolved in the blood (PaO_2).

$$CaO_2 = ([Hb] \times 1.34 \times SaO_2) + (0.003 \times PaO_2) \qquad (1)$$

Vascular disruption secondary to fracture creates a hypoxic gradient of injury wherein the pO_2 at the center of the wound is very low (38,83–86). The depth of the pO_2 nadir is related to the severity of the bony and soft-tissue vascular disruption (38,83–86). In vivo this hypoxic, high-lactate, low-pH fracture microenvironment induces the transcription of a number of genes necessary for fracture repair (87,91). Moreover, the milieu promotes inflammatory cell, fibroblast, endothelial cell, and osteoblast chemotaxis and activation (88,90,92). For example, in our laboratory, we have demonstrated that hypoxia increases osteoblast vascular endothelial growth factor (VEGF), IGF-2, TGF-β1 TGF-β type I receptor, and collagen I and III expression while it simultaneously decreases the expression of tissue inhibitor of metalloproteinase-1 (TIMP-1) (93–97). Moreover, we have found that hypoxia regulates osteoblast proliferation and differentiation (94). Taken together these data suggest that hypoxia induce osteoblast-derived growth factors and ECM molecule expression that, we hypothesize, are important for initiating early genetic/cellular cascades that eventually lead to successful fracture healing.

While we have limited our discussion of hypoxia to osteoblast biology, the effects of oxygen tension on other cell types should not be overlooked. In particular, oxygen tension has profound effects on angiogenic and osteogenic stem cell differentiation/function. For example, in a low-oxygen environment, osteoblastic precursors are shunted down chondrogenic pathways, which impairs or delays fracture healing (98–101).

B. Blood Supply

Re-establishing an adequate blood supply is essential for successful fracture healing. Injury-mediated vascular disruption with inadequate vascular restoration (e.g., aged, nutritionally depleted, diabetic, smoking patients) leads to delayed unions and nonunions (102). While all fractures cause local vascular injury, soft-tissue loss, and hematoma formation, high-energy degloving fractures often lead to large-volume tissue necrosis, substantial vessel thrombosis, and profound local hypoperfusion. How do fractures, including the devastating high-energy fractures, successfully recruit a new blood supply? Does the fracture microenvironment (hypoxia, lactate, pH) simply call out to local and systemic angioblastic cells? The answer is unknown, but successful angiogenesis remains intertwined in successful fracture healing. Study after study illustrates that new blood flow permits new bone formation in fracture-healing models. For example, in tibia fracture models, ligating two of the three lower-leg vessels decreases perfusion and increases delayed unions by 30% (103). Moreover, many vascular watershed bony areas such as the femoral head, proximal pole of the scaphoid, distal tibia, and talar body are particularly vulnerable to postfracture avascular necrosis and impaired healing (6).

Still, the mechanism for new vessel ingrowth remains elusive. We know that mechanical loading promotes neoangiogenesis in long-bone fracture-healing models, but we do not know how (104,105). Do microenvironment stimuli attract local medullary microvascular endothelial cells and pericytes or bone marrow-derived precursors (27–30,90)? Do fractures with larger intercalary gaps demand more mesenchymal cell trafficking to establish new blood flow? Does profound interruption of the local blood supply impede the migration of pluripotential cells (84,85). Will adoptive angioblastic therapy or bone marrow stimulation improve fracture healing? Fortunately, craniofacial bone is well perfused with an elaborate collateral soft-tissue vascular network; however, to reduce out fracture complications, we must learn from the appendicular paradigm and conduct new hypothesis-driven craniofacial bony research.

C. Infections

Soft-tissue or bony infections (osteomyelitis) can lead to delayed unions and nonunions. Reviewing over 1400 mandibular fractures, Mathog et al. demonstrated that 72% (18 out of 25) of nonunions were associated with osteomyelitis (106). Infections increase local energy expenditure, expand the penumbra of normal tissue necrosis, and contribute to small-vessel thrombosis (6,107). Infections can also directly inhibit osteoblast proliferation and lead to fibrous union (106).

D. Fracture Gap Apposition

As the length of the intercalary fracture gap increase, the risk of delayed unions and nonunions increases (108–111). To investigate this phenomenon, researchers have used critical size defect (CSD) fracture-healing models. When the gap size is small, the healing rate is inversely proportional to the intercalary distance (Fig. 3). As intercalary distance increases to subcritical levels, delayed unions begin to occur more frequently. Finally, as the intercalary fracture gap reaches a critical distance (i.e., CSD), the fracture will no longer heal during the lifetime of the animal or, more precisely, during the period of investigation (110). For example, using a sheep metatarsus fracture model, Claes et al. investigated how the intercalary distances and interfragmental movement affected the fracture healing. Three different sizes of intercalary distance (1, 2, and 6 mm) were created, and applied with 7% or 31% interfragmental strain, respectively. The callouses of the metatarsus were evaluated radiographically and the regenerative strengths were evaluated using three-point bending test 9 days after the surgery. They found that there were significant reductions of the bending stiffness with increased size of the gap (from 1 to 6 mm). As gap sizes increased beyond 2 mm, the fractures became more susceptible to interfragmental movement and strain; there were no proportional increased callous volumes with increasing strain level. The larger gaps impair new-vessel intercalary bridging and this, of course, impairs new bone formation (110). In addition, we hypothesize that larger-size gaps may exceed the supply of angioblastic and/or osteoblastic precursors or the center of larger gaps may simply exceed the maximal distance that precursor can migrate from the bone edges or surrounding tissues. Moreover, larger gaps are associated with larger intercalary strain (more than 15%) (31); therefore, mesenchymal precursors may be forced to differentiate into fibrous tissue or fibrocartilage, setting up conditions for nonunion formation (see Fig. 2). Finally, larger interfragmental gaps are almost always associated with disruption of the periostium. Loss of periosteal continuity allows the soft tissues to move into the fracture gap and

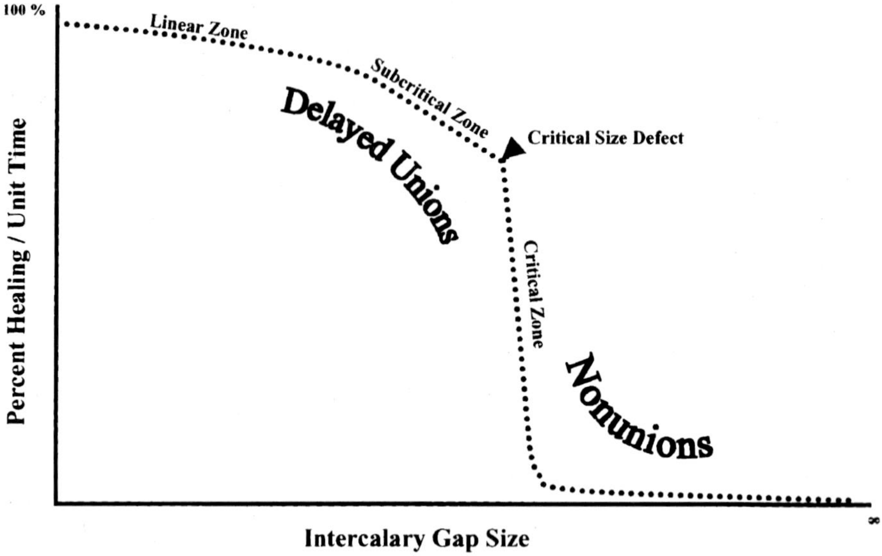

Figure 3 Idealized representation of the fracture healing–intercalary gap dynamic. When the gap size is small (e.g., Kerf of an osteotomy or nondisplaced fracture), the healing rate is inversely proportional to the intercalary distance (Linear Zone). As intercalary distance increases (e.g., displaced fracture), delayed unions begin to occur more frequently (Subcritical Zone). Finally, as the intercalary fracture gap reaches a critical distance (indicated by the arrowhead), the fracture will no longer heal (Critical Zone) and, instead, it forms a nonunion.

physically impair new-vessel ingrowth. Irrespective of the mechanism, a larger gap impairs angiogenesis and, consequently, new bone formation, so precise anatomical reduction and end-fragment apposition are critical for successful fracture healing.

E. Immobilization

Interfragmental movement has important implications on fracture healing; stresses and strains determine the fate of intercalary tissue (see Fig. 2). Micromotion stimulates new vessel formation, but excessive motion (gap strain $\geq$15%) prunes budding capillaries, inhibits osteogenesis, and leads to nonunion (32,112,113). Moreover, micromotion stimulates blood flow and periosteal callus formation and, ultimately, it improve fracture healing (32).

While rigid fixation promotes primary fracture healing, most titanium and Vitallium fixation systems are overengineered. So, how can we maximize fracture fixation without causing stress shielding? In the long bones, intramedullary (IM) nails facilitate micromotion, but they destroy the endosteal blood supply leading to healing through periosteal callous pathways; however, IM nailing has little application in the craniofacial skeleton. Fine-wire external fixation causes little damage to the endosteal blood supply, provides sufficient stability, and facilitates primary fracture healing (8). In craniofacial fracture management, plates and screws are commonly used for the fixation (114–116). Bioresorbable plates and screws, the new generation of fixation materials, can be shaped to fit the local area without concern for removing the devices. This will further perfect the fixation and limit damaging the soft-tissue envelope (114–116).

VI. SYSTEMIC STRATEGIES TO IMPROVE FRACTURE HEALING

Systemic therapies to improve fracture healing are predicated on increasing the body's own regenerative capacity. On the simplest level, this involves providing adequate nutrition to maintain patient health and maximize healing. although surgeons still debate the best assessment of a patient's nutrition status, most concede that body weight less than 80–85% of ideal weight and serum albumin concentration less than 3.0g/100mL are indicators of impaired wound healing (117). The true transferrin level is also an excellent independent indicator of recent nutrition status (117). Optimizing these parameters with special diet, tube feeds, or even total parental nutrition (TPN) may be the first step to maximizing the patient's native ability to heal.

Preoperative and postoperative smoking cessation is also essential for optimizing bony repair. Glassman et al. found a statistically significant correlation between smoking cession and nonunion rates in spinal fusion cases (118). The authors demonstrated that smoking cessation reduced nonunion rates from 22.2% (persistent smoker) to 20.2% (stopped $\leq$1 month prior to surgery) to 19.6% (stopped $>$1 month prior to surgery). More remarkably, in the best-case scenario, if the patients did not smoke for at least 6 months after fracture fixation, the nonunion rates dramatically declined to 17.1% (the nonsmokers' nonunion rate in this study was 14.2%) (118).

Since anemia, low SaO_2 and low PaO_2 cause the CaO_2 to decline and impair fracture healing [see Eqn. (1)], optimizing oxygen-carrying capacity is crucial for optimal healing. However, is there an optimal fracture-healing hematocrit? The answer is complex limited space prevents an adequate discussion, but most surgeons find a hematocrit of 30% acceptable (119). Can we improve fracture healing by hematocrit doping beyond 30%? First, the body can adjust to a low hematocrit and temporally maintain the local oxygen tension at a relatively stable level: the metabolic consequences may cause increasing blood flow to the fracture site with "rightward shifting" of the O_2 disassociation curve and increased O2 released to the wound site. Furthermore, what about improving fracture healing by increasing the PaO_2? Interestingly, Ueng et al. demonstrated that hyperbaric oxygen (HBO) therapy effectively improves bone mineral density and torsional strength in the healing fractures of cigarette smokers compared to untreated smokers (120).

A variety of factors can be used systemically to improve fracture healing (recombinant proteins are discussed separately below). For example, Jahng and Kim ovariectomized rats and then created closed bilateral tibial fractures 3 months later (121). The fractures were stabilized with intramedullary Kirschner wires and the animals were treated with recombinant human (rh)PTH or saline once a day for 30 consecutive days postfracture. The authors demonstrated that rhPTH therapy improved morphometric and biomechanical parameters of fracture healing in dose-dependent manner. Jahng and Kim's findings suggest that rhPTH therapy may improves fracture healing, for example, in postmenopausal osteoporotic patients; however, more studies are needed to validate this point.

Patients on chronic corticosteroids have impaired wound and fracture healing (122). Vitamin A has been shown to partly reverse the suppressive effects of steroids by increasing pro-angiogenic/osteogenic cytokines at the soft-tissue wound site (122). Although the effects of vitamin A on fracture healing have not been reported, we would hypothesize that the systemic administration of vitamin A should improve fracture healing through similar pathways; however, this hypothesis remains unproven. Finally, despite the pro-osteogenic effects of almost a dozen hormones, the U.S. Food and Drug Administration (FDA) has not approved hormonal therapy to enhance fracture healing in humans (61–68).

VII. MECHANICAL STRATEGIES TO IMPROVE FRACTURE HEALING

Imposing adequate amounts of mechanical stimulation will enhance fracture healing. Goodship et al. applied cyclical interfragmentary micromotions to the fracture callous using a femoral-fracture-healing model, and assessed the healing by radiography, bone densitometry, fracture stiffness index, and material testing postmortem (123). They found that the intermediate-loading group (40 mm/s) yielded the best results by the criteria they tested, and more or less mechanical stimulation resulted in less optimal healing. In addition, applying mechanical stimulation at the early stages of the fracture-healing process (around 1 week postfracturing) was more effective than later interventions in stimulating healing (123). However, the form of mechanical stimulation is of critical importance, since we have shown in a rat mandibular distraction osteogenesis model that grossly "pumping" the regenerate (i.e., lengthening and contracting the distraction gap during the distraction) does not yield greater bone formation (124). This result was likely because the mechanical forces used were suboptimal for new bone induction (too high or too low) or at inappropriate intervals.

A number of noninvasive methods are used to mechanically stimulate bone formation. Many of these new techniques have been applied to complicated lone-bone nonunions. While these methods have not been reported in the craniofacial literature, mechanical stimulation may become an important part of post-operative craniofacial care. Some of the more common techniques include low-intensity ultrasound, pulsed electromagnetic field, and extracorporeal shock wave therapies.

Low-intensity ultrasound is thought to mechanically stimulate fracture healing through high-frequency acoustic pressure waves. Therapy is usually instituted during the first week postfracture; the standard ultrasound intensity never exceeds 30 mW/cm^2 and is routinely applied for 20 min/day (125). Animal studies have demonstrated that low-intensity ultrasound improves callous formation and accelerates none healing (126–128). Numerous clinical studies have demonstrated that ultrasound improves fresh-fracture healing and stimulates nonunion healing (128). In a recent meta-analysis, Busse et al. examined randomized studies on the effects of low-intensity ultrasound on fracture-healing rates (129). Pooling 158 fractures for analysis, the authors demonstrated that time to fracture healing was 64 days shorter in the group receiving low-intensity ultrasound therapy compared to the control group. Although low-intensity ultrasound is FDA-approved for the treatment of fresh long-bone fractures, its efficacy on craniofacial fracture healing remains unknown (130).

When bone is subjected to mechanical force, fluid is pushed through the canalicular system. This fluid flow generates electric potentials that are thought to play an important role in mechanotransduction and bone formation/remodeling (130,131). Investigators have attempted to mimic these electric potentials by applying pulsed electromagnetic fields to the fracture site. A number of studies have demonstrated that pulsed electromagnetic field therapy is efficacious in both animal models and clinical studies. For example, Sarker et al. used pulsed electromagnetic field therapy to improve facture callous formation and healing in a stabilized midshaft rat tibia fracture model (132). Abeed et al. reported a series of 16 patients with nonunions treated with capacitative coupled electrical stimulation (133). Using a 63 kHz with 6-V peak-to-peak sine wave signal strength treatment protocol, the authors applied an electromagnetic field across tow 40-mm-diameter steel discs placed directly on the skin adjacent to the fracture site. After an average of 15 weeks, 11 of 16 patients healed with electromagnetic therapy. Interestingly, all patients with a fracture gap size $\leq$80 mm had complete healing of their nonunions. Finally, in a dramatic illustration of the power of pulsed electromagnetic field therapy, Scott et al. (134) reported a randomized double-blind study on 23 patients. The authors demonstrated that 60% of nonunions treated with capacitative coupling healed. In marked contrast, no control patients healed. While electromagnetic therapy seems conspicuously efficacious and the technology has been approved by the FDA, treatment protocols are not yet widely accepted.

Extracorporeal shock waves were first applied clinically for the treatment of kidney stones; however, orthopedic surgeons have begun using extracorporeal shock wave therapy for the treatment of delayed unions and nonunions. Similar to low-intensity ultrasound and pulsed electromagnetic field therapy, extracorporeal shock is designed to stimulate fracture healing by increasing growth factor production, cellular proliferation and chemotaxis, neo-angiogenesis, and extracellular matrix deposition. Several researchers have explored the efficacy of extracorporeal shock in animal models and clinical studies (135–146). For example, in a prospective study, Rompe et al. examined the effects of high-energy extracorporeal shock wave therapy (3000 impulses of an energy flux density of 0.6 mJ/mm^2) on tibial and femoral diaphyseal and metaphyseal fractures and osteotomies that had not healed for at least 9 months after injury or surgery (142). Patients were followed at 4-week intervals beginning 8 weeks after the initiation of treatment. The authors reported no complications, but found roentgenographic evidence of bony consolidation in 31 of 43 cases after an average of 4 months of therapy. They concluded that high-energy shock wave therapy was effective in stimulating bone healing in patients with diaphyseal or metaphyseal nonunion of the femur or tibia. Schaden et al. reported on a series of 115 nonunion or delayed fracture-healing patients treated with high-energy shock wave therapy and physical therapy (144). Despite some minor local reactions such as swelling, hematomas, and petechial hemorrhages, the authors found that after a single treatment, 75.7% patients had roentgenographic evidence of bony consolidation. These dramatic results suggest that extracorporeal shock wave therapy should be tested in double-blind prospective randomized trials as a noninvasive treatment option for patients with delayed unions and nonunions.

VIII. RECOMBINANT GROWTH FACTOR STRATEGIES TO IMPROVE FRACTURE HEALING

A vast amount of literature demonstrates that recombinant growth factors augment fracture healing (147–155). Recombinant growth factors may be delivered systemically or locally, alone or as part of a matrix/scaffold composite, dissolved in saline or packaged in a liposomal particle. Dozens of proangiogenic and pro-osteogenic recombinant growth factors have been investigated, but most can be grouped into five categories: (1) members of the TGF superfamily (e.g., TGF-β1, activin A, or bone morphogenetic proteins (BMPs)); (2) the FGF family (e.g., FGF-2); (3) the IGF family (IGF-1 and 2); (4) the platelet-derived growth factor family (e.g., PDGF-BB); and (5) growth hormone.

Growth factor therapy is conceptually designed to replace or augment the expression of naturally occurring fracture site cytokines. For example TGF-βs, IGF-1, BMP-2, –4 and, –7, and FGF-2 are upregulated in fracture sites (156–158). Some evidence suggests that circulating growth factors can accelerate fracture healing (159–163). For example, Bidner et al. demonstrated that cultured osteoblasts exposed to serum from patients with severe head injuries had greater growth factor and mitogenic activity than control subjects, supporting a humoral mechanism for the phenomenon of enhanced bone healing in severe head injury patients (160). Moreover, studies conducted mainly in animal long-bone models further demonstrate that systemically administered FGF-2 and GH enhance bone formation and accelerate bone regenerate consolidation (153–155). Interestingly, the osteogenic effects of circulating growth factors are not confined to the fracture site. Skeletal injuries lead to enhanced bone formation at other noninjured sites, supporting the notion that systematic growth factors have diffuse effects throughout the skeleton (153–164). For example, systemic administration of PDGF, an osteoblast mitogen, was shown to increase bone density and strength in long bones as well as the vertebrae of noninjured rats (165). This suggests that systemic administration of recombinant growth factors may be applicable not only to skeletal fractures but also to generalized conditions such as osteoporosis. While investigators have delivered fracture-specific recombinant proteins systemically in animal models, this route is associated with prohibitive clinical toxicity (166–169).

Although systemic toxicity is problematic, local administration may alleviate some of the hazards. Sakai et al. investigated the effects of recombinant activin A (r-activin A), an osteogenic member of the TGF-β superfamily, on fracture healing using a rat fibular fracture model. R-activan A was administered locally to the fibular fracture site once a day for 2 weeks with doses ranging from 0.4 to 10 μg/day. Results demonstrated that r-activin increased callus formation in an dose-dependent manner and led to significantly improved mechanical strength compared to controls (148). In a separate study, the direct application of rhFGF-2 to fracture sites yielded equally encouraging results (149). Recombinant proteins have been used locally to repair a variety of craniofacial defects: calvarial, zygomatic, periodontal, alveolar, and mandibular tissues (170–179).

While even local recombinant protein administration may have untoward effects, carrier matrices can overcome this obstacle. For example, Ripamonti et al. treated nonhuman primate critical-size calvarial defects with a carrier matrix containing osteogenic protein-1 (BMP-7) (180). By day 30, the authors demonstrated extensive endocranial and pericranial bone formation that enveloped the implanted hydroxyapatite (HR) carrier. At this time point, the interval porous spaces contained only a vascular network, without any evidence of new bone formation. By 90 and 365 days after implantation, however, there was extensive remodeling and bone had completely penetrated the central pore spaces. In addition to HR, investigators have used a variety of alpha-hydroxy acid-based polymer carriers. For example, Higuchi et al. used polylactide/polyglycolide (PLA/PGA) copolymers impregnated with rhBMP-2 to improve histomorphometric indices of mandibular fracture healing (150).

In addition to matrix scaffolding materials, recombinant growth factors have also been added to biodegradable hardware (151,152,181). The concept is simple: provide pro-osteogenic factors to the fracture site via a biodegradable osteofixation system; however, the application is difficult. Previous studies have demonstrated that PLA/PGA copolymer osteofixation constructs are significantly weakened by the addition of therapeutic factor such as antibiotics of bioactive glass 13–93 (182–183). Therefore, researchers speculate that recombinant growth factors may significantly reduce the mechanical integrity of the biodegradable fixation systems. Whether this reduction is clinically significant, however, remains unanswered. While comparisons between the growth-factor-loaded bioabsorbable plating systems and topographically similar metallic counterparts may provide some insight into the relative pullout strength of the different materials, the overengineering of metallic screws may still preclude meaningful clinical conclusions (184–186). Therefore, we must wait for in vivo studies to determine the true functional strength and efficacy of these the growth-factor-loaded biodegradable systems.

Although recombinant growth therapy has been successful, many questions remain unanswered. What is the optimal local concentration for any particular growth factor? How can we consistenly deliver therapeutic levels to *all* fracture sites? Will highly vascular craniofacial bone impart different pharmacokinetics to growth factor protocols established for long-bone fractures? How can we overcome the short recombinant protein serum half-life and tremendous production expense? What are the short- and long-term effects of circulating recombinant growth factors on endocrine hormone levels? How can we improve carrier matrices and growth-factor-loaded biodegradable plating systems? Can growth factors be used in combinations with cell-based applications? Regardless of the nuances and caveats of these questions and others, recombinant growth-factor-mediated therapy remains a landmark advance in fracture healing history.

IX. GENE TRANSFER STRATEGIES TO IMPROVE FRACTURE HEALING

The basic strategy of gene transfer for fracture repair is to utilize the native cellular machinery to produce factors that can enhance or accelerate osseous healing. This may involve supplementing cells in the fracture microenvironment with proangiogenic or pro-osteogenic genes to initiate cascades that will improve cellular recruitment, differentiation, and extracellular matrix production. At present, researchers are still attempting to manufacture better gene transport vehicles to improve delivery efficiency to the target tissues, increase cell surface attachment and internalization, and guide intracellular trafficking to enhance nuclear uptake and expression. While many new gene delivery vehicles exist, currently, investigators commonly rely on viral and nonviral vectors to deliver gene products to the fracture site.

A. Viral Vectors

Through natural selection numerous viruses have evolved to successfully infect and efficiently exploit human intracellular machinery. These viruses have developed excellent cell surface attachment and internalization mechanisms that enable them to deliver their DNA/RNA and achieve high-level viral protein production. Capitalizing on this efficient machinery, biologists have gutted and redesigned permissive viruses to carry biologically active gene products. Today, replication-deficient viruses can selectively transfect dividing and/or nondividing cells and evade primary immune detection by eliminating intracellular viral protein production. A number of recombinant viral vectors are available for craniofacial fracture repair [adenoviruses, adenoassociated viruses, lentiviruses, herpes simplex virus (HSV), and naked DNA]. However, adenoviruses have several distinct advantages over other available viral vectors, making them the most frequently studied as candidate vectors for osseous repair. Adenoviruses efficiently infect and express their transgenes in a wide variety of cell types, including dividing and nondividing cells. Since the adenoviral DNA does not integrate into the host genome, the enormous transgene expression is short-lived. Although this might be a disadvantage in the treatment of chronic conditions such as osteoporosis, transient transgene expression is ideally suited for the treatment of fractures that require only short-term expression to stimulate repair. Finally, adenoviruses are easy to manipulate, have a large transgene insert capacity (8 kb), and can be produced in high titers (10^{10}–10^{12} Virion/mL)(187).

A number of studies in long bones have demonstrated the potential efficacy adenoviruses in fracture repair. For example, Baltzer et al. created segmental femoral defects in New Zealand white rabbits and introduced adenovirus vectors containing BMP-2 or luceferase control (188). Healing was accessed histologically, radiographically, and biomechanically. The BMP-2-adenovirus-treated defects showed complete healing at 7 weeks, while those treated with control adenovirus remained unhealed. Radiographically, the BMP-2-adenovirus-treated defects had statistically more bone formation than controls at 12 weeks. In addition, material testing demonstrated significantly increased bending strength at 12 weeks. Similarly, Alden et al. demonstrated successful repair of mandibular defects using BMP-2 and BMP-9 adenoviral constructs compared to β-galactosidase-treated mandibles (189).

Adenoviral gene transfer techniques combined with cell-based strategies have also proven effective. Lieberman et al. successfully treated 8-mm femoral defects with bone marrow cells transfected with BMP-2-producing adenovirus (190). They treated defects with either BMP-2-transfected bone marrow cells, bone marrow cells transfected with β-galactosidase-producing adenovirus, bone marrow cells without transfection, recombinant BMP-2, or demineralized bone matrix. At 8 weeks, only those defects treated with BMP-2-producing cells or recombinant BMP-2 healed radiographically. However, when examined histologically, the regenerate bone treated with the BMP-2-adenovirus-transfected bone marrow was denser and more robust than that of recombinant BMP-2-treated specimens.

In our laboratory, we have used adenoviral vehicles to investigate the mechanisms impairing adult calvarial healing. We have found that the adult dura mater is deficient in growth factors such as FGF-2 and TGF-β1 compared to juvenile dura mater (51–53). In attempting to "turn back the biological clock," we transfected adult dura mater with a TGF-β1-overexpression adenovirus. We used media from wild-type and transgenic adult dura mater to then condition adult osteoblasts. We were particularly surprised to find that overexpression of TGF-β1 in mature dura mater led to a 31-fold increase in adult osteoblast bone nodule surface area compared to adult osteoblasts conditioned with media from wild-type adult dural cells (51). Even more surprisingly, in a separate preliminary study, we found treatment of adult osteoblasts with conditioned media from TGF-β1-transfected adult dura mater led to an absolute bone nodule surface area that surpassed young osteoblasts conditioned with wild-type juvenile dura mater (51). In other words, with the introduction of a single gene, we have already begun to make adult dura mater appear "phenotypically juvenile."

B. Nonviral Gene Transfer

Nonviral methods of gene transfer include injection of naked deoxyribonucleic acid (DNA), particle bombardment, or "gene gun" therapy, electroporation, calcium phosphate, diethylaminoethyl-dextran, liposomes, and gene-activated matrices (GAM). Presently, direct DNA injection, particle bombardment, electroporation, calcium phosphate, and diethylaminoethyl-dextran are impractical for fracture repair owing to their low transfection efficiencies. For example, extraordinarily high gene gun transfer efficiency is just 13% (191). Therefore, we will limit our discussion to liposomes and GAMs.

Liposomes are multilayer lipid vesicles ranging from 30 nm to several micrometers in size (192). Cationic liposomes (positive charge) form noncovalent complexes with plasmid DNA. By neutralizing the negatively charged DNA and decreasing electrostatic repulsion, DNA plasmids more easily pass through the negatively charged cell membranes. Multiple cationic lipid systems have been developed based on mono- or multiple-cationic amino groups [e.g., DOTAP (*N*-1[-(2,3-dioleoyloxy)propyl]-*N*,*N*,*N*-trimethylammoniumethyl sulphate) or DOTMA (*N*-[1-(2,3-dioleoyloxy) propyl]-*N*,*N*,*N*-trimethylammonium chloride)] (193). Most of the cationic lipids have similar in vitro transfection efficiencies, but each system seems to preferentially transfect specific cell lines. With few exceptions, neutral lipids such as DOPE (dioleoylphosphatidyl-ethanolamine) improve in vitro transfection efficiency (194). Unfortunately, cationic liposomal in vivo transfection efficiency has remained relatively low (only 1/200 of adenoviral efficiency) (195). Moreover, peripheral liposomal infusate must be prepared in low-volume, high-concentration, aggregate-free mixtures. Recent reports have just narrowly overcome these technically challenging requirements: nonionic surfactants (Tween 80) and/or polycations (polylysine or protomine) can increase lipid/DNA complex concentrations and simultaneously decrease complex diameter ($\sim$100 nm) to produce homogeneous suspensions acceptable for systemic administration (196–197).

Despite low in vivo transfection rates, cationic lipid-based delivery systems have several advantages (198). Liposome/DNA complexes are easy to prepare and there are no limits to the size or number of genes that can be delivered. In addition, because lipid carrier systems lack foreign proteins, they evoke minimal immune response. Furthermore, the cationic lipid systems have no risk of insertional mutagenesis (possible with retroviruses) or wild-type breakthrough (possible with adenoviruses). Finally, recent clinical studies suggest that liposomes can be safely administered to humans (199).

How can liposomes be utilized for craniofacial fracture repair? One potential way is to use highly selective arterial infusions to deliver liposomal-based inductive therapy directly to the target tissues. For example, liposomal/DNA suspensions may be selectively introduced into the inferior alveolar artery to perfuse the fracture/osteotomy of a reconstructed or distracted mandible. However, since liposomes injected through the vasculature eventually course to lung, liver, spleen, heart, and kidney, investigators have tried to reduce nonspecific reticuloendothelial clearance using oligodextran surfactants (200).

Others have tried to redesign the oligosaccharide structure to modify the surface geometry of the liposomal complex to decrease its clearance (200). Another approach is to improve liposomal targetting by coating the complex surface with monoclonal antibodies or peptides [e.g., arginine-glycine-aspartic acid (RGD)] to improve binding specificity. For example, Bednarski et al. have taken lipid-mediated gene transfer and RGD sequences in a new direction by coating solid lipid nanoparticles (SLN) with peptidomimetic sequences. This RGD coating enables SLN to traffic to actively forming vessels (e.g., tumor vasculature or a newly healing fracture) expressing $a_v\beta_3$ and $a_v\beta_5$ integrins (201–202). We have recently used ^{111}In-labeled RGD-coated SLN as an initial step toward characterizing neoangiogenesis in a rat mandibular osteotomy/distraction osteogenesis model (unpublished data). However, the gene delivery/engineering efficacy and safety of these novel lipid transfer techniques remain unproven.

GAM is a biodegradable scaffold engineered to contain biologically active cDNAs driven off mammalian expression vectors. When GAMs are placed into a fracture or wound site, immigrating cells pick up the plasmids and express the transgenes (203). Since the GAM system delivers genes instead of recombinant proteins, researchers have reported longer expression times (weeks vs. hours) (203,204). For example, using GAM to transfer 1.0 mg of plasmid DNA into a canine bone defect model, investigators detected picogram levels of recombinant peptide over a 2-week period (203). GAMs may be designed as lyophilic implants or sponges, injectable gels or pastes, or atomized for medical device coating (205).

The GAM system has already been used effectively to stimulate healing in critically sized long-bone defects in rats, dogs, and sheep (206).

Fang et al. implanted into 5-mm femoral defects GAM containing plasmid coding for BMP-4, parathyroid hormone (hPTH-34), or both (207). Each treatment group had increased bone formation, but GAM containing both the BMP-4 and parathyroid hormone plasmids resulted in faster bone formation than GAM containing either plasmid alone. In similar studies by Bonadio et al. utilizing a canine model, radiographic analysis demonstrated that GAM, consisting of a collagen sponge containing parathyroid hormone plasmid, implanted into 1-cm gaps (203). They found that this method was safe, had gene expression for at least 6 weeks, and improved bone formation in a dose-dependent and time-dependent manner. To date, however, GAM has not been applied to the craniofacial skeleton. Since much of the craniofacial skeleton bears relatively modest mechanical loads, structurally reinforced GAM systems may be used for zygomatic, orbital rim, and skull fractures. Several clinical trials are underway, and we will soon know the safety profile of GAM in humans (208).

X. CELL-BASED STRATEGIES TO IMPROVE FRACTURE HEALING

At least four cell-based approaches are used to enhance fracture repair: (1) conductive strategies; (2) cellular applications requiring in vivo self-assembly; (3) acellular scaffolds that require in vivo cellular recruitment; and (4) cells preseeded onto scaffolds.

A. Conductive Strategies

Guided tissue regeneration (GTR) is based on the principle that different cellular components have varying rates of migration into a wound during healing. By mechanically hindering the rapid migration of soft-tissue cells into a bone defect, presumably slower-migrating preangiogenic or preosteogenic cells may preferentially repopulate the intercalary space. In practice, this is accomplished by placing a membrane barrier [expanded polytetrafluorethylene (e-PTFE) is commonly used] around an osseous defect. Several authors have demonstrated improved bone formation in defects using this technique. For example, Dahlin et al. reported that the use of Teflon membrane barriers around mandibular defect in rats improved osseous healing. They found that defects covered in Teflon exhibited compete healing at 6 weeks while control defects had little or no osseous healing even after 22 weeks (209). GTR-generated bone healing has also been reported in mandibular defects in monkeys, in zygomatic arch osteotomy defects of rabbits, and in calvarial defects in rats and rabbits (209–217). Currently, GTR is used for the treatment of periodontal intrabony defects, class II furcation defects, gingival recession defects, and alveolar bone defects in conjunction with dental implant (218–222). Current research in GTR is focused on developing absorbable material for GTR, such as polygycolic acid (PGA) products. In vitro studies demonstrates that these materials not only act as barriers to fibroblast cell migration, but may have intrinsic osteoinductive properties similar to the ceramics discussed below. The use of guided tissue regeneration, in conjunction with other cell-based strategies, may provide invaluable for improving the capacity for endogenous osseous healing.

B. Cellular Applications Requiring In Vivo Self-Assembly

Percutaneous or intraoperative local administration of cell suspensions delivers progenitor or lineage-committed cells directly to the wound site. However, without scaffolding it seems hard to imagine that cells could assume aggregate function, attract a blood supply, and build a higher-order structure. Nevertheless, in 1993, Niedzwiedzki et al. were able to percutaneously transplant ex vivo expanded, bone-marrow-derived MSCs into a rabbit radial defect (223). The authors found that fractures treated with MSCs healed faster and had greater amounts of compact bone compared to untreated fractures. Despite Niedzwiedzki's success, cellular suspensions have not been used locally to treat craniofacial bone defects.

While the events that regulate the migration of progenitor cells to a site of bony injury remain unknown, there is evidence that bone-marrow-derived angioblastic cells can traffic to healing wounds (28–30,224,225). More recent reports suggest that bone-marrow-derived osteoblastic precursors can engraft at fracture sites following intravenous administration (42). Therefore, it is conceivable that angioblastic and/or osteoblastic marrow-derived MSCs administered systemically could traffic to an area of injury. Although we would hypothesize that these mechanisms already exist endogenously, the systemic administration of MSCs may prove beneficial for patients with suppressed bone marrow function (e.g., patients on chemotherapy or elderly patents). Moreover, the introduction of gene-modified MSCs may enhance angioblastic and/or osteoblastic precursor trafficking and assembly at sites of injury. While these hypotheses remain to be proven, the intense vascularity of the craniofacial skeleton seems an excellent starting point for systemically administered MSC-based therapeutic strategies.

C. Acellular Scaffolds

Numerous bone-scaffolding materials have been described, but most can be classified based on their component materials: natural polymers, synthetic polymers, and minerals. Although all three categories of materials have been used for craniofacial tissue engineering, we limit our discussion to mineral-based osteoconductive calcium phosphate ceramics (CPCs). The chemical anisotropic materials most often utilized to construct polycrystalline ceramics are hydroxyapatite (HA) and tricalcium phosphate (TCP). These ceramics have been targeted because they have the native composition of bone, mechanical features similar to bone, controlled absorption, and biologically active properties that are believed to facilitate osteogenic differentiation of MSCs (226). When they are transplanted as acellular scaffolds, their chemical properties promote recruitment of osteoprogenitor cells, vascular invasion, and bone formation.

Physical structure and chemical composition determine the properties of CPCs. Physical structure is the most important factor governing the osteoconductive nature of the scaffold. For example, the porosity of a scaffold influences fibrovascular infiltration and, in turn, determines the extent of bony ingrowth (227). In addition, the interconnectivity, or pore-to-pore continuity, is important in determining CPC properties. Highly interconnected porous ceramics, formed using the replamineform technique, improve both bone ingrowth and support of scaffold-tissue interactions compared to "dead end" pores (228). However, these benefits of increased interconnectivity must be balanced with decreased amount of scaffolding support for effective cell seeding of implants (229).

The calcium-to-phosphate ratio determines the stability and absorbability of CPCs. High-calcium-to-phosphate ceramics such as hydroxyapatite (HA) are slow-absorbing ceramics that are highly stable in vivo (230). There are now HA implants derived from the coral of marine invertebrates. These HA implants have the advantage of porosity that has similar structure to cancellous bone. Using a simple hydrothermal exchange reaction, the coral's calcium carbonate ($CaCO_3$) is converted into the more mechanically stable hyroxyapatite $[Ca_{10}(P_4)]_6(OH)_2$ with complete preservation of the internal porous microstructure (226,231,232). The other advantage of the coral-derived HA implants is that they appear to be absorbed at a more rapid rate than traditional HA implants (233).

The tricalcium phosphates, with their lower calcium-to-phosphate ratio, have the principal advantage of faster absorption owing to their higher solubility. However, overly rapid reabsorption can occur resulting in mechanical failure due to inadequate bone formation. There are now biphasic or composite calcium phosphates, which combine various ratios of HA and TCP yielding intermediate levels of absorption. Both HA and TCP have been used in a wide range of animal and clinical studies with good results when applied to the treatment of small defects where there is good contact with the host bone and minimal shear stress (226,234).

In craniofacial reconstruction, there have been a number of case reports where HA implants were used successfully for orbital roof reconstruction, calvarial defects filling, and cranioplasty (235–241).

D. Cells Preseeded onto Scaffolds

Cells can easily be seeded onto either HA or TCP implants, and several cell types can be used (embryonic stem cells, mesenchymal stem cells, lineage-committed cells). Numerous studies have shown that seeding with bone marrow stromal MSCs results in increased levels of osteogenesis and new vascular ingrowth within the implant infrastructure when implanted in vivo (226–242). Of critical importance is seeding adequate numbers of cells on these scaffolds, since seeding less than the critical amount results in failure of adequate bone formation (243).

Cells have been seeded onto natural (e.g., collagen, alginate, agarose, hyaluronic acid derivatives, chitosan, and fibrin glue), synthetic [e.g., polyglycolide (PGA), polylactides (PLLA, PDLA), polycaprolactone (PCL), and polydioxanone (PDS)], and mineral [polycrystalline ceramics (HA and TCP)] scaffolds. The inability to create in vitro vascular ingrowth and perfuse these constructs has profoundly restricted their design. Diffusional limitations of mass transfer have also curtailed efforts to engineer highly vascular tissues. For example, in vitro bone construct thickness has been limited to 250–500 μm (244,245).

Despite these limitations, Schleiphake et al. were able to use cell-seeded scaffolds to repair critically sized mandibular defects in sheep (246). They enhanced mandibular segmental defects using autogenous osteoprogenitor cells seeded on a porous calcium phosphate scaffold. Using a sheep model, they seeded cylindrical scaffolds of pyrolized bovine bone (35 mm long, 13 mm diameter) with osteoprogenitor cells harvested from the treated sheep's iliac crest. Seeded implant or unseeded implant controls were then placed into 35-mm mandibular defects. After 5 months, they found histologically significantly more bone formation in the implants seeded with cells than in unseeded controls (34.4% vs. 10.4%).

XI. CONCLUSIONS

The future of craniofacial fracture healing lies in continued rigorous clinical and basic science research. For example, by characterizing the molecular and cellular differences between juvenile and adult dura mater, we have already learned that we can turn back the clock on adult dura mater and make it appear "phenotypically juvenile." This observation may one day lead to more advanced molecular array analysis of gene expression cascades during calvarial healing. Similar analyses of long-bone fractures have led to the application of novel recombinant proteins and gene-modified fracture protocols. However, many issues still remain unresolved. For example, little is known about the biomechanical transduction of stresses on angiogenic and osteogenic cells within the fracture gap. Although this biomechanical transfer of force appears to be a central event leading to a well-orchestrated cascade of events mediating bony healing, little is known about how cells perceive this force, interpret it, and transmit intracellular messages. Understanding the molecular mechanisms guiding successful fracture healing has important clinical implications as it is a fundamental step toward the evolution of targeted therapeutic interventions designed to accelerate osseous healing. Indeed, the development of novel recombinant proteins, gene transfer techniques, minimally invasive approaches, and the identification of objective endpoints will propel the field of craniofacial fracture biology by reducing complications (e.g., delayed union and nonunion) and optimizing patient outcomes.

ACKNOWLEDGMENTS

This work was supported by NIH Grants RO1 DE13028, R01 DE13194, and RO1 DE14526.

REFERENCES

1. Olerud S, Danckwardt-Lilliestrom G. Fracture healing in compression osteosynthesis: an experimental study in dogs with an avascular, diaphyseal, intermediate fragment. Acta Orthop Scand Suppl 1971; 137:1–44.
2. Allgower M, Spiegel PG. Internal fixation of fractures: evolution of concepts. Clin Orthop 1979; 138:26–29.
3. Milner JC, Rhinelander FW. Compression fixation and primary bone healing. Surg Forum 1968; 19:453–456.
4. Lane WA. . The Operative Treatment of Fractures. London: Medical Publishing1913.
5. Greenbaum MA, Kanat IO. Current concepts in bone healing: review of the literature. J Am Podiatr Med Assoc 1993; 83:123–129.
6. Buckwalter JA, Einhorn TA, Bolander ME, Cruess RL. Healing of musculoskeletal tissues. In: Rockwood CA, Green DP, Buckholz RW, Heckman JD, eds. Rockwood and Green's Fractures in Adults. Philadelphia: Lippincott-Raven Publishing1996:182–261.
7. Marsh DR, Li G. The biology of fracture healing: optimising outcome. Br Med Bull 1999; 55:856–869.

8. Marsh D. Concepts of fracture union, delayed union, and nonunion. Clin Orthop 1998:S22–30.
9. Watson-Jones R, Coltart WD. The classic: Slow union of fractures with a study of 804 fractures of the shafts of the tibia and femur, by R Watson-Jones and WD Coltart. Clin Orthop 1982; 168:2–16.
10. Watson-Jones R. The classic: "Fractures and Joint Injuries" by Sir Reginald Watson-Jones, taken from "Fractures and Joint Injuries," by R Watson-Jones. Clin Orthop 1974. Vol. II. 4th ed. Baltimore: Williams and Wilkins Company, 1955. 105:4–10.
11. Harkess J, Ramsey WC, Harkess, JW. Principles of fractures and dislocations. Rockwood CA, Green DP, Buckholz RW, Heckman JD. Rockwood & Green's Fracture in Adult. Vol. 1 Hagerstown, MD: Lippincott Williams & Wilkins, 1996:3–13.
12. Roux W. Terminologie der Entwicklungsmechanik der Tiere und Pflansen. Leipzig: Wilhelm Engelmann1912.
13. Benninghoff A. Experimentelle Untersuchungen Uber den Einfluss verschiedenartiger Beanspruchung auf den Knorpel. Verh anat Ges 1924; 33:194.
14. Pauwels. F. Biomechanics of the Locomotor Apparatus. Berlin: Springer-Verlag1980.
15. Perren SM, Cordey, J. The concept of interfragmentary strain. In: HK IU, ed. Current Concepts of Internal Fixation of Fractures. New York: Springer-Verlag1980:63–77.
16. Perren SM. Physical and biological aspects of fracture healing with special reference to internal fixation. Clin Orthop 1979:175–196.
17. Giori NJ, Ryd L, Carter DR. Mechanical influences on tissue differentiation at bone-cement interfaces. J Arthroplast 1995; 10:514–522.
18. Giori NJ, Beaupre GS, Carter DR. Cellular shape and pressure may mediate mechanical control of tissue composition in tendons. J Orthop Res 1993; 11:581–591.
19. Carter DR, Blenman PR, Beaupre GS. Correlations between mechanical stress history and tissue differentiation in initial fracture healing. J Orthop Res 1988; 6:736–748.
20. Carter DR, Giori, N. Effect of mechanical stress on tissue differentiation in the bony implant bed. In: Davies J, ed. The Bone-Biomaterial Interface. Toronto: University of Toronto Press1991:367–379.
21. Blenman PR, Carter DR, Beaupre GS. Role of mechanical leading in the progressive ossification of a fracture callus. J Orthop Res 1989; 7:398–407.
22. Carter DR, Beaupre GS, Giori NJ, Helms JA. Mechanobiology of skeletal regeneration. Clin Orthop 1998:S41–55.
23. Carter DR, Orr TE, Fyhrie DP, Schurman DJ. Influences of mechanical stress on prenatal and postnatal skeletal development. Clin Orthop 1987:237–250.
24. Azuma Y, Ito M, Harada Y, Takagi H, Ohta T, Jingushi S. Low-intensity pulsed ultrasound accelerates rat femoral fracture healing by acting on the various cellular reactions in the fracture callus. J Bone Miner Res 2001; 16:671–680.

25. Baker AB, Sanders JE. Angiogenesis simulated by mechanical loading. Microvasc Res 2000; 60:177–181.
26. Lewinson D, Maor G, Rozen N, Rabinovich I, Stahl S, Rachmiel A. Expression of vascular antigens by bone cells during bone regeneration in a membranous bone distraction system. Histochem Cell Biol 2001; 116:381–388.
27. Kasid A, Morecki S, Aebersold P, Cornetta K, Culver K, Freeman S, Director E, Lotze MT, Blaese RM, Anderson WF. Human gene transfer: characterization of human tumor-infiltrating lymphocytes as vehicles for retroviral-mediated gene transfer in man. Proc Natl Acad Sci USA 1990; 87:473–477.
28. Kalka C, Masuda H, Takahashi T, Kalka-Moll WM, Silver M, Kearney M, Li T, Isner JM, Asahara T. Transplantation of ex vivo expanded endothelial progenitor cells for therapeutic neovascularization. Proc Natl Acad Sci USA 2000; 97:3422–3427.
29. Asahara T, Murohara T, Sullivan A, Silver M, van der Zee R, Li T, Witzenbichler B, Schatteman G, Isner JM. Isolation of putative progenitor endothelial cells for angiogenesis. Science 1997; 275:964–967.
30. Rafii S. Circulating endothelial precursors: mystery, reality, and promise. J Clin Invest 2000; 105:17–19.
31. Claes LE, Heigele CA. Magnitudes of local stress and strain along bony surfaces predict the course and type of fracture healing. J Biomech 1999; 32: 255–266.
32. Wallace AL, Draper ERC, Strachan RK, McCarthy ID, Hughes PF. The vascular response to fracture micromovement. Clin Orthop 1994; 301:281–290.
33. Loboa E, Fang, TD, Warren, SM, Lindsey, DP, Fong, KD, Longaker, MT, Carter, DR. Personal communication, 2002.
34. Taylor AE. Capillary fluid filtration: Starling forces and lymph flow. Circ Res 1981; 49:557–575.
35. Gan L, Miocic M, Doroudi R, Selin-Sjogren L, Jern S. Distinct regulation of vascular endothelial growth factor in intact human conduit vessels exposed to laminar fluid shear stress and pressure. Biochem Biophys Res Commun 2000; 272:490–496.
36. Fong KD. Equibiaxial strain affects calvarial osteoblast biology. Unpublished data, 2002.
37. Chen KD, Li YS, Kim M, Li S, Yuan S, Chien S, Shyy JY. Mechanotransduction in response to shear stress: roles of receptor tyrosine kinases, integrins, and Shc. J Biol Chem 1999; 274:18393–18400.
38. Grundes O, Reikeras O. Blood flow and mechanical properties of healing bone: femoral osteotomies studied in rats. Acta Orthop Scand 1992; 63:487–491.
39. Aronson J. Temporal and spatial increases in blood flow during distraction osteogenesis. Clin Orthop 1994; g:124–131.
40. Rowe NM, Mehrara BJ, Luchs JS, Dudziak ME, Steinbrech DS, Illei PB, Fernandez GJ, Gittes GK, Longaker MT. Angiogenesis during mandibular distraction osteogenesis. Ann Plast Surg 1999; 42:470–475.

41. Hausman MR, Schaffler MB, Majeska RJ. Prevention of fracture healing in rats by an inhibitor of angiogenesis. Bone 2001; 29:560–564.
42. Hou Z, Nguyen Q, Frenkel B, Nilsson SK, Milne M, van Wijnen AJ, Stein JL, Quesenberry P, Lian JB, Stein GS. Osteoblast-specific gene expression after transplantation of marrow cells: implications for skeletal gene therapy. Proc Natl Acad Sci USA 1999; 96:7294–7299.
43. Glaser MA, Blaine ES. Fate of cranial defects secondary to fracture and surgery. Radiology 1940; 34:671–684.
44. Buckwalter JA, et al. Musculoskeletal Tissue and the Musculoskelotal System. In: Weistein S, Buckwalter JA, eds. Turek's Orthopedics: Principles and their application. Philadelphia: JB Lippincott, 1944:13–67.
45. Buckwalter JA, Cooper RR. Bone structure and function. Instr Course Lect 1987; 36:27–48.
46. Buckwalter TA, Woo SL, Goldberg VM, et al. Soft tissue aging and musculoskeletal function. J Bone Joint Surg 1993; 75A:1533–1548.
47. Tonna EA, Cronkite EP. The periosteum: autoradiographic studies on cellular proliferation and transformation utilizing tritiated thymidine. Clin Orthop Rel Res 1963; 30:218–233.
48. Fernandez-Ferrero S, Ramos F. Dyshaemopoietic bone marrow features in healthy subjects are related to age. Leuk Res 2001; 25:187–189.
49. Zharhary D. Age-related changes in the capability of the bone marrow to generate B cells. J Immunol 1988; 141:1863–1869.
50. Eren R, Zharhary D, Abel L, Globerson A. Age-related changes in the capacity of bone marrow cells to differentiale in thymic organ cultures. Cell Immunol 1988; 112:449–455.
51. Cowen C. Personal communication, 2002.
52. Greenwald JA, Mehrara BJ, Spector JA, Chin G, Steinbrech DS, Saadeh PB, Luchs J, Paccione MF, Gittes GK, Longaker MT. Biomolecular mechanisms of calvarial bone induction: immature vs. mature dura mater. Plast Reconstr Surg 2000; 105:1382–1392.
53. Greenwald JA, Mehrara BJ, Spector JA, Fagenolz PJ, Saddeh PB, Steinbrech DS, Gittes GK, Longaker MT. Immature vs. mature dura mater. II. Differential expression of genes critical to calvarial re-ossification. Plast Reconstr Surg 2000; 106:630–638.
54. Jensen JE, Jensen TG, Smith TK, Johnston DA, Dudrick SJ. Nutrition in orthopaedic surgery. J Bone Joint Surg Am 1982; 64:1263–1272.
55. Cuthbertson DP, Fell GS, Smith CM, Tilstone WJ. Metabolism after injury. I. Effects of severity, nutrition, and environmental temperature on protein potassium, zinc, and creatine. Br J Surg 1972; 59:926–931.
56. Cuthbertson DP, Fell GS, Tilstone WJ. Nutrition in the post-traumatic period. Nutr Metab 1972; 14:92–109.
57. Hayda RA, Brighton CT, Esterhai JL Jr. Pathophysiology of delayed healing. Clin Orthop 1998:S31–40.
58. Macey LR, Kana SM, Jingushi S, Terek RM, Borretos J, Bolander ME. Defects of early fracture-healing in experimental diabetes. J Bone Joint Surg Am 1989; 71:722–733.

59. Gooch HL, Hale JE, Fujioka H, Balian G, Hurwitz SR. Alterations of cartilage and collagen expression during fracture healing in experimental diabetes. Connect Tissue Res 2000; 41:81–91.
60. Funk JR, Hale JE, Carmines D, Gooch HL, Hurwitz SR. Biomechanical evaluation of early fracture healing in normal and diabetic rats. J Orthop Res 2000; 18:126–132.
61. Gennari C. Calcium and vitamin D nutrition and bone disease of the elderly. Public Health Nutr 2001; 4:547–559.
62. Bak B, Andreassen TT. The effect of growth hormone on fracture healing in old rats. Bone 1991; 12:151–154.
63. Hsu JD, Robinson RA. Studies on the healing of long-bone fractures in hereditary pituitary insufficient mice. J Surg Res 1969; 9:535–536.
64. Koskinen EV, Ryoppy SA, Lindholm TS. Bone formation by induction under the influence of growth hormone and cortisone. Isr J Med Sci 1971; 7:378–380.
65. Misol S, Samaan N, Ponseti IV. Growth hormone in delayed fracture union. Clin Orthop 1971; 74:206–208.
66. Ewald F, Tachdjian MO. The effect of thyrocalcitonin on fractured humeri. Surg Gynecol Obstet 1967; 125:1075–1080.
67. Udupa KN, Gupta LP. Role of vitamin A in the repair of fracture. Indian J Med Res 1966; 54:1122–1130.
68. Steier A, Gedalia I, Schwarz A, Rodan A. Effect of vitamin D_2 and fluoride on experimental bone fracture healing in rats. J Dent Res 1967; 46:675–680.
69. Simmons DJ, Kunin AS. Autoradiographic and biochemical investigations of the effect of cortisone on the bones of the rat. Clin Orthop 1967; 55:201–215.
70. Herbsman H, Kwon K, Shaftan GW, Gordon B, Fox LM, Enquist IF. The influence of systemic factors on fracture healing. J Trauma 1966; 6:75–85.
71. Cruess RL, Sakai T. Effect of cortisone upon synthesis rates of some components of rat bone matrix. Clin Orthop 1972; 86:253–259.
72. Schmitz MA, Finnegan M, Natarajan R, Champine J. Effect of smoking on tibial shaft fracture healing. Clin Orthop 1999:184–200.
73. Cobb TK, Gabrielsen TA, Campbell DC 2nd, Wallrichs SL, Ilstrup DM. Cigarette smoking and nonunion after ankle arthrodesis. Foot Ankle Int 1994; 15:64–67.
74. Haug RH, Schwimmer A. Fibrous union of the mandible: a review of 27 patients. J Oral Maxillofac Surg 1994; 52:832–839.
75. Brown CW, Orme TJ, Richardson HD. The rate of pseudarthrosis (surgical nonunion) in patients who are smokers and patients who are nonsmokers: a comparison study. Spine 1986; 11:942–943.
76. van Adrichem LN, Hovius SE, van Strik R, van der Meulen JC. The acute effect of cigarette smoking on the microcirculation of a replanted digit. J Hand Surg [Am] 1992; 17:230–234.
77. Sarin CL, Austin JC, Nickel WO. Effects of smoking on digital blood-flow velocity. JAMA 1974; 229:1327–1328.
78. Ma L, Chow JY, Cho CH. Cigarette smoking delays ulcer healing: role of constitutive nitric oxide synthase in rat stomach. Am J Physiol 1999; 276:G238–248.

79. Ma L, Chow JY, Liu ES, Cho CH. Cigarette smoke and its extract delays ulcer healing and reduces nitric oxide synthase activity and angiogenesis in rat stomach. Clin Exp Pharmacol Physiol 1999; 26:828–829.
80. Volm M, Koomagi R, Mattern J. Angiogenesis and cigarette smoking in squamous cell lung carcinomas: an immunohistochemical study of 28 cases. Anticancer Res 1999; 19:333–336.
81. Liu XD, Zhu YK, Umino T, Spurzem JR, Romberger DJ, Wang H, Reed E, Rennard SI. Cigarette smoke inhibits osteogenic differentiation and proliferation of human osteoprogenitor cells in monolayer and three-dimensional collagen gel culture. J Lab Clin Med 2001; 137:208–219.
82. Ramp WK, Lenz LG, Galvin RJ. Nicotine inhibits collagen synthesis and alkaline phosphatase activity, but stimulates DNA synthesis in osteoblast-like cells. Proc Soc Exp Biol Med 1991; 197:36–43.
83. Heppenstall RB, Grislis G, Hunt TK. Tissue gas tensions and oxygen consumption in healing bone defects. Clin Orthop 1975; 106:357–365.
84. Rhinelander FW, Baragry RA. Microangiography in bone healing. I. Undisplaced closed fractures. J Bone Joint Surg 1962; 44A:1273–1298.
85. Rhinelander FW, Phillips RS, Steel WM, Beer JC. microangiography and bone healing. II. Displaced closed fractures. J Bone Joint Surg 1968; 50A: 643–667.
86. Wray JB, Goodman HO. Post fracture vascular changes and healing process. Arch Surg 1963; 87:801–804.
87. Kaartinen V, Voncken JW, Shuler C, Warburton D, Bu D, Heisterkamp N, Groffen J. Abnormal lung development and cleft palate in mice lacking TGF-beta 3 indicates defects of epithelial-mesenchymal interaction. Nat Genet 1995; 11:415–421.
88. Knighton DR, Hunt TK, Scheuenstuhl H, Halliday BJ, Werb Z, Banda MJ. Oxygen tension regulates the expression of angiogenesis factor by macrophages. Science 1983; 221:1283–1285.
89. Knighton DR, Fiegel VD. Regulation of cutaneous wound healing by growth factors and the microenvironment. Invest Radiol 1991; 26:604–611.
90. Brighton CT, Hunt RM. Early histological and ultrastructural changes in medullary fracture callus. J Bone Joint Surg [Am] 1991; 73:832–847.
91. Parfitt AM. Osteonal and hemi-osteonal remodeling: the spatial and temporal framework for signal traffic in adult human bone. J Cell Biochem 1994; 55:273–286.
92. Knighton DR, Silver IA, Hunt TK. Regulation of wound-healing angiogenesis—effect of oxygen gradients and inspired oxygen concentration. Surgery 1981; 90:262–270.
93. Steinbrech DS, Longaker MT, Mehrara BJ, Saadeh PB, Chin GS, Gerrets RP, Chau DC, Rowe NM, Gittes GK. Fibroblast response to hypoxia: the relationship between angiogenesis and matrix regulation. J Surg Res 1999; 84:127–133.
94. Steinbrech DS, Mehrara BJ, Saadeh PB, Chin G, Dudziak ME, Gerrets RP, Gittes GK, Longaker MT. Hypoxia regulates VEGF expression and cellular proliferation by osteoblasts in vitro. Plast Reconstr Surg 1999; 104:738–747.

95. Steinbrech DS, Mehrara BJ, Saaden PB, Greenwald JA, Spector JA, Gittes GK, Longaker MT. Hypoxia increases insulin-like growth factor gene expression in rat osteoblasts. Ann Plast Surg 2000; 44:529–534.
96. Steinbrech DS, Mehrara BJ, Saadeh PB, Greenwald JA, Spector JA, Gittes GK, Longaker MT. VEGF expression in an osteoblast-like cell line is regulated by a hypoxia response mechanism. Am J Physiol 2000; 278:C853–860.
97. Warren SM, Steinbrech DS, Mehrara BJ, Saadeh PB, Greenwald JA, Spector JA, Bouletreau PJ, Longaker MT. Hypoxia regulates osteoblast gene expression. J Surg Res 2001; 99:147–155.
98. Basett CAL HI. Influence of oxygen concentration and mechanical factors in differentiation of connective tissues in vivo. Nature (Lond) 1961; 190:460–461.
99. Hunter S, Caplan AI. Control of cartilage differentiation. In: Hall B, ed. Cartilage Development, Differentiation and Growth. Vol. II New York: Academic Press1983:87–119.
100. Ketenjian AY, Jafri AM, Arsenis C. Studies on the mechanism of callus cartilage differentiation and calcification during fracture healing. Orthop Clin North Am 1978; 9:43–65.
101. Lane JM, Suda M, von der Mark K, Timpl R. Immunofluorescent localization of structural collagen types in endochondral fracture repair. J Orthop Res 1986; 4:318–329.
102. Brinker MR, Bailey DE Jr. Fracture healing in tibia fractures with an associated vascular injury. J Trauma 1997; 42:11–19.
103. Dickson K, Katzman S, Delgado E, Contreras D. Delayed unions and nonunions of open tibial fractures: correlation with arteriography results. Clin Orthop 1994:189–193.
104. Sarmiento A, Schaeffer JF, Beckerman L, Latta LL, Enis JE. Fracture healing in rat femora as affected by functional weight-bearing. J Bone Joint Surg Am 1977; 59:369–375.
105. Kirchen ME, O'Connor KM, Gruber HE, Sweeney JR, Fras IA, Stover SJ, Sarmiento A, Marshall GJ. Effects of microgravity on bone healing in a rat fibular osteotomy model. Clin Orthop 1995:231–242.
106. Mathog RH, Toma V, Clayman L, Wolf S. Nonunion of the mandible: an analysis of contributing factors. J Oral Maxillofac Surg 2000; 58:746–752; discussion 752–743.
107. Adinoff AD. Hollister JR. Steroid-induced fractures and bone loss in patients with asthma. N Engl J Med 1983; 309:265–268.
108. Egger EL, Gottsauner-Wolf F, Palmer J, Aro HT, Chao EY. Effects of axial dynamization on bone healing. J Trauma 1993; 34:185–192.
109. Aro HT, Kelly PJ, Lewallen DG, Chao EY. The effects of physiologic dynamic compression on bone healing under external fixation. Clin Orthop 1990:260–273.
110. Claes L, Augat P, Suger G, Wilke HJ. Influence of size and stability of the osteotomy gap on the success of fracture healing. J Orthop Res 1997; 15:577–584.
111. Claes LE, Wilke HJ, Augat P, Rubenacker S, Margevicius KJ. Effect of dynamization on gap healing of diaphyseal fractures under external fixation. Clin Biomech (Bristol, Avon) 1995; 10:227–234.

112. Kenwright J, Goodship AE. Controlled mechanical stimulation in the treatment of tibial fractures. Clin Orthop, 1989; 241:36–47.
113. Kenwright J, Richardson JB, Cunningham JL, et al. Axial movement and tibial fractures: a controlled randomized trial of treatment. J Bone Joint Surg 1991; 73B:654–659.
114. Hobar PC. Methods of rigid fixation. Clin Plast Surg 1992; 19:31–39.
115. Frodel JL Jr, Marentette LJ. Lag screw fixation in the upper craniomaxillofacial skeleton. Arch Otolaryngol Head Neck Surg 1993; 119:297–304.
116. Suuronen R, Haers PE, Lindqvist C, Sailer HF. Update on bioresorbable plates in maxillofacial surgery. Facial Plast Surg 1999; 15:61–72.
117. Fischer JE. Metabolism in surgical patients protein, carbohydrate, and fat utilization by oral and parenteral routes. In: Townsend K, ed. Sabiston Textbook of surgery. St. Louis: W.B. Saunders, 2001:100–130.
118. Glassman SD, Anagnost SC, Parker A, Burke D, Johnson JR, Dimar JR. The effect of cigarette smoking and smoking cessation on spinal fusion. Spine 2000; 25:2608–2615.
119. Daly J, Barie PS, Dudrick SJ. Preparation of the Patient. In: Nyhus L, Baker RJ, Fischer, JE, eds. Mastery of Surgery. Vol I. Boston, New York, Toronto, London: Little, Brown, 1997:22–49.
120. Ueng SW, Lee SS, Lin SS, Wang CR, Liu SJ, Tai CL, Shih CH. Hyperbaric oxygen therapy mitigates the adverse effect of cigarette smoking on the bone healing of tibial lengthening: an experimental study on rabbits. J Trauma 1999; 47:752–759.
121. Jahng JS, Kim HW. Effect of intermittent administration of parathyroid hormone on fracture healing in ovariectomized rats. Orthopedics 2000; 23:1089–1094.
122. Wicke C, Halliday B, Allen D, Roche NS, Scheuenstuhl H, Spencer MM, Roberts AB, Hunt TK. Effects of steroids and retinoids on wound healing. Arch Surg 2000; 135:1265–1270.
123. Goodship AE, Cunningham JL, Kenwright J. Strain rate and timing of stimulation in mechanical modulation of fracture healing. Clin Orthop 1998: S105–115.
124. Greenwald JA, Luchs JS, Mehrara BJ, Spector JA, Mackool RJ, McCarthy JG, Longaker MT. "Pumping the regenerate": an evaluation of oscillating distraction osteogenesis in the rodent mandible. Ann Plast Surg 2000; 44:516–521.
125. Warden SJ, Bennell KL, McMeeken JM, Wark JD. Acceleration of fresh fracture repair using the sonic accelerated fracture healing system (SAFHS): a review. Calcif Tissue Int 2000; 66:157–163.
126. Dyson M, Brookes M. Stimulation of bone repair by ultrasound. Ultrasound Med Biol 1983; Suppl 2: 61–66.
127. Hadjiargyrou M, McLeod K, Ryaby JP, Rubin C. Enhancement of fracture healing by low intensity ultrasound. Clin Orthop 1998:S216–229.
128. Spadaro JA, Albanese SA. Application of low-intensity ultrasound to growing bone in rats. Ultrasound Med Biol 1998; 24:567–573.

129. Busse JW, Bhandari M, Kulkarni AV, Tunks E. The effect of low-intensity pulsed ultrasound therapy on time to fracture healing: a meta-analysis. Cmaj 2002; 166:437–441.
130. Hannouche D, Petite H, Sedel L. Current trends in the enhancement of fracture healing. J Bone Joint Surg Br 2001; 83:157–164.
131. Duncan RL, Turner CH. Mechanotransduction and the functional response of bone to mechanical strain. Calcif Tissue Int 1995; 57:344–358.
132. Sarker AB, Nashimuddin AN, Islam KM, Rabbani KS, Rahman M, Mushin AU, Hussain M. Effect of PEMF on fresh fracture-healing in rat tibia. Bangladesh Med Res Counc Bull 1993; 19:103–112.
133. Abeed RI, Naseer M, Abel EW. Capacitively coupled electrical stimulation treatment: results from patients with failed long bone fracture unions. J Orthop Trauma 1998; 12:510–513.
134. Scott, et al. A prospective, double-blind trial of electrical capacitive coupling in the treatment of non-union of long bones. J Bone Joint Surg Ann 1995; 77(5):809.
135. Augat P, Claes L, Suger G. In vivo effect of shock-waves on the healing of fractured bone. Clin Biomech (Bristol, Avon) 1995; 10:374–378.
136. Beutler S, Regel G, Pape HC, Machtens S, Weinberg AM, Kremeike I, Jonas U, Tscherne H. [Extracorporeal shock wave therapy for delayed union of long bone fractures—preliminary results of a prospective cohort study]. Unfallchirurg 1999; 102:839–847.
137. Heinrichs W, Witzsch U, Burger RA. [Extracorporeal shock-wave therapy (ESWT) for pseudoarthrosis: a new indication for regional anesthesia]. Anaesthesist 1993; 42:361–364.
138. Haupt G. Use of extracorporeal shock waves in the treatment of pseudarthrosis, tendinopathy and other orthopedic diseases. J Urol 1997; 158:4–11.
139. Ikeda K, Tomita K, Takayama K. Application of extracorporeal shock wave on bone: preliminary report. J Trauma 1999; 47:946–950.
140. McCormack D, Lane H, McElwain J. The osteogenic potential of extracorporeal shock wave therapy. an in-vivo study. Ir J Med Sci 1996; 165:20–22.
141. Orhan Z, Alper M, Akman, Y, Yavuz O, Yalciner A. An experimental study on the application of extracorporeal shock waves in the treatment of tendon injuries: preliminary report. J Orthop Sci 2001; 6:566–570.
142. Rompe JD, Rosendahl T, Schollner C, Theis C. High-energy extracorporeal shock wave treatment of nonunions. Clin Orthop 2001:102–111.
143. Rompe JD, Kullmer K, Vogel J, Eckardt A, Wahlmann U, Eysel P, Hopf C, Kirkpatrick CJ, Burger R, Nafe B. [Extracorporeal shock-wave therapy: experimental basis, clinical application]. Orthopade 1997; 26:215–228.
144. Schaden W, Fischer A, Sailler A. Extracorporeal shock wave therapy of nonunion or delayed osseous union. Clin Orthop 2001:90–94.
145. Thiel M. Application of shock waves in medicine. Clin Orthop 2001:18–21.
146. Vogel J, Rompe JD, Hopf C, Heine J, Burger R. [High-energy extracorporeal shock-wave therapy (ESWT) in the treatment of pseudarthrosis]. Z Orthop Ihre Grenzgeb 1997; 135:145–149.

147. Kawaguchi H, Nakamura K, Tabata Y, Ikada Y, Aoyama I, Anzai J, Nakamura T, Hiyama Y, Tamura M. Acceleration of fracture healing in nonhuman primates by fibroblast growth factor-2. J Clin Endocrinol Metab 2001; 86:875–880.
148. Sakai R, Miwa K, Eto Y. Local administration of activin promotes fracture healing in the rat fibula fracture model. Bone 1999; 25:191–196.
149. Kato T, Kawaguchi H, Hanada K, Aoyama I, Hiyama Y, Nakamura T, Kuzutani K, Tamura M, Kurokawa T, Nakamura K. Single local injection of recombinant fibroblast growth factor-2 stimulates healing of segmental bone defects in rabbits. J Orthop Res 1998; 16:654–659.
150. Higuchi T, Kinoshita A, Takahashi, K, Oda S, Ishikawa I. Bone regeneration by recombinant human bone morphogenetic protein-2 in rat mandibular defects: an experimental model of defect filling. J Periodontol 1999; 70:1026–1031.
151. Tielinen L, Manninen M, Puolakkainen P, Pihlajamaki H, Pohjonen T, Rautavuori J, Tormala P. Polylactide pin with transforming growth factor beta 1 in delayed osteotomy fixation. Clinc Orthop 1988:312–322.
152. Tielinen L, Manninen M, Puolakkainen P, Patiala H, Pohjonen T, Rautavuori J, Rokkanen P. Combining transforming growth factor-beta(1) to a bioabsorbable self-reinforced polylactide pin for osteotomy healing: an experimental study on rats. J Orthop Sci 1999; 4:421–430.
153. Raschke M, Kolbeck S, Bail H, Schmidmaier G, Flyvbjerg A, Lindner T, Dahne M, Roenne IA, Haas N. Homologous growth hormone accelerates healing of segmental bone defects. Bone 2001; 29:368–373.
154. Nakamura T, Hanada K, Tamura M, Shibanushi T, Nigi H, Tagawa M, Fukumoto S, Matsumoto T. Stimulation of endosteal bone formation by systemic injections of recombinant basic fibroblast growth factor in rats. Endocrinology 1995; 136:1276–1284.
155. Hao Y, Dai K, Guo L, Wang Y, Tang T. Effects of recombinant human growth hormone (r-hGH) on experimental osteoporotic fracture healing. Chin J Traumatol 2001; 4:102–105.
156. Spector JA, Luchs JS, Mehrara BJ, Greenwald JA, Smith LP, Longaker MT. Expression of bone morphogenetic proteins during membranous bone healing. Plast Reconstr Surg 2001; 107:124–134.
157. Tavakoli K, Yu Y, Shahidi S, Bonar F, Walsh WR, Poole MD. Expression of growth factors in the mandibular distraction zone: a sheep study. Br J Plast Surg 1999; 52:434–439.
158. Dryl D, Grabowska SZ, Citko A, Palka J, Antonowicz B, Rogowski F. Insulin-like growth factor-I (IGF-I) in serum and bone tissue during rat mandible fracture healing. Rocz Akad Med Bialymst 2001; 46: 290–299.
159. Bab I, Pass-Even L, Gazet D, al e. Osteogenesis in vivo diffusing chamber cultures of bone marrow cells. J Bone Min Res 1988; 4:373.
160. Bidner SM, Rubins IM, Desjardins JV, Zukor DJ, Goltzman D. Evidence for a humoral mechanism for enhanced osteogenesis after head injury. J Bone Joint Surg Am 1990; 72:1144–1149.

161. Perkins R, Skirving AP. Callus formation and the rate of healing of femoral fractures in patients with head injuries. J Bone Joint Surg Br 1987; 69: 521–524.
162. Smith R. Head injury, fracture healing and callus. J Bone Joint Surg Br 1987; 69:518–520.
163. Spencer RF. The effect of head injury on fracture healing: a quantitative assessment. J Bone Joint Surg Br 1987; 69:525–528.
164. Einhorn TA, Simon G, Devlin VJ, Warman J, Sidhu SP, Vigorita VJ. The osteogenic response to distant skeletal injury. J Bone Joint Surg Am 1990; 72:1374–1378.
165. Mitlak BH, Finkelman RD, Hill EL, Li J, Martin B, Smith T, D'Andrea M, Antoniades HN, Lynch SE. The effect of systemically administered PDGF-BB on the rodent skeleton. J Bone Miner Res 1996; 11:238–247.
166. Kaufman HL, Swartout BG, Horig H, Lubensky I. Combination interleukin-2 and interleukin-12 induces severe gastrointestinal toxicity and epithelial cell apoptosis in mice. Cytokine 2002; 17:43–52.
167. Motzer RJ, Rakhit A, Schwartz LH, Olencki T, Malone TM, Sandstrom K, Nadeau R, Parmar H, Bukowski R. Phase I trial of subcutaneous recombinant human interleukin-12 in patients with advanced renal cell carcinoma. Clin Cancer Res 1998; 4:1183–1191.
168. Prussick R. Adverse cutaneous reactions to chemotherapeutic agents and cytokine therapy. Semin Cutan Med Surg 1996; 15:267–276.
169. Papini M, Bruni PL. Cutaneous reactions to recombinant cytokine therapy. J Am Acad Dermatol 1996; 35:1021–1022.
170. Marchac D, Renier D. Craiosynostosis. World J Surg 1989; 13:358–365.
171. Bosch C, Melsen B, Gibbons R, Vargervik K. Human recombinant transforming growth factor-beta 1 in healing of calvarial bone defects. J Craniofac Surg 1996; 7:300–310.
172. Ripamonti U, Crooks J, Petit JC, Rueger DC. Periodontal tissue regeneration by combined applications of recombinant human osteogenic protein-1 and bone morphogenetic protein-2: a pilot study in Chacma baboons (*Papio ursinus*). Eur J Oral Sci 2001; 109:241–248.
173. Hunt DR, Jovanovic SA, Wikesjo UM, Wozney JM, Bernard GW. Hyaluronan supports recombinant human bone morphogenetic protein-2 induced bone reconstruction of advanced alveolar ridge defects in dogs: a pilot study. J Periodontol 2001; 72:651–658.
174. Stewart KJ, Weyand B, van't Hof RJ, White SA, Lvoff GO, Maffulli N, Poole MD. A quantitative analysis of the effect of insulin-like growth factor-1 infusion during mandibular distraction osteogenesis in rabbits. Br J Plast Surg 1999; 52:343–350.
175. Thaller SR, Dart A, Tesluk H. The effects of insulin like growth factor I on critical sized calvarial defects in Sprague Dawley rats. Ann Plas Surg 1993; 31:429–433.
176. Thaller SR, Hoyt J, Tesluk H, Holmes R. The effect of insulin growth factor-1 on calvarial sutures in a Sprague-Dawley rat. J Craniofac Surg 1993; 4: 35–39.

177. Thaller SR, Hoyt J, Tesluk H, Holmes R. Effect of insulin-like growth factor-1 on zygomatic arch bone regeneration: a preliminary histological and histometric study. Ann Plast Surg 1993; 31:421–428.
178. Thaller SR, Lee TJ, Armstrong M, Tesluk H, Stern JS. Effect of insulin-like growth factor type 1 on critical-size defects in diabetic rats. J Craniofac Surg 1995; 6:218–223.
179. Thaller SR, Salzhauer MA, Rubinstein AJ, Thion A, Tesluk H. Effect of insulin-like growth factor type I on critical size calvarial bone defects in irradiated rats. J Craniofac Surg 1998; 9:138–141.
180. Ripamonti U, Crooks J, Rueger DC. Induction of bone formation by recombinant human osteogenic protein-1 and sintered porous hydroxyapatite in adult primates. Plast Reconstr Surg 2001; 107:977–988.
181. Ashammakhi N, Peltoniemi H, Waris E, Suuronen R, Serlo W, Kellomaki M, Tormala P, Waris T. Developments in craniomaxillofacial surgery: use of self-reinforced bioabsorbable osteofixation devices. Plast Reconstr Surg 2001; 108:167–180.
182. Tiainen et al. Bioabsorbable ciprofloxacine-containing and plain self-reinforced polyactide-polyglycolide 80/20 screws: pull-out strength properties in human cadaver parietal bones. J Craniofac Surg, In press, 2002.
183. Leinonen. Holding power of bioabsorbable ciprofloxacin-containing self-reinforced poly-L/DL-lactide 70/30 bioactive glass 13 miniscrews in human cadaveric bone. J Craniofac Surg. In press, 2002..
184. Pietrzak WS. Principles of development and use of absorbable internal fixation. Tissue Eng 2000; 6:425–433.
185. Pietrzak WS. Critical concepts of absorbable internal fixation. J Craniofac Surg 2000; 11:335–341.
186. Pietrzak WS, Eppley BL. Resorbable polymer fixation for craniomaxillofacial surgery: development and engineering paradigms. J Craniofac Surg 2000; 11:575–585.
187. Warren SM, Fong KD, Longaker MT, et al. Tools and techniques for craniofacial tissue engineering. Submitted, 2002.
188. Baltzer AW, Lattermann C, Whalen JD, Wooley P, Weiss K, Grimm M, Ghivizzani SC, Robbins PD, Evans CH. Genetic enhancement of fracture repair: healing of an experimental segmental defect by adenoviral transfer of the BMP-2 gene. Gene Ther 2000; 7:734–739.
189. Alden TD, Beres EJ, Laurent JS, Engh JA, Das S, London SD, Jane JA Jr, Hudson SB, Helm GA. The use of bone morphogenetic protein gene therapy in craniofacial bone repair. J Craniofac Surg 2000; 11: 24–30.
190. Lieberman JR, Le LQ, Wu L, Finerman GA, Berk A, Witte ON, Stevenson S. Regional gene therapy with a BMP-2-producing murine stromal cell line induces heterotopic and orthotopic bone formation in rodents. J Orthop Res 1998; 16:330–339.
191. Shillitoe EJ, Noonan S, Hinkle CC, Marini FC, 3rd, Kellman RM. Transduction of normal and malignant oral epithelium by particle bombardment. Cancer Gene Ther 1998; 5:176–182.

192. Banerjee R. Liposomes: applications in medicine. J Biomater Appl 2001; 16:3–21.
193. Campbell RB, Balasubramanian SV, Straubinger RM. Phospholipid-cationic lipid interactions: influences on membrane and vesicle properties. Biochim Biophys Acta 2001; 1512:27–39.
194. Colosimo A, Serafino A, Sangiuolo F, Di Sario S, Bruscia E, Amicucci P, Novelli G, Dallapiccola B, Mossa G. Gene transfection efficiency of tracheal epithelial cells by DC-chol-DOPE/DNA complexes. Biochim Biophys Acta 1999; 1419:186–194.
195. Fortunati E, Bout A, Zanta MA, Valerio D, Scarpa M. In vitro and in vivo gene transfer to pulmonary cells mediated by cationic liposomes. Biochim Biophys Acta 1996; 1306:55–62.
196. Sorgi FL, Bhattacharya S, Huang L. Protamine sulfate enhances lipid-mediated gene transfer. Gene Ther 1997; 4:961–968.
197. Kim TW, Chung H, Kwon IC, Sung HC, Jeong SY. Optimization of lipid composition in cationic emulsion as in vitro and in vivo transfection agents. Pharm Res 2001; 18:54–60.
198. Fielding RM. Liposomal drug delivery: advantages and limitations from a clinical pharmacokinetic and therapeutic perspective. Clin Pharmacokinet 1991; 21:155–164.
199. Nabel GJ, Nabel EG, Yang ZY, Fox BA, Plautz GE, Gao X, Huang L, Shu S, Gordon D, Chang AE. Direct gene transfer with DNA-liposome complexes in melanoma: expression, biologic activity, and lack of toxicity in humans. Proc Natl Acad Sci USA 1993; 90:11307–11311.
200. Lestini BJ, Sagnella SM, Xu Z, Shive MS, Richter NJ, Jayaseharan J, Case AJ, Kottke-Marchant K, Anderson JM, Marchant RE. Surface modification of liposomes for selective cell targeting in cardiovascular drug delivery. J Control Release 2002; 78:235–247.
201. Bednarski M. Personal communication, 2002.
202. Sipkins DA, Cheresh DA, Kazemi MR, Nevin LM, Bednarski MD, Li KC. Detection of tumor angiogenesis in vivo by alphaVbeta3-targeted magnetic resonance imaging. Nat Med 1998; 4:623–626.
203. Bonadio J, Smiley E, Patil P, Goldstein S. Localized, direct plasmid gene delivery in vivo: prolonged therapy results in reproducible tissue regeneration. Nat Med 1999; 5:753–759.
204. Giannobile WV. Periodontal tissue engineering by growth factors. Bone 1996; 19:23S-37S.
205. Bonadio J. Tissue engineering via local gene delivery. J Mol Med 2000; 78:303–311.
206. Goldstein SA. In vivo nonviral delivery factors to enhance bone repair. Clin Orthop 2000; 379S:113–119.
207. Fang J, Zhu YY, Smiley E, Bonadio J, Rouleau JP, Goldstein SA, McCauley LK, Davidson BL, Roessler BJ. Stimulation of new bone formation by direct transfer of osteogenic plasmid genes. Proc Natl Acad Sci USA 1996; 93:5753–5758.

208. Bianco P, Robey PG. Stem cells in tissue engineering. Nature 2001; 414: 118–121.
209. Dahlin C, Linde A, Gottlow J, Nyman S. Healing of bone defects by guided tissue regeneration. Plast Reconstr Surg 1988; 81:672–676.
210. Kostopoulos L, Karring T. Guided bone regeneration in mandibular defects in rats using a bioresorbable polymer. Clin Oral Implants Res 1994; 5:66–74.
211. Dahlin C, Gottlow J, Linde A, Nyman S. Healing of maxillary and mandibular bone defects using a membrane technique: an experimental study in monkeys. Scand J Plast Reconstr Surg Hand Surg 1990; 24:13–19.
212. Kostopoulos L, Karring T. Augmentation of the rat mandible using guided tissue regeneration. Clin Oral Implants Res 1994; 5:75–82.
213. Kostopoulos L, Karring T. Role of periosteum in the formation of jaw bone: an experiment in the rat. J Clin Periodontal 1995; 22:247–254.
214. Kostopoulos L, Lioubavina N, Karring T, Uraguchi R. Role of chitin beads in the formation of jaw bone by guided tissue regeneration: an experiment in the rat. Clin Oral Implants Res 2001; 12:325–331.
215. Kostopoulos L, Karring T, Uraguchi R. Formation of jawbone tuberosities by guided tissue regeneration: an experimental study in the rat. Clin Oral Implants Res 1994; 5:245–253.
216. Lundgren D, Nyman S, Mathisen T, Isaksson S, Klinge B. Guided bone regeneration of cranial defects, using biodegradable barriers: an experimental pilot study in the rabbit. J Craniomaxillofac Surg 1992; 20:257–260.
217. Mundell RD, Mooney MP, Siegel MI, Losken A. Osseous guided tissue regeneration using collagen barrier membrane. J Oral Maxillofac Surg 1993; 51:1004–1012.
218. Karring T, Cortellini P. Regenerative therapy: furcation defects. Periodontology 2000; 19:115–137.
219. Pini Prato G, Clauser C, Cortellini P, Tinti C, Vincenzi G, Pagliaro U. Guided tissue regeneration versus mucogingival surgery in the treatment of human buccal recessions: a 4-year follow-up study. J Periodontol 1996; 67:1216–1223.
220. Buser D, Bragger U, Lang NP, Nyman S. Regeneration and enlargement of jaw bone using guided tissue regeneration. Clin Oral Implants Res 1990; 1:22–32.
221. Dahlin C, Andersson L, Linde A. Bone augmentation at fenestrated implants by an osteopromotive membrane technique: a controlled clinical study. Clin Oral Implants Res 1991; 2:159–165.
222. Mellonig JT, Nevins M. Guided bone regeneration of bone defects associated with implants: an evidence-based outcome assessment. Int J Periodon Restor Dent 1995; 15:168–185.
223. Niedzwiedzki T, Dabrowski Z, Miszta H, Pawlikowski M. Bone healing after bone marrow stromal cell transplantation to the bone defect. Biomaterials 1993; 14:115–121.
224. Takahashi T, Kalka C, Masuda H, Chen D, Silver M, Kearney M, Magner M, Isner JM, Asahara T. Ischemia- and cytokine-induced mobilization of bone marrow-derived endothelial progenitor cells for neovascularization. Nat Med 1999; 5:434–438.

225. Peichev M, Naiyer AJ, Pereira D, Zhu Z, Lane WJ, Williams M, Oz MC, Hicklin DJ, Witte L, Moore MA, Rafii S. Expression of VEGFR-2 and AC133 by circulating human CD34(+) cells identifies a population of functional endothelial precursors. Blood 2000; 95:952–958.
226. Ohgushi H, Caplan AI. Stem cell technology and bioceramics: from cell to gene engineering. J Biomed Mater Res 1999; 48:913–927.
227. Daculsi G, Passuti N. Effect of the macroporosity for osseous substitution of calcium phosphate ceramics. Biomaterials 1990; 11:86–87.
228. Lemons JE. Ceramics: past, present, and future. Bone 1996; 19:121S-128S.
229. Dennis JE, Haynesworth SE, Young RG, Caplan AI. Osteogenesis in marrow-derived mesenchymal cell porous ceramic composites transplanted subcutaneously: effect of fibronectin and laminin on cell retention and rate of osteogenic expression. Cell Transplant 1992; 1:23–32.
230. Fleming JE Jr, Cornell CN, Muschler GF. Bone cells and matrices in orthopedic tissue enginering. Orthop Clin North Am 2000; 31:357–374.
231. Vuola J, Goransson H, Bohling T, Asko-Seljavaara S. Bone marrow induced osteogenesis in hydroxyapatite and calcium carbonate implants. Biomaterials 1996; 17:1761–1766.
232. Shors EC. Coralline bone graft substitutes. Orthop Clin North Am 1999; 30:599–613.
233. Pollick S, Shors EC, Holmes RE, Kraut RA. Bone formation and implant degradation of coralline porous ceramics placed in bone and ectopic sites. J Oral Maxillofac Surg 1995; 53:915–922; discussion 922–913.
234. Block JE, Thorn MR. Clinical indications of calcium-phosphate biomaterials and related composites for orthopedic procedures. Calcif Tissue Int 2000; 66:234–238.
235. Allard RH, Swart JG. Orbital roof reconstruction with a hydroxyapatite implant. J Oral Maxillofac Surg 1982; 40:237–239.
236. Zide MF, Kent JN, Machado L. Hydroxylapatite cranioplasty directly over dura. J Oral Maxillofac Surg 1987; 45:481–486.
237. Yamashima T. Cranioplasty with hydroxylapatite ceramic plates that can easily be trimmed during surgery: a preliminary report. Acta Neurochir (Wien) 1989; 96:149–153.
238. Yamashima T. Reconstruction of surgical skull defects with hydroxylapatite ceramic buttons and granules. Acta Neurochir (Wien) 1988; 90:157–162.
239. Yamashima T. Modern cranioplasty with hydroxylapatite ceramic granules, buttons, and plates. Neurosurgery 1993; 33:939–940.
240. Matukas VJ, Clanton JT, Langford KH, Aronin PA. Hydroxylapatite: an adjunct to cranial bone grafting. J Neurosurg 1988; 69:514–517.
241. Waite PD, Morawetz RB, Zeiger HE, Pincock JL. Reconstruction of cranial defects with porous hydroxylapatiteblocks. Neurosurgery 1989; 25:214–217.
242. Bruder SP, Fox BS. Tissue engineering of bone: cell based strategies. Clin Orthop 1999:S68–83.
243. Blokhuis TJ, Termaat MF, den Boer FC, Patka P, Bakker FC, Haarman HJ. Properties of calcium phosphate ceramics in relation to their in vivo behavior. J Trauma 2000; 48:179–186.

244. Ishaug SL, Crane GM, Miller MJ, Yasko AW, Yaszemski MJ, Mikos AG. Bone formation by three-dimensional stromal osteoblast culture in biodegradable polymer scaffolds. J Biomed Mater Res 1997; 36: 17–28.
245. Martin I, Padera RF, Vunjak-Novakovic G, Freed LE. In vitro differentiation of chick embryo bone marrow stromal cells into cartilaginous and bone-like tissues. J Orthop Res 1998; 16:181–189.
246. Schliephake H, Knebel JW, Aufderheide M, Tauscher M. Use of cultivated osteoprogenitor cells to increase bone formation in segmental mandibular defects: an experimental pilot study in sheep. Int J Oral Maxillofac Surg 2001; 30:531–537.

8

The Use of Biomaterials in Craniofacial Trauma

Mutaz B. Habal
The Tampa Bay Craniofacial Center, University of South Florida and University of Florida, Tampa, Florida, U.S.A.

Ralph E. Holmes and Steven R. Cohen
Sharp Childrens' Hospital, San Diego, California, U.S.A.

I. INTRODUCTION

The standard of care today in the treatment of patients with simple or extensive craniofacial trauma involves the utilization of multiple biomaterials. The biomaterials used are inert, producing minimal inflammatory reaction to adjacent tissues and no biological response. The goal in the use of biomaterials is to maximize the positive final outcome of treatment for the patient and minimize complications that may ensue from the patient's condition. This chapter outlines the applications of biomaterials and their utility for the trauma surgeon treating various problems in the craniofacial region. This work is by no means inclusive of all biomaterials used in craniofacial practice but addresses those most frequently encountered in treatment of craniofacial trauma today.

Today, the application and utility of biomaterials are essential for standard-of-care treatment of patients with extensive craniofacial trauma. It is, therefore, imperative that surgeons using biomaterials have a comprehensive knowledge and understanding of the implications and effects of these materials when used in living biological systems. The biochemistry and composition vary from system to system, so the details of the variables become as important as the mechanics of application. By definition, most biomaterials in use today are inert. They do not initiate any major inflammatory response or reaction and are easy for the practicing surgeon treating facial trauma to use.

In the past, controversy arose regarding the nature of the application of biomaterials in trauma patients because of the high degree of contamination found in traumatic wounds. The difference in the use of biomaterials in elective craniofacial surgery and its application in traumatic injuries is related to considerations of clean versus clean/contaminated or grossly contaminated wounds of the craniofacial skeleton. It was thought that the use of biomaterials in clean/contaminated (type II) or grossly contaminated (type III) wounds should be delayed, and immediate application limited to the clean conditions such as type I wounds. Other issues involving the use of biomaterials in traumatic injury were related to open versus closed wounds and the situation of internal contamination from the internal paranasal sinuses. These concerns compelled surgeons to defer the use of all biomaterials in craniofacial surgery related to primary trauma, and it had become a principle that such biomaterials should only be used in the former-type wounds rather than the latter two types. These concerns were alleviated as early as the 1970s. The presence of a good blood supply to the head and neck area may be the factor that differentiates trauma surgery in the craniofacial region from that in other regions of the body.

Biomaterials used today in craniofacial trauma are divided into two categories: biomaterials used in immediate trauma repair and those used for delayed reconstruction. Biomaterials are also used operatively for immediate skeletal fixation and for delayed recreation and reconstruction of craniofacial structures. In secondary reconstruction of traumatic defects, biomaterials are used as contour-fitting materials, and these procedures are most often deferred until after immediate surgical repair. Fixation of the craniofacial skeleton has undergone a major evolution in the past 20 years. However, our search continues for the ideal fixation device. The future of all skeletal fixation devices lies in the use of new biomaterials and new combinations of these materials. In addition, the use of contour-fitting biomaterial will eventually follow the same process as in the past: that of the time element involved in the body's ability to incorporate these materials as a component that is not easily differentiated from adjacent tissue.

The last important concept that we need to review in this chapter is that of regeneration as it affects the use of biomaterials in the craniofacial region. Biomaterial implants have the ability to allow surrounding bone to regenerate new bone while using the applied material as a scaffold. A knowledge of the longevity of all the applied biomaterials is essential, as well as an understanding of the processes that are involved in either total elimination by hydrolysis, incorporation, or regeneration (1,2).

II. SAFETY CONSIDERATIONS

The applications and use of the biomaterials in any biological system are always associated with a major question: Are those biomaterials safe to use or are they capable of causing harm? It is also important to know if there are any by-products that will be, under any circumstances, harmful. Safety issues are the fundamental focus of the Food and Drug Administration (FDA) and its European equivalents. These agencies study all biomaterials that are used for medical purposes, their efficacy, and the animal studies required before the premarket studies (PMS) are designed to collect data from clinical applications. Data are then analyzed, and if the biomaterial is found to be safe and efficacious, it is then released for marketing to doctors' offices and hospitals for use in human patients. All the biomaterials referred for discussion in this chapter have passed through this process and its final applications.

III. FIXATION OF THE CRANIOFACIAL SKELETON

A review of the history of skeletal fixation is helpful to the understanding of the situations in which we work today. Skeletal fixation in the craniofacial region has gone through many advances in the past few decades. Most of these advances have followed major international conflicts involving the complex treatment of large numbers of casualties.

Initially, fractures of the craniofacial skeleton were treated without fixation by allowing the bones to heal in open soft tissue, then performing the repair at a later time. Fractures were also treated with closed reduction after manipulation. The next development was the use of an external apparatus for fixation. This method was useful until the external fixation was removed and the repaired structures collapsed again.

Internal fixation then came into practice and required the use of rigid fixation. Use of the plating system began at the turn of the century, with use of stainless steel plates. The use of Vitallium and titanium plating followed. In the latter part of the last century, the use of resorbable plating systems evolved and they have advanced to their present status today. Resorbable plating systems remain the state of the art for skeletal fixation.

The evolution of biocompatible resorbable polymers offers surgeons of today a new array of options for craniofacial skeletal fixation. Some of the potential benefits of resorbable polymers include greater ease and accuracy of contour adaptation, clear radiographic presentation owing to the absence of x-ray scatter, elimination of the need for secondary surgeries for device removal, and reduced risk of stress shielding of the underlying bone. Known as polyesters, these copolymers have chemical, physical, material, mechanical, and biological properties different from those of metal fixation devices. Knowledge of these differences will facilitate the utilization of resorbable implants in fixation for craniofacial trauma.

Among the bioresorbable polyester craniomaxillofacial fixation devices approved for clinical use by the FDA, copolymers of lactides and glycolides are available. The first copolymer of L-lactide and glycolide (LactoSorb, W. Lorenz, Jacksonville, FL) was approved by the FDA in 1996. The lactide in LactoSorb is a homopolymer of the levo form. The ratio of the L-lactide monomer to the glycolide monomer is 82:18 in poly (L-lactide-co-glycolide), to take advantage of glycolide's rapid degradation time. Strength declines to approximately 70% by 6–9 weeks and resorption is complete by 12 months.

Approved, more recently, in 1998 is a copolymer produced from a mixture of 70% L-lactide monomer and 30% D,L-lactide monomer (MacroPore, MacroPore Biosurgery, Inc., San Diego, CA). This 70:30 ratio in poly (L-lactide-co-D,L-lactide) DLLA retains approximately 70% of its initial strength after 9 months, and approximately 50% after 12 months, with resorption completed by 24–36 months. Additional resorbable polyesters from Bionx, Leibinger (delta system and the new delta system); Synthes (resorbable system); KLS Martin (resorb-X); and Iona (two systems) are all FDA approved and available for surgeons to use. The differences among these systems are the ratios of the copolymers used in the compositions that affect their longevity, a consideration of importance to surgeons. The deciding factor in which system to use is the individual surgeon's preference and ease in clinical application.

In view of these considerations, the primary focus in this chapter will be on the use of poly (L-lactide-co-D,L-lactide) for skeletal repair and fixation, owing to the extensive clinical experiences of the authors and to the commonalities this system shares with other systems that use similar materials in different compositions. The acronym (DLLA), L-La/D,L-La copolymer, will also be utilized to designate a copolymer of the two monomers, L-lactide and D,L-lactide.

IV. PHYSICAL PROPERTIES

Poly (L-lactide), which has a high crystallinity, is characterized by its strength and long degradation time. Conversely, a polymer created from D,L-lactide has little strength and degrades rapidly. Combining L-lactide and D,L-lactide results in a copolymer with the intermediate characteristics of strength for 6–9 months and resorption in 24–36 months. In addition, the copolymer is optically clear and noncrystalline, resulting in minimal foreign body reactions by tissue. It should be noted that, even within a given copolymer, strength and degradation characteristics can vary according to the degree of polymerization. Therefore, the manufacturer must maintain this within the desired range. A common measure of the degree of polymerization is called intrinsic viscosity (IV) and, for any given polymer, the IV correlates with molecular weight. To measure IV the polymer is dissolved in a standardized, known amount of chloroform and then passed through a viscometer. The length of time that it takes for passage is used to calculate the At sufficiently high temperatures all materials change from hard to soft and finally to liquid. The temperature at which a material changes from hard to soft is known as the glass transition temperature (Tg). For 70:30 poly (L-lactide-co-D,L-lactide) the Tg is 55°C [131°F], thus allowing heat to be utilized for contouring these implants.

Contouring an orbital floor liner illustrates this property. After a template is made of the orbital floor, the template is held against the orbital floor liner (Fig.1A), then placed in a water bath and heated above Tg (Fig. 1B). The floor liner becomes soft in a few seconds and simply drapes over the template when lifted from the water bath (Fig. 1C). In a few more seconds the floor liner cools below Tg and can be removed from the template. The liner is then ready to be placed in the patient (Fig. 1D). It is useful to note that 70:30 poly (L-lactide-co-D,L-lactide) has shape memory, and if placed back in the water bath it will return to its original contour, thus providing additional opportunities to recontour it. If only a portion of an implant needs to be recontoured, only that portion need be placed back in the water bath. Cyclic heating of 70:30 poly (L-lactide-co-D,L-lactide) to 70°C can be performed multiple times with no change in material strength or IV.

V. CHEMICAL PROPERTIES

When lactic acid undergoes polymerization, ester bonds are formed and H_2O is released. Therefore, lactidec copolymers are also known as polyesters. Resorption of lactide copolymers takes place as a reversal of this process, with sorption of H_2O and scission of the ester linkages. This bulk hydrolysis of lactide copolymer implants continues until single lactic acid molecules are released, which are then motabolized into glucose or into CO_2 and H_2O via the Krebs tricarboxylic acid cycle.

A variety of factors are known to affect the rate to lactide copolymer resorption (Table 1). A higher IV or molecular weight means there are more

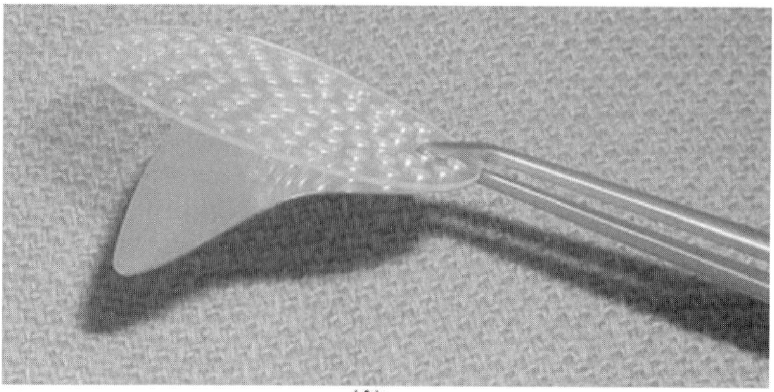

(A)

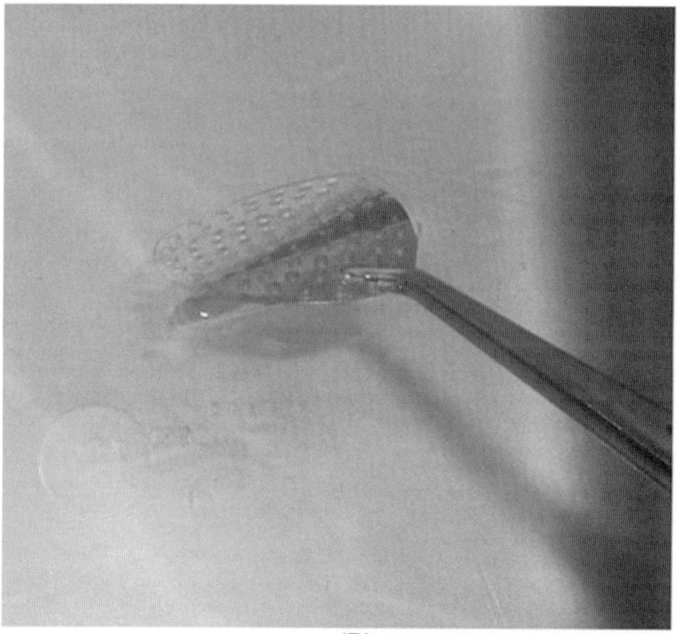

(B)

Figure 1 Contouring resorbable copolymer by warming above Tg with a water bath. (A) Orbital floor template and 70:30: L-La/D,L-La copolymer mesh is held together. (B) Dipped into water bath where the copolymer softens and drapes over the template. (C) Withdrawn from the water bath where the copolymer cools. (D) The copolymer is separated having the desired template contour.

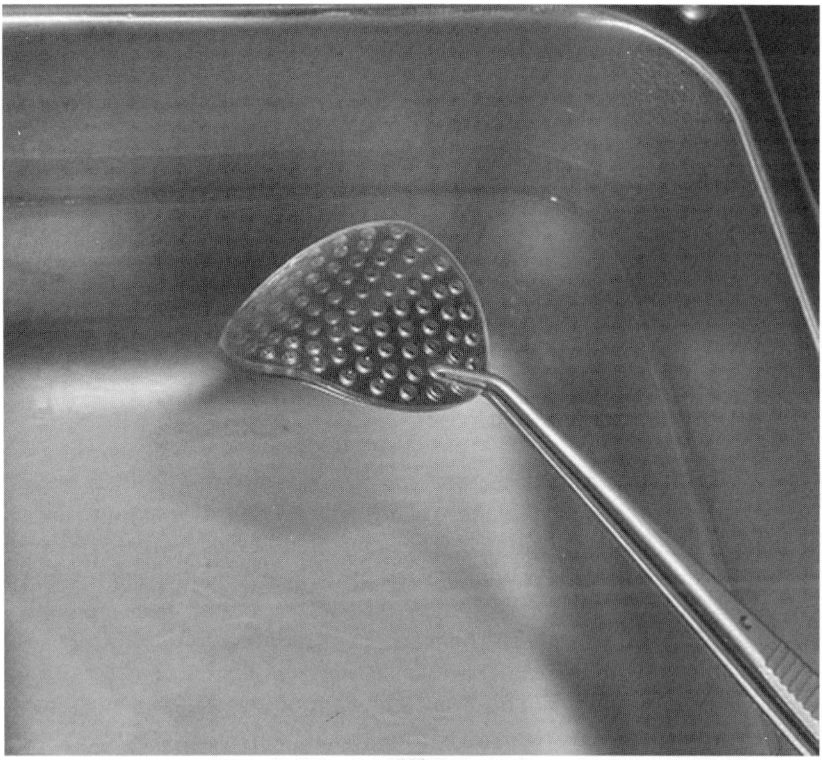

(C)

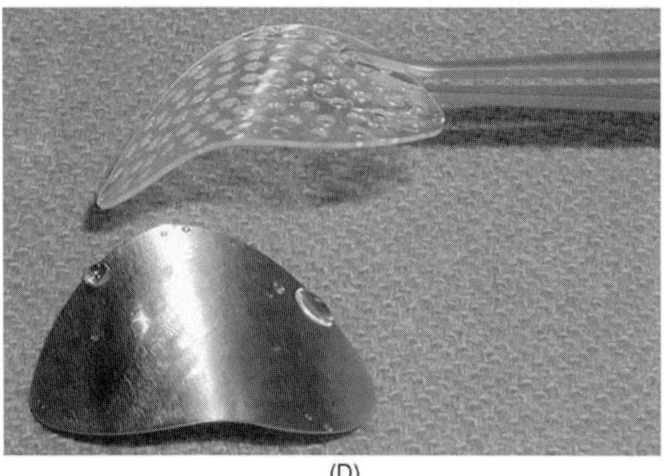

(D)

Figure 1 (*continued*)

Table 1 Factors Affecting Lactide Copolymer Resorption

Molecular weight
Size of implant
Surface area (porosity)
Molar ratio (copolymers)
Vascularity
Functional activity
Crystallinity
Manufacturing process
Sterilization process

ester linkages that undergo scission, and this process results in a longer resorption time. A larger implant size or volume will also require more scission before implant resorption can be completed. If the polymer is packed more tightly in an orderly crystalline pattern, there is less space for H_2O access and resorption will take longer than for noncrystialline implants. Since hydrolysis occurs both on the implant surface and within its interior, implant porosity will increase surface area, facilitate H_2O access, and decrease resorption time. The molecular configuration of copolymers may alter resorption time. Greater vascularity of the implant host site, as well as flexural bending from functional loading, appears to be associated with an increased rate of hydrolysis.

VI. TOXICOLOGY

The Toxicology of lactides has been of minimal concern, owing to the relatively small volumes of implant material, slow degradation rates, and short serum half-lives. The serum half-life of the levo form is 15 min; for the D,L form it is 22 min. The normal resting blood lactate level is 1.1–2.8 mm/L. After muscular activity it will rise 10-fold to 10–23 mm/L. If the assumption is made that degradation occurs over 2 months, with first-order kinetics and a half-life of 74 h, a 100-g implant would release 0.18 mm/L of lactide acid in the first minute, far less than the changes resulting from muscular activity. Two of the largest sheets of 70:30 L-La/D,L-La copolymer weigh only 18 g, and degradation actually takes place over a much longer, 18–36-month time interval. Even with first-order kinetics starting instantly, 18 g of lactide copolymer would result in an increase in blood lactate levels of only 1.1%.

VII. HISTOLOGY

The histological responses to 70:30 L-La/D,L-La copolymer have been well studied. There is an initial acute inflammatory response following implantation. By 72 h there is a narrow zone of fibrinous exudate, edematous granulation tissue, and a modest degree of fibroblast proliferation. By 7–14 days the granulation tissue has matured into a thin, cellular, fibrovascular capsule (3,4). Measurements of in vivo tissue pH adjacent to 70:30 L-La/D,L-La copolymer implants have detected no change during degradation (5,6).

VIII. MECHANICAL PROPERTIES

The mechanical properties of 70:30 L-La/D,L-La copolymer, bone, and steel are listed in Table 2. The tensile strength of lactide is approximately 30% of the strength of bone. With a tensile strength of 70 MPa, lactide materials can readily be designed to accommodate the failure loads for non-weight-bearing bones. When designed as 1.0-mm-thick plates, the tensile strength is approximately 190 N, or 45 lb (Table 3). When metal screws are overtorqued, the threads strip the bone. When lactide screws are overtorqued, the heads shear off. The sheer strength of 2.0-mm screws is approximately

Table 2 Mechanical Properties of 70:30 Poly (L-Lactide-co-D,L-Lactide)

Material	Tensile strength (MPa)	Young's modulus (MPa)
(L-Lactide-co-D,L-lactide)	~70	~4,000
Bone	~200	~20,000
Steel	~1,000	~200,000

Table 3 Tensile Strength of 1.0-mm-Thick Plates of 70:30 Poly(L-Lactide-co-D,L-Lactide)

Sample	Peak load (N)	Elongation (mm)
1	192.8	1.5
2	184.1	1.1
3	196.3	1.3
4	192.3	1.7

Source: Unpublished data, MacroPore Biosurgery, Inc., San Diego, CA.

Table 4 Shear Strength of 2.0-mm-Diameter Screws of 70:30 Poly (L-Lactide-co-D,L-Lactide)

Sample	Peak load (N)	Elongation (mm)
1	84.6	1.4
2	83.5	1.2
3	90.6	1.2

Source: Unpublished data, MacroPore Biosurgery, Inc., San Diego, CA.

85 N, of 20 lb (Table 4). As the 70:30 L-La/D,L-La copolymer undergoes hydrolysis, its mechanical strength will decrease. At 3 months, strength remains near 100%, decreasing to 90% at 6 months, 70% at 9 months, 50% at 12 months, and 0% by 18 months.

IX. PLATE SELECTION FOR FRACTURE FIXATION

As with all fixation systems, clinical experience eventually determines the choice of implant design that is most likely to produce a successful outcome. As a starting point, it is recommended that the surgeon select a copolymer design one size larger than the titanium system currently employed (Table 5). An example from the authors' experience is the substitution of titanium with PLA for genioplasty (Fig. 2A). A traditional metal plate with two holes on each side and 2.0-mm screws would normally have been used (Fig. 2B); however, this patient insisted on resorbable over metal fixation. To assure adequate stability, the 70:30 L-La/D,L-La copolymer plate was contoured from a piece of 1.0-mm-thick mesh with four holes on each side and attached with 2.4-mm screws (Fig. 2C). While this design may be excessive in strength, it is appropriate to be conservative until clinical experience is acquired.

Table 5 Comparison of Copolymer and Titanium Plate Size for Fracture Fixation

For titanium plate size	Use this copolymer plate size
1.3 mm titanium	1.5 mm L-La/D,L-La copolymer
1.5 mm titanium	2.0 mm L-La/D,L-La copolymer
2.0 mm titanium	2.4 mm L-La/D,L-La copolymer
2.4 mm titanium	2.7 mm L-La/D,L-La copolymer

Table 6 Five Years' Experience with the Bioresorbable Plating System (MH)

Category	No. of patient	Plates	Screws	Panels	$\bar{\varepsilon}$
Congenital	176	923	2405	121	3449
Trauma	65	103	368	35	506
Tumor	54	294	653	46	993
Cosmetic reconstruction	29	0	58	0	58
Total	324	1320	3484	202	5006

Follow up in months: (1–42), arithmetic mean 22. No major complications.

X. CLINICAL EXPERIENCE

The following is a review of the authors' clinical experience with biomaterial use in craniofacial fixation.

A. Resorbable Fixation: Zygomatic and Midface Fractures

The natural extension of surgical experience with metal plates is to use resorbable plates of similar designs, such as in malar fracture fixation (Fig. 3A,B). The principles of exposure and reduction of fractures remain unchanged when resorbable plates are employed (Fig. 4A,B). The holes for lactide screws require tapping and maximal screw insertion torque. The plates can be precontoured by dipping in a hot-water bath and, after insertion of one or two screws, be further contoured by using a flat heat applier (Fig. 5), a gauze sponge dipped in the warm-water bath, or by dripping warm water onto the plate. Resorbable plates are easily trimmed in situ using a cautery tip attachment (Fig. 6). Resorbable mesh may be used in place of metal mesh, such as in an orbital floor fracture (Fig. 7). Resorbable mesh is easily trimmed with scissors. It is helpful to leave the leading edge of the mesh uncut so it can be inserted with less likelihood of engaging adjacent soft tissues. Fragments of bone can be incorporated into either resorbable plates (Fig. 8A,B) or meshes (Fig. 9A,B).

With increased experience, it became apparent to the authors that resorbable mesh offered more sites for fixation and provided greater strength when contoured in three dimensions. By allowing custom shapes to be cut with multiple mesh spaces for screw or tack fixation, the surgeon is freed from the geometrical restrictions of limited selection for metal plate designs. Combined with the speed and ease of adapting mesh to three-dimensional contours using warm water (Fig. 10A,B) it is not surprising that the use of resorbable mesh with screw or tack fixation has become even more prevalent than resorbable plates in our craniofacial and midfacial reconstructions.

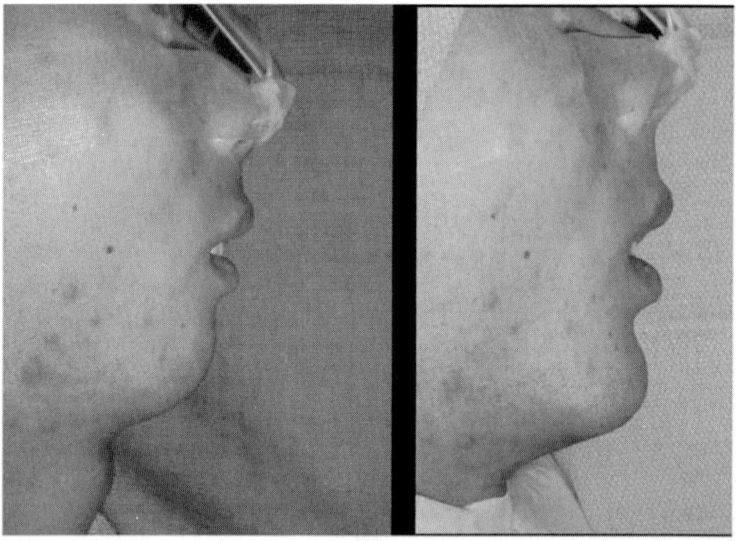

(A)

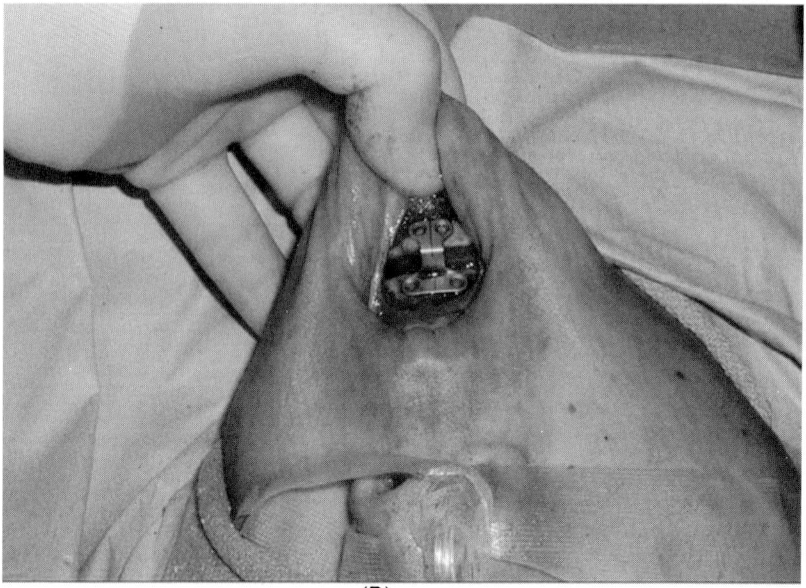

(B)

Figure 2 Plate selection for bone fixation. (A) Pre- and postop genioplasty in patient who requested copolymer rather than titanium fixation. (B) With metal fixation, thin plate with 2-hole fixation is adequate. (C) With copolymer fixation, thicker plate with 4-hole fixation is desirable until clinical experience is acquired.

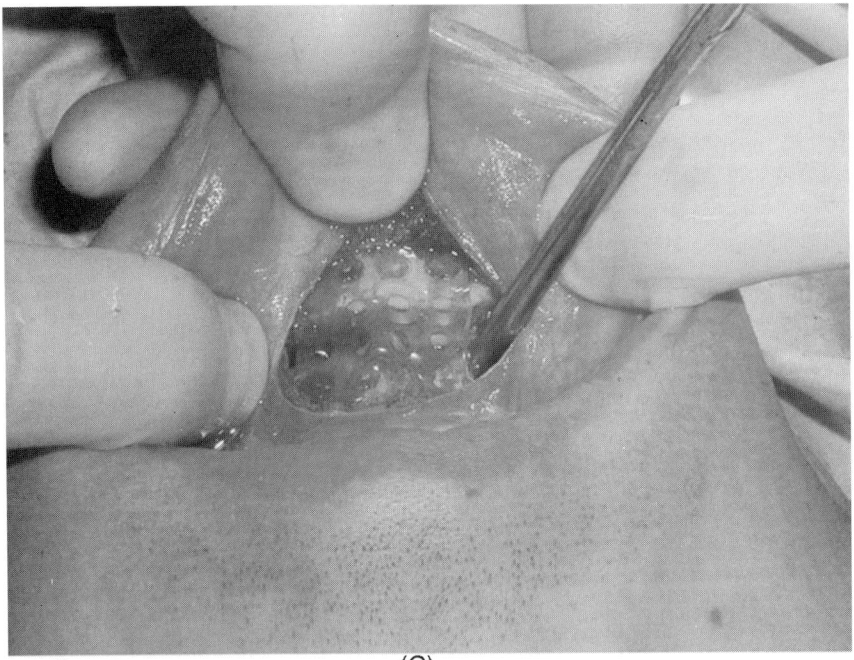

(C)

Figure 2 *(continued)*

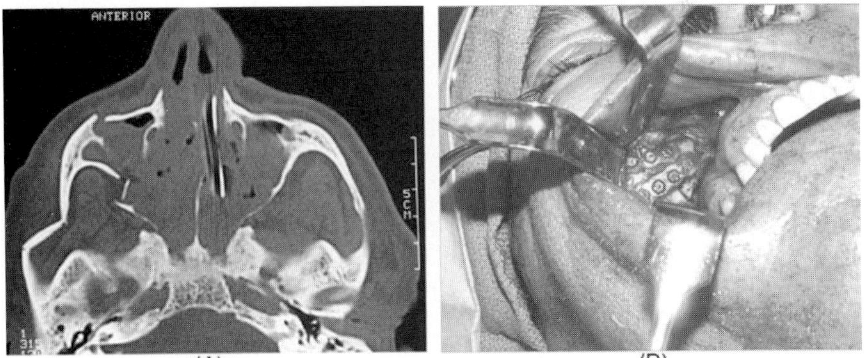

(A) (B)

Figure 3 Resorbable fixation of right malar fracture. (A) X-ray of right malar complex fracture. (B) Resorbable plates spanning fracture site with screw fixation.

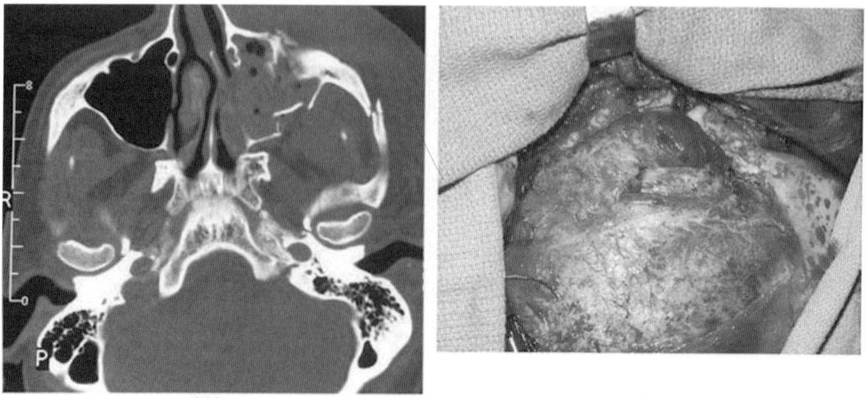

(A) (B)

Figure 4 Resorbable fixation of left malar fracture. (A) X-ray of left malar complex fracture with unstable arch. (B) Hemicoronal exposure with resorbable plate fixation of lateral orbital rim and zygomatic arch.

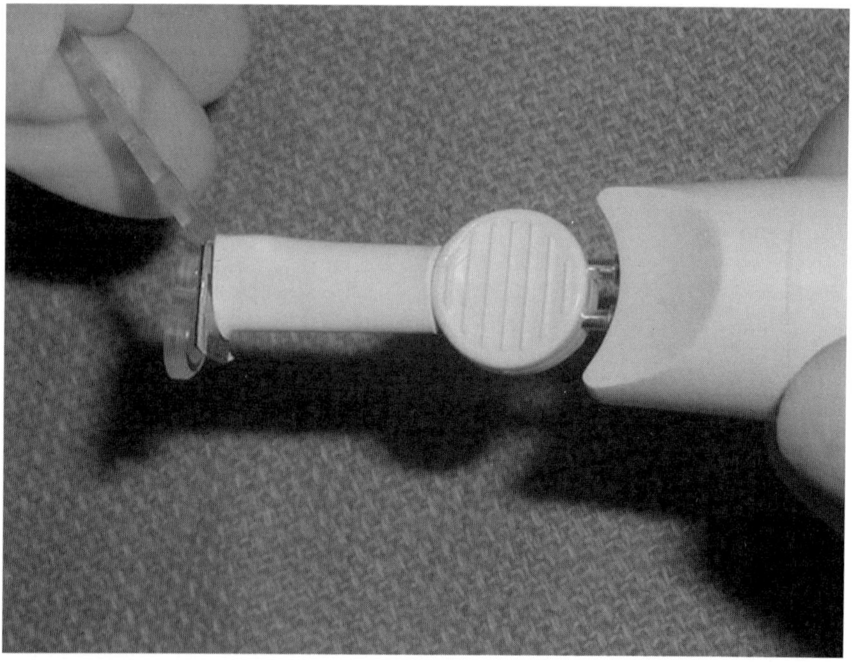

Figure 5 Contouring of resorbable plate using a flat heat applier (PowerPen, MacroPore Biosurgical, Inc.).

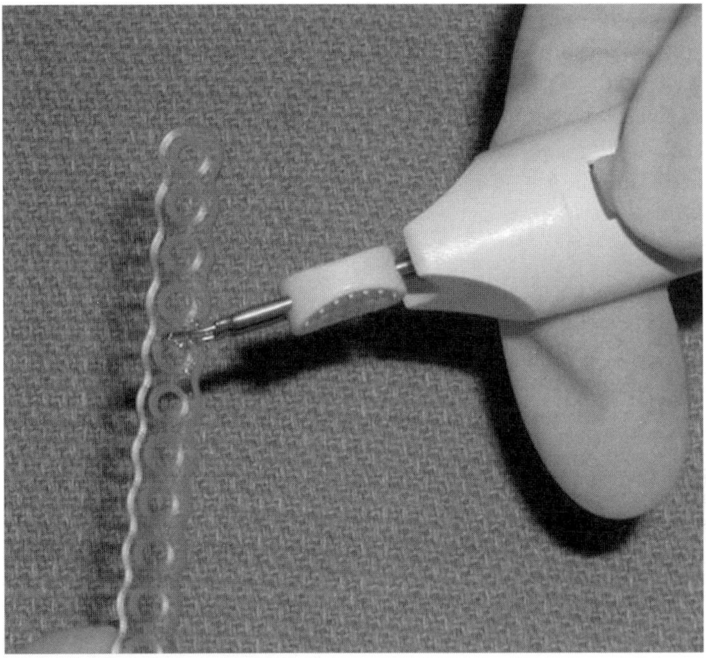

Figure 6 Trimming of resorbable plate using a cautery tip attachment (PowerPen, MacroPore Biosurgical, Inc.).

B. Resorbable Fixation: Fronto-orbital Fractures

The properties of resorption and the ease of contouring have enabled complex fixation requirements of fronto-orbital fractures to be readily accomplished. With use of the resorbable mesh as a template, accuracy of bone fragment fixation can be facilitated. In a 2-year-old girl kicked in the forehead by a horse, the neurosurgeon outlined his planned craniotomy (Fig. 11A). Prior to making the bone cuts, a sheet of resorbable mesh was contoured over the fracture site to match the normal right forehead. The fragments were then reduced into this template on the back table, fixated with tracks, and then returned to the patient after completion of the neurosurgical repair (Fig. 11B). Additional tacks placed around the mesh periphery secured the reduction, restoring this girl's forehead symmetry (Fig. 11C).

When trauma results in boney defects, easily contoured resorbable mesh can be shaped into a template for the bone graft reconstruction. In an 11-year-old girl, anterior cranial base fractures (Fig. 12A) were sustained in a motor vehicle accident. Following acute debridement she was transferred for definitive care of her cerebrospinal fluid leaks and fronto-orbital

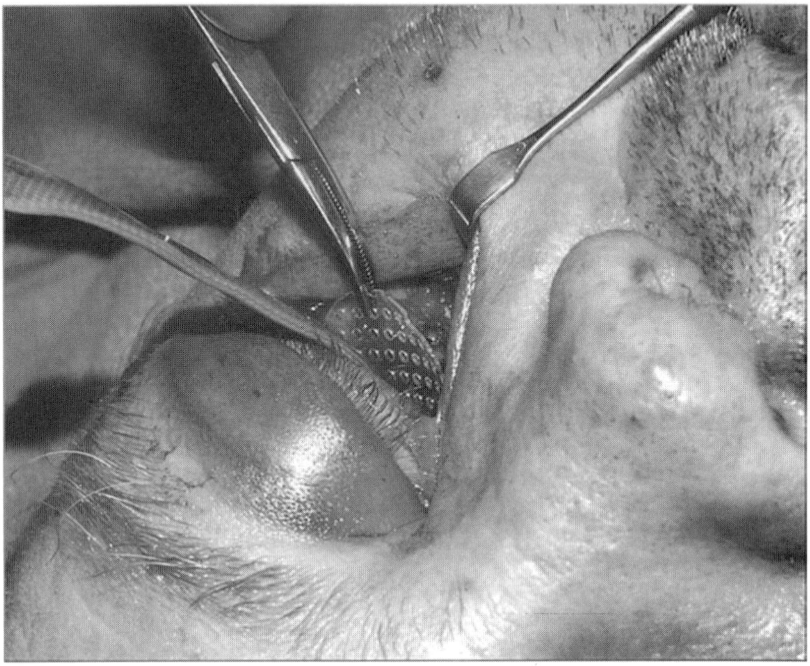

Figure 7 Placement of resorbable mesh to reconstruction orbital floor blowout fracture.

bone defects (Fig. 12B). To provide neurosurgical access to the anterior cranial base, the remaining frontal bone flap and orbital rim were removed (Fig. 12C). Contoured resorbable meshes were then used to rebuild the fronoto-orbital construct from split cranial bone grafts from the flap, along with the portions of the orbital rim that had been removed (Fig. 12D). A good fronto-orbital contour was achieved after the construct was fixated around its periphery (Fig. 12E,F).

C. Resorbable Fixation of Secondary Craniofacial Trauma Reconstruction

Perhaps no area of secondary craniofacial trauma reconstruction has been as challenging as the cranio-orbital fractures of the complex curvatures and multiple planes involved in the frontal bone, the orbital rims, and orbital roof. The availability of easily contoured, large resorbable sheets makes it possible to form templates using in situ anatomy for ex vivo back

(A)

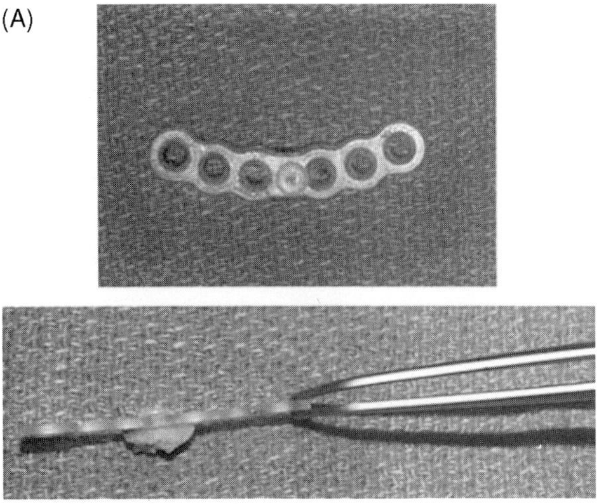

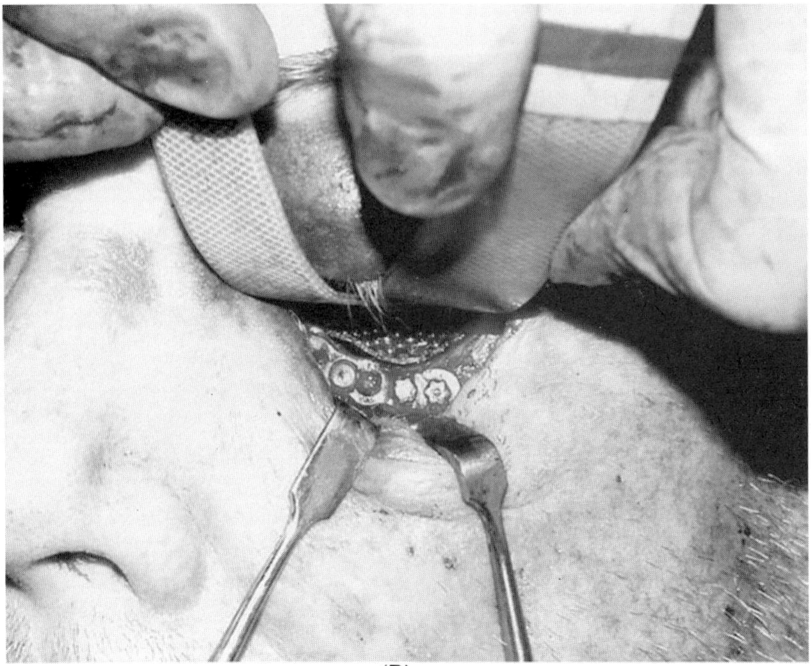

(B)

Figure 8 Reduction of loose bony fragments in orbital rim. (A) Front and side views of small bony orbital rim fragment tacked to plate. (B) Orbital rim fixated with plate holding small bony fragment.

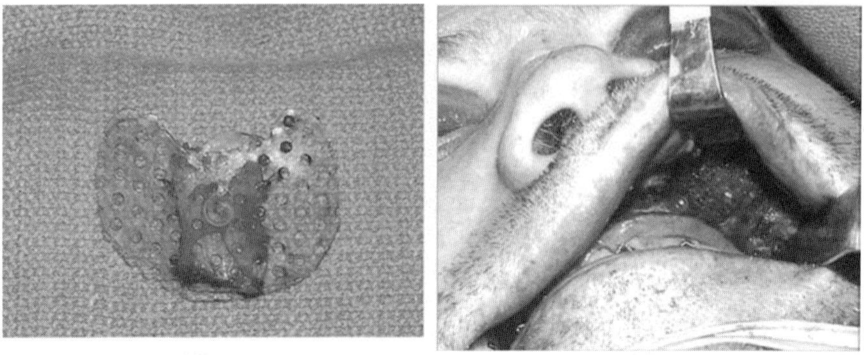

(A) (B)

Figure 9 Reduction of loose bone fragments in anterior maxillary wall. (A) Anterior maxillary wall fragment tacked to contoured mesh with relief for infraorbital nerve. (B) Mesh with fragment tacked into position to restore anterior maxillary wall.

table assembly of the bone graft reconstruction. In a 59-year-old man kicked in the right fronto-orbital area by a horse, osseous debridement was carried out at the time of initial neurosurgical repair (Fig. 13A). Three months later he underwent reconsturction of his defect, which included absence of the frontal bone; supraorbital, lateral, and medial orbital rims; and orbital roof (Fig. 13B). A full-thickness bone flap from the right parietal skull was split,

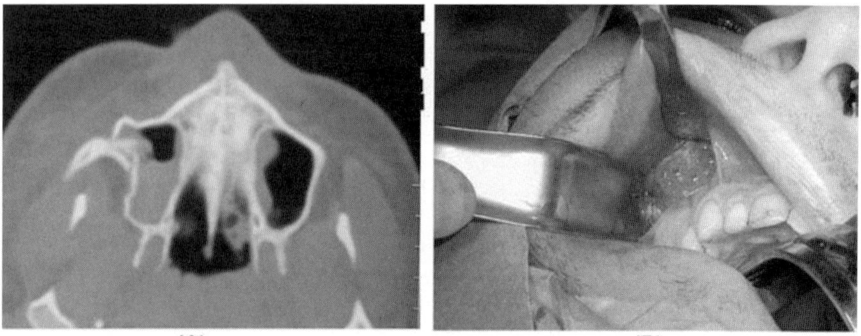

(A) (B)

Figure 10 Contoured mesh fixation of right malar fracture. (A) X-ray of right malar fracture. (B) MacroPore mesh contoured across maxilla and around maxillary buttress, then fixated using mesh holes, to provide added rigidity of 3-dimensionally contoured mesh.

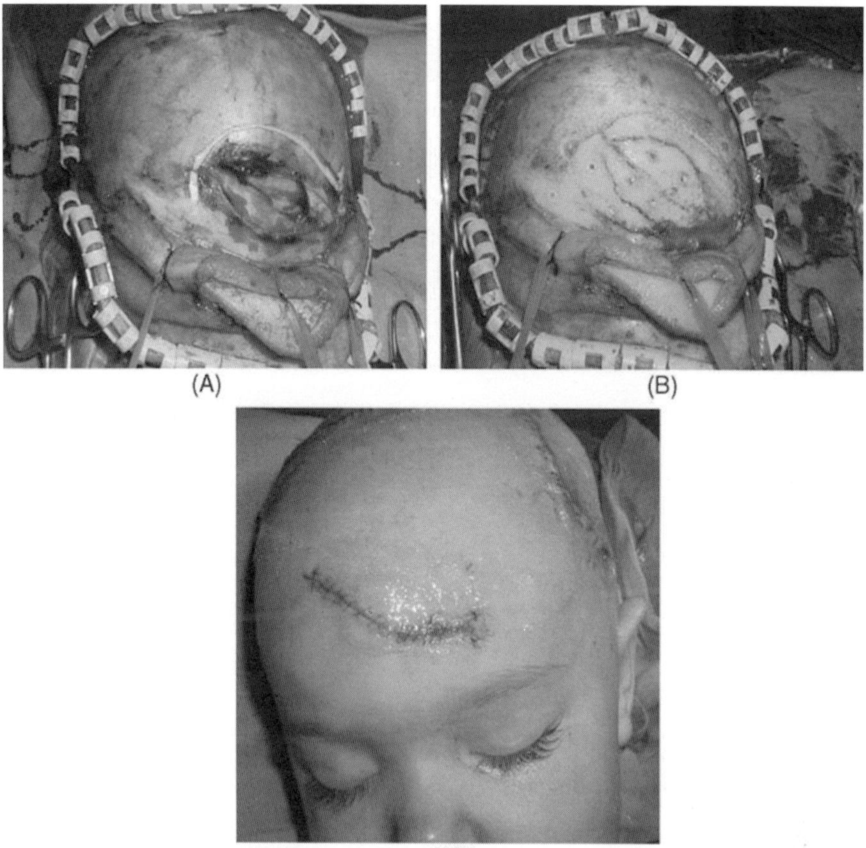

(A) (B) (C)

Figure 11 Reconstruction of frontal fractures in 2-year-old kicked by horse. (A) Intraoperative view of depressed fractures and planned craniotomy after precontouring MacroPore mesh. (B) Fracture fragments reduced and fixated into mesh template, then fixated around periphery. (C) Restoration of normal forehead contour.

and the inner table was replaced and fixated with a resorbable mesh that was contoured before the craniotomy. A template of the desired orbitocranical defect was formed using a sheet of 0.75-mm-thick Macro Pore mesh, and the cranial bone graft was then cut to fit into the mesh template and fixated with tacks (Fig. 13C). The construct was fitted into the defect and secured around the periphery with additional tacks (Fig. 13D). Three months later

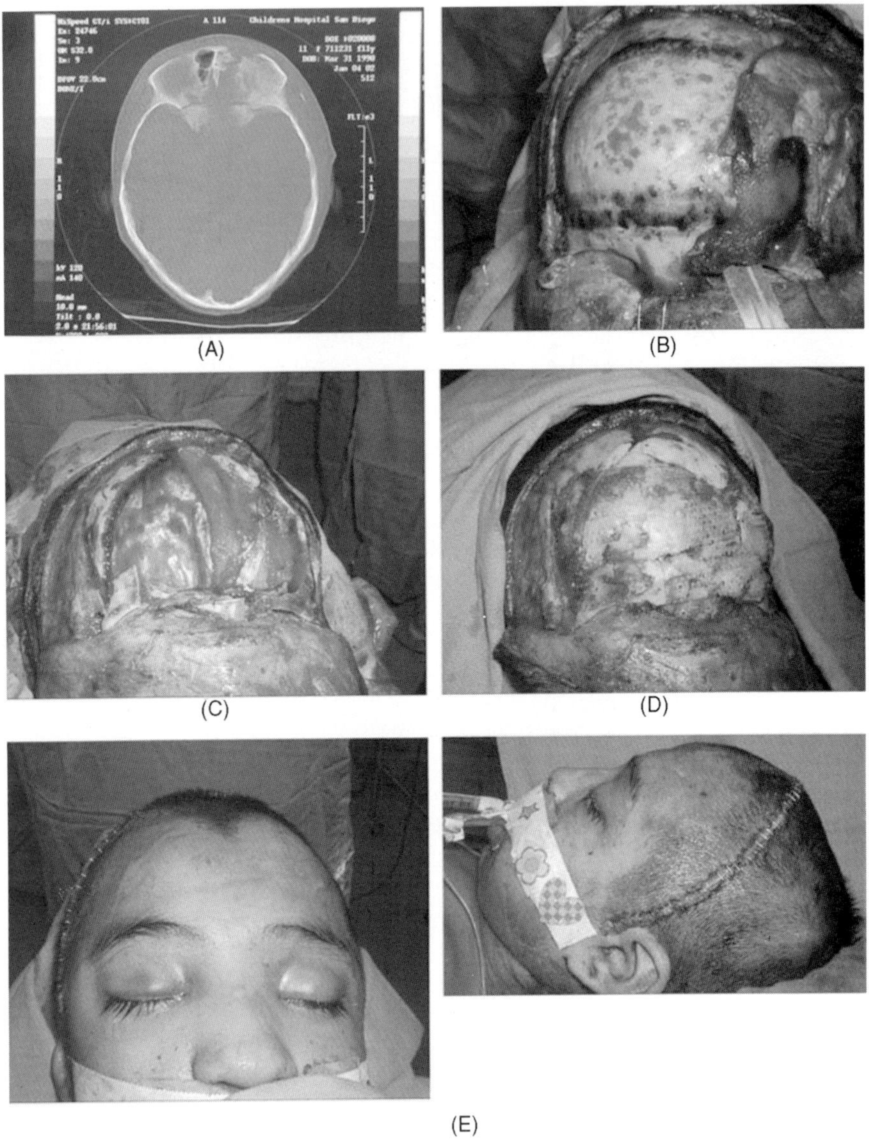

Figure 12 Reconstruction of complex fronto-orbital fractures in 11-year-old after motor vehicle injury. (A) X-ray showing fractures of left orbit and anterior skull base. (B) Left fronto-orbital defect and planned craniotomy. (C) Bone removal to provide neurosurgical access. (D) Construct of split cranial bone and orbital rim in contoured MacroPore mesh fixated around periphery. (E) Frontal and lateral views of reconstructed fronto-orbital contour.

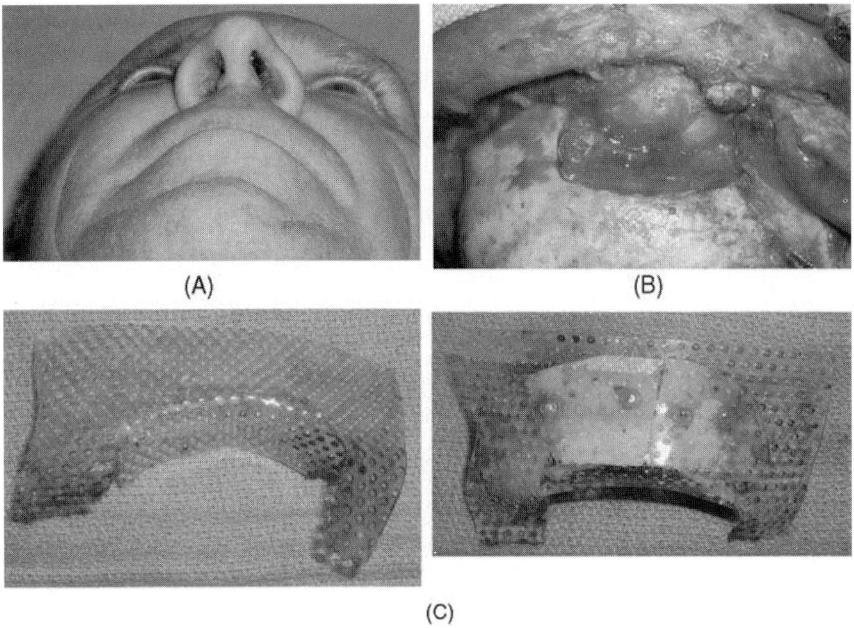

Figure 13 Secondary reconstruction of the orbito-cranial complex. (A) A 59-year-old patient with traumatic loss of right frontal bone, orbital rims and roof. (B) Intra-operative view showing globe and posterior table with loss of rims, roof and anterior table. (C) A sheet of MacroPore mesh has been contoured into a template for the desired reconstruction and split cranial bone has been cut, reduced into the template, and fixated with tacks. (D) Frontal and lateral views of templated bone graft construct placed into defect and tacked around periphery. (E) Frontal and lateral views 6-mos postop showing excellent reconstruction of orbito-cranial contours just prior to ptosis correction.

the cranio-orbital contour was excellent, the patient's preoperative diplopia completely resolved, and a ptosis correction was scheduled to complete the reconstruction (Fig. 13E).

XI. EVOLUTION

Our experience is primarily with a pediatric craniofacial population, in a practice that stresses treatment of the traumatic injuries of the craniofacial skeleton. However, our application of the techniques of fixation is similar to controlled osteotomies, noncontrolled osteotomies, as well as multiple

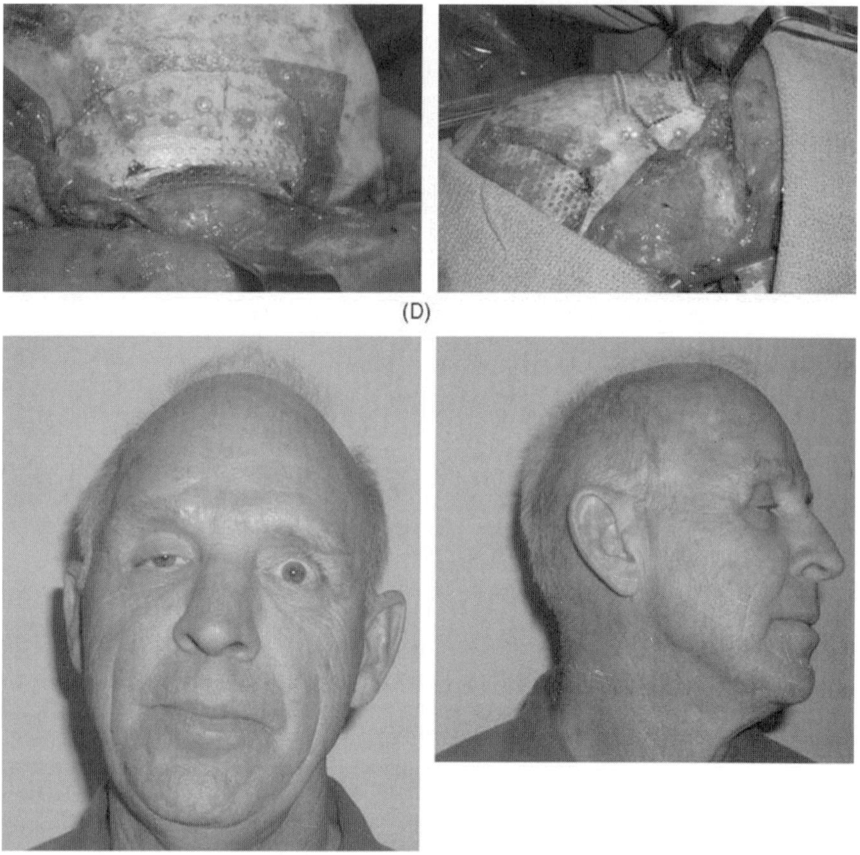

(D)

(E)

Figure 13 (*continued*)

craniofacial fractures. Over time our initial utilization of preformed plate design has been replaced by the use of sheets of mesh, which are easily cut to fit the requirements of repair for a given fracture. This choice is a matter of preference. With complex reconstructions, we have found that easily contoured resorbable mesh permits quick creation of templates that guide bone graft assembly to a precise and accurate reconstruction. We anticipate that techniques will continue to evolve as more experience is gained with the properties of resorbable copolymers used for craniofacial fracture fixation and reconstruction.

XII. OTHER BIOMATERIALS UTILITY

The above descriptions of biomaterials reflect those that are used most often in clinical practice. Today many surgeons prefer the use of metallic implants, particularly titanium, for the correction of facial fractures. Two points, however, must be stressed. First, in children, it is the standard of care to use bioresorbable plates and screws to mechanically stabilize the craniofacial skeleton, and it is impermissible to do otherwise. These patients have a higher possibility of screw migration, growth disturbances, and a need for unnecessary secondary operations. Second, for the adult population, repeated surgeries may also be avoided with the use of bioresorbable plating systems.

Other biomaterials are used to a lesser extent in patients with craniofacial trauma. Their use is limited to delayed reconstruction and, very rarely, such biomaterials are applied in the primary care of patients with multiple facial injuries. Fixation of the skeleton in the correction of facial fractures is the primary use for bioresorbable copolymers. When a defect in the craniofacial areas must to be reconstructed, bone grafting is the treatment of choice. However, if that treatment is not an option or will precipitate a major disability of the patient, the surgeon should be knowledgeable in the applications of those biomaterials in use and familiar with the indications and contraindications of all such biomaterials.

A. Polymethylmethacrylate

The use of methylmethacrylate was popular after World War II. However, analyzing that experience, we have learned that such biomaterial should not be used in type II wounds or in any contaminated areas of the craniofacial skeleton. Infection and fistulization often result, even when the biomaterial utilized for the repair has been present for over 30 years. The utility of the application of methylmethacrylate is in covering large defects in the skull. It is also used to protect the brain when skull defects are present. The reported incidence of infection varies owing to the longevity of use and because of the transient nature of the population in this country. The lack of standardized records, continuity of care, and information reporting contribute to the inaccuracy of existing data. Methylmethacrelate is also used to correct contour abnormalities in patients with trauma. The same principles apply for the avoidance of use in contaminated areas and type II and III wounds. This biomaterial application should always follow a list of strict indications and contraindications to achieve the best possible outcome for trauma patients. Finally, reconstruction of large defects in the skull may achieve the immediate purpose for the desired result, but the patient will end up with a shatter effect if the area is subjected to other blunt trauma. Reinforcement with metallic mesh did not alleviate that issue.

B. Silicones

Silicone rubber in the form of room temperature vulcanizing silicone (RTV) or prefabricated silicone components was used in skull repair, but was found to have no added value. Use of silicone was very popular in the early 1970s, and served in reconstruction to fill defects in areas of traumatic injury or for contour abnormalities. The applications for silicone today are limited. This material is capable of causing major complications in dynamic sites owing to its ability to erode the underlying bone.

C. Polyetherurethan Terephthalate and Med Pore

Both materials are used in a similar fashion to silicone but have less utility in trauma patients. We have extensive experience in the use of the polyurethane mesh as a contour and enhancer for bone regeneration for large defects in the skull. However, large sheets of bioresorbable biomaterial have replaced its use by obviating the need for a secondary surgery to remove the implant (7), (Fig. 14).

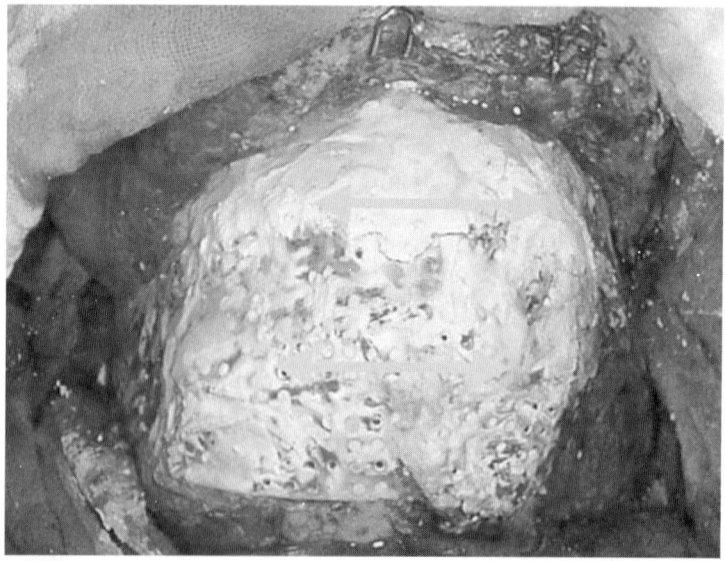

Figure 14 Application of bone substitute to correct a contour defect.

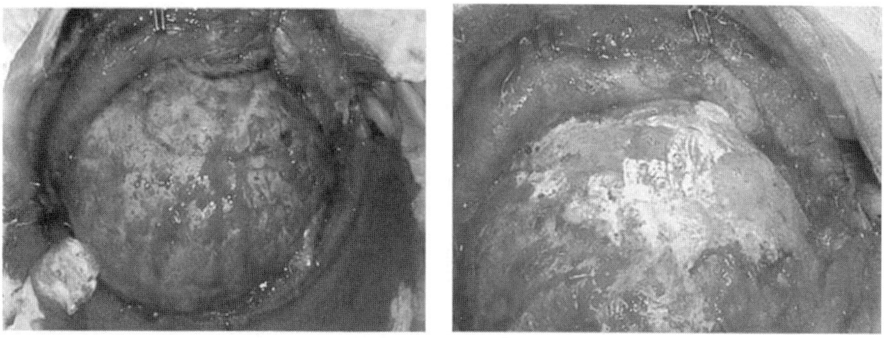

A B

Figure 15 (A) Application of bioinductive biomaterial implant to correct contour abnormalities in the forehead; (B) after the application is complete.

D. Bone Substitutes

To complete this discussion, we must also note the various bone substitutes that are in use today and available in most operating rooms. Bone substitutes react with the surrounding tissues to make the application more

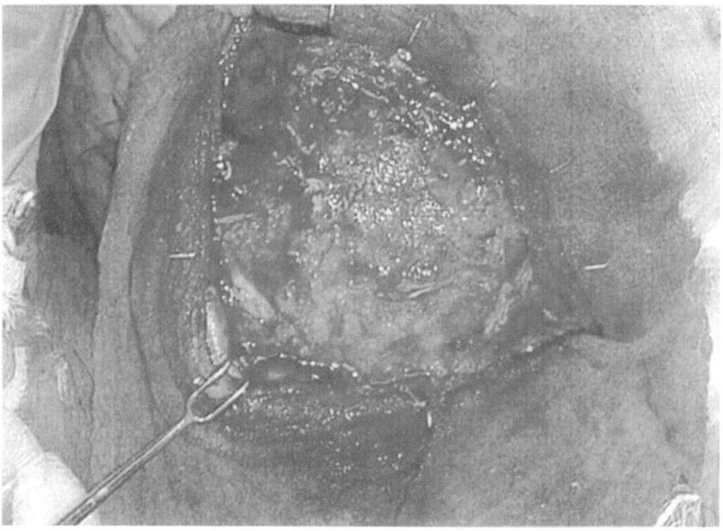

Figure 16 Bioinductive biomaterial in contour abnormalities of the temporal parietal region.

appropriate. Their main use is for filling defects that need a scaffold (8). These biomaterials do not stand shear force, even after they consolidate, and are mechanically unstable. A second, more useful, application is for contour abnormalities (Fig. 15).

We are not going to put a recommendation on any one of these biomaterials, but we will list them in a systematic way that will help those interested to know the difference between each component (9) (Fig. 16).

1. Biomaterials in Bone Substitutes

1. Osteoinductive: Demineralized bone implants vary from 17% to 99%. Use should be species specific, so that is no crossing of species boundaries.
   Dynagraft 17%
2. Osteoconductive: Calcium sulfate, calcium phosphate, and calcium carbonate combinations.
   Norian
   Mimex
   Bonepaste
3. Bioactive and interactive: Composition is changed when in contact with the biological stystem.
   Bioglas
4. Tissue engineering: Active cells and active scaffold will be needed here. Scaffolds used vary from hydroxyapatite to coolagen to most of the degradable carriers. The stem cells used must be autologus. Such uses in trauma patients are under study today and have limited applications.

REFERENCES

1. Habal MB. Absorbable platting system-discussion of, resorbable plate fixation in pediatric craniofacial surgery. Plast Reconstr Surg 1997; 100:8–11.
2. Habal MB, Pieterzak WS. Key points in the fixation of the craniofacial skeleton with absorbable biomaterial. J Craniofac Surg 1999; 10:491–499.
3. Kulkarni RK, Pani KC, Neuman C, Leonard F. Polylactic acid for surgical implants. Arch Surg 1966; 93:839–843.
4. Gogolewski S, Jovanovic M, Perren SM, Dillon JG, Hughes MK. Tissue response and in vivo degradation of selected polyhydroxyacids: polylactides, poly(3-hydroxybutyrate), and poly(3-hydroxybutyrate-co-3-hydroxyvalerate). J Biomed Mater Res 1993; 27:1135–1148.
5. Van der Elst M, Dijkema AR, Klein CP, patka P, Haarman HJ. Tissue reaction on PLLA versus stainless steel interlocking nails for fracture fixation: an animal study. Biomaterials 1995; 16:103–106.

6. Mainil-Varlet P, Rahn B, Gogolewski S. Long-term in vivo degradation and bone reaction to various polylactides. Biomaterials 1997; 18:257–266.
7. Habal MB. Absorbable, invisible and flexible plating system for the craniofacial skeleton. J Craniofac Surg 1997; 8:121–126.
8. Habal MB, Reddi AH. Bone Grafts and Bone Substitutes. New York: WB Saunders, 1992.
9. Tharanon W, Sinn DP, Hobar PC, Sklar FH, Salomon J. Surgical outcomes using bioabsorbable plating systems in pediatric craniofacial surgery. Craniofac Surg 1998; 9:441–444.

9

Endoscopic Approaches in the Treatment of Facial Fractures

Mark Martin and Chen Lee
McGill University, Montreal, Quebec, Canada

William Y. Hoffman
University of California at San Francisco, San Francisco, California, U.S.A.

I. INTRODUCTION

Treatment of facial fractures has progressed through several distinct phases during the twentieth century. Early in the last century facial fractures were treated using limited interventions, relying mostly on closed-reduction techniques, owing to the technical constraints that affected surgery in general at the time. Fractures that involved tooth-bearing segments were reduced and then stabilized by using various maxillomandibular fixation techniques. These techniques could not, of course, effect precise three-dimensional reduction of displaced and comminuted fractures. They did allow fracture healing to occur in maximal-intercuspal position (MIP), so that a more predictable coordination of the mandibular and maxillary dental arches was achieved even though malunion at distant fracture sites was a common problem. Displacement at distant fracture sites was still possible owing to movements occurring through the craniomandibular joints, proximal mandibular fractures, and fractured midface buttresses. Malunions in these complex midface fractures that had been treated closed often resulted in elongated, retruded facies because of displacement at these fracture sites, which was due to both the force of impact and the functional forces of the masticatory and cervical musculature. In an attempt to control the observed tendency for fracture displacement and facial elongation, the American surgeon Adams in 1942 introduced his suspension wiring techniques to secure the mobile arch-bearing segments to the cranial base (1). Although these techniques did reduce the tendency toward facial lengthening, the effect was uncontrolled and shortened, retruded facies were often the result. Advances in antimicrobial therapy and anesthetic techniques permitted innovative surgeons to further develop Milton's concept of securing lower and midfacial fractures to the stable cranial base via open techniques.

Luhr's pivotal suggestion in 1968 that facial fractures could be accurately fixed using small plates and screws was a key advance, but was not put into widespread use until the 1980s (2). During this decade plate and screw fixation was popularized due largely to the impressive results displayed by Manson in Baltimore and Gruss in Toronto (3,4). Manson and Gruss can be credited with the development and dispersion of a systematic approach to open reduction and internal fixation (ORIF) of facial fractures through a series of articles detailing techniques and analysis of results. Wide exposure of all fracture sites, accurate anatomical reduction, rigid internal fixation, and immediate bone grafting of critical defects became the standard of care. Anatomical repair of the facial skeleton became the standard of care in most areas of the facial skeleton except for a few areas where controversy remained, namely the mandibular condyle and zygomatic arch. Soon surgeons began to recognize, however, that the extensive exposures utilized in these approaches had deleterious effects on the soft tissues. Soft-tissue descent after extensive subperiosteal dissection was noted and discussed by Phillips (5). The sequelae of the bicoronal and transcutaneous lid incisions became increasingly apparent.

Late in the twentieth century surgeons treating facial fractures began to focus their efforts on refining their techniques to improve the risk-benefit profile of their interventions. Minimally invasive approaches had revolutionised many surgeries in general surgery, gynecology, thoracic surgery, and orthopedics. A lack of natural optical cavities surrounding the usual sites of facial bone fracture delayed the introduction of this technology to these injuries, even though the ability to conduct fracture repair through minute incisions would be of great advantage in the craniofacial region for aesthetic reasons. Endoscopic approaches to aesthetic brow deformity and to flap harvest were some of the first applications to appear in the plastic surgical literature, and these are now considered viable techniques (6–9). In 1998 Jacobovicz et al. were the first to report the application of endoscopic assistance to ORIF of mandibular condyle fractures (10). Reports detailing endoscopic approaches to the zygoma also had begun to appear in the literature (11,12). Endoscopic assistance in the treatment of orbital and frontal sinus fractures is now garnering increasing interest. This chapter reviews the application of the endoscope to surgical management of fractures of the condyle and zygomatic arch in detail, and discusses the development of endoscopic techniques to treat frontal sinus and orbital fractures.

II. MANDIBULAR CONDYLE FRACTURES

A. Rationale

Controversy continues to surround the subject of mandibular condyle fractures, with about 100 articles concerning the treatment of these injuries appearing in the English literature over the last half century (13). These injuries are common, accounting for between 21% and 52% of all mandibular fractures (14). The controversy revolves around the decision to treat these fractures in an open or a closed fashion. Although the orthopedic principles of anatomical reduction and adequate fixation have achieved acceptance in the treatment of fractures in the rest of the craniofacial skeleton, hesitation remains in applying these principles to condylar injuries. Instead closed techniques have remained the standard of care in many centers. These methods have been loosely referred to as "closed reductions" even though reduction of the fracture cannot be expected, and a malunion is the usual result (15). Prolonged periods of MMF and various protocols using elastic guidance are instead used to force a neuromuscular adaptation to the new biomechanically disadvantaged craniomandibular joint. As in all surgical interventions, a risk-benefit analysis must be considered regarding condylar fracture surgery. The main reasons for reluctance to open these fractures are: (1) the perception that these fractures respond well to closed treatment (16–19), (2) the reluctance to produce significant facial scarring in the pursuit of subtle benefits, and (3) the risk of facial nerve injury from transcutaneous dissection, which would be devastating for patient and surgeon alike (20).

Well-conducted clinical studies have only recently begun to appear that detail the problems associated with closed treatment of condylar fractures and the benefits of ORIF. Silvennoinen et al. analyzed a series of patients treated with closed techniques and discovered an impressive 39% complication rate (14). Several recent studies have compared the results of open versus closed treatment and suggest definite benefits of anatomical reduction of condylar fractures (21–23). In spite of these new studies, widespread adoption of open techniques has not been realized due to the aforementioned concerns regarding facial scarring and the risk of facial nerve injury. In 1998 Jacobovicz et al. reported on endoscopically assisted open reduction and internal fixation (EAORIF) of mandibular condyle fractures (10). The guiding principle behind this approach was to achieve the proven benefits of anatomical reduction and rigid internal fixation of the fracture, while reducing the surgical sequelae of the open approach to an acceptable level.

B. Surgical Anatomy

The craniomandibular joint is unique in the body in being ginglymoathrodial and bilateral in nature. Normal incisal opening begins with rotation in the superior joint space, and then proceeds to translation in the inferior joint space. Translation occurs as the condyle passes down the articular eminence, which has an average slope of 35 degrees (condylar inclination) in the sagittal plane. The medial wall of the mandibular fossa has an average slope of approximately 15 degrees (Bennett angle), which is important in precise guidance of excursive movements. The intervening articular disc aids in regulating these intricate movements.

In condylar fractures the proximal segment normally flexes anteriorly under the influence of the lateral pterygoid muscle. Displacement at the fracture site results in shortening of posterior mandibular height as the pterygomasseteric sling telescopes the distal fragment cephalad over the proximal fragment. Neuromuscular adaptation can often force the mandible into MIP when the condyle is allowed to heal in a malunion in this configuration. Patients, however, spend the vast majority of their time not in MIP, but rather in a habitual rest position where a normal freeway space (FWS) of several millimetres exists between the teeth. In this natural rest position, and during function, the muscles of mastication and the remainder of the soft-tissue envelope of the mandible seek to reseat the condyle into the mandibular fossa. This reseating reveals the loss of posterior mandibular height through a loss of sagittal projection through the pogonion due to clockwise rotation, chin-point deviation toward the malunion in the transverse plane, worsening deviation on functional opening, and limitation of opening due to interference with ipsilateral translation. We have also observed painful hypermobility of the contralateral joint after malunions. Thus an ability to achieve MIP through effort is not an adequate indication for choosing closed treatment. Alterations in mandibular posture at rest and deviations in function are more relevant aesthetically.

Numerous transcutaneous incisions have been championed in the literature, attesting perhaps to the lack of an ideal approach. All are associated with a risk of facial nerve transection or blunt traction injury, and all will leave a sizable facial scar. The retromandibular vein may be encountered and this thin-walled vessel may be the source of brisk hemorrhage. A nerve stimulator may be useful in identifying branches of this highly variable nerve; however, even identifying these branches surgically may lead to temporary palsies, which is disturbing to all concerned.

C. Indications

Various authors have offered a multitude of relative and absolute indications for opening condyle fractures, although scientifically validated criteria for differentiating fractures at relatively greater or lesser risk of sequelae cannot be found in the literature. The oft-cited list of indications offered by Zide and Kent relates mainly to unusual fractures that are extremely rare in our center and we do not find this list helpful clinically (24). We choose to classify condylar fractures into head (intracapsular), neck, and subcondylar. The significance of this classification is that fractures of the condylar head (intracapsular) are not amenable to EAORIF but fortunately are not usually associated with significant loss of ramal height. The main problem following intracapsular fractures relates to the development of degenerative joint changes over time.

Condylar neck fractures may be treatable by EAORIF as long as there is sufficient bone stock to place at least two bicortical screws in the proximal fragment. Subcondylar fractures are generally suitable for EAORIF as long as significant comminution is not present as the technique relies on an identifiable fracture line to guide reduction and interfragmentary friction to maintain reduction during fixation (25). Subcondylar fractures are further divided into medial and lateral override patterns according to the direction of proximal fragment displacement relative to the distal fragment. Lateral override fractures are generally much easier to manipulate into reduction, and thankfully comprise a large majority of adult subcondylar fractures (90% in our series). Displacement refers to separation of the fracture ends, whereas dislocation refers to a position of the condylar head outside its normal location in the mandibular fossa (26). We do not operate on nondisplaced fractures as these may be expected to do well when treated closed and monitored closely for loss of reduction. We feel there is abundant evidence that fractures of the growing condyle do well when treated closed, owing to the remarkable remodelling ability of the preadolescent condylar head, and do not open these fractures in the absence of exceptional indications (27–29). In light of the expected high incidence of complications when treating displaced neck and subcondylar fractures closed, the expected benefits of anatomical ORIF, and the low morbidity of the endoscopic approach, we offer EAORIF to a wider scope of patients than we would transcutaneous ORIF. Patients with significantly displaced or dislocated fractures of the mandibular neck or subcondylar region with some combination of associated loss of posterior ramal height, loss of sagittal projection, malocclusion, deviant chin position at rest or in function, and without medical contraindications for surgery are offered EAORIF after a discussion of possible risks and benefits.

D. Diagnosis

Clinically, condylar fracture patients typically present with a history of trauma, complaints of pre-auricular pain, and often malocclusion. On examination typical findings include: malocclusion in the form of ipsilateral posterior prematurities and contralateral posterior open bite; pre-auricular tenderness; intra-aural tenderness, ecchymosis, and possible laceration; retrotympanic hematoma; intraoral ecchymosis; deviation of the chin point to the ipsilateral side at rest and on opening; and a loss of sagittal projection of the pogonion.

Although panoramic radiographs may identify condylar fractures and provide an efficient overview of coincident dentoalveolar pathology, they are insufficient to accurately guide the surgeon in selecting EAORIF over other modes of treatment. Thin-slice (1.5 mm) computed-tomography scannning in the axial and coronal planes provides excellent detail regarding fracture displacement, condylar dislocation, comminution, and medial versus lateral override displacement and is ideal in guiding patient selection and is our study of choice in all suspected condylar fracture patients. Three-dimensional reformatting involves no extra radiation dosing, is routinely available at most centers, and provides the surgeon with a good overview of the fracture pattern, which is of use in predicting the necessity for any special operative maneuvers preoperatively (Fig. 1).

E. Endoscopic Equipment

Equipment specifically designed for endoscopic repair of condyle fractures will soon be commercially available (Synthes Maxillofacial, West Chester, PA). While these instruments are desirable, this technique can be completed using standard endoscopic equipment designed for aesthetic surgery of the face. The instruments used in our technique are adapted from those designed for other purposes. The endoscope is a 4-mm-diameter, 30-degree-angle scope (Karl Storz, Tuttlingen, Germany). The optical cavity must be maintained through mechanical retraction, and toward this end we have found the 4-mm-endoscope-mounted retractor (Isse Dissector Retractor, Karl Storz, Tuttlingen, Germany) to be very useful. A video system (Olympus America Inc., Lake Success, NY) consisting of a three-chip camera (Olympus XLS), camera converter (Olympus 3C-TV), and monitor (OEV 201) is used to display the endoscopic image.

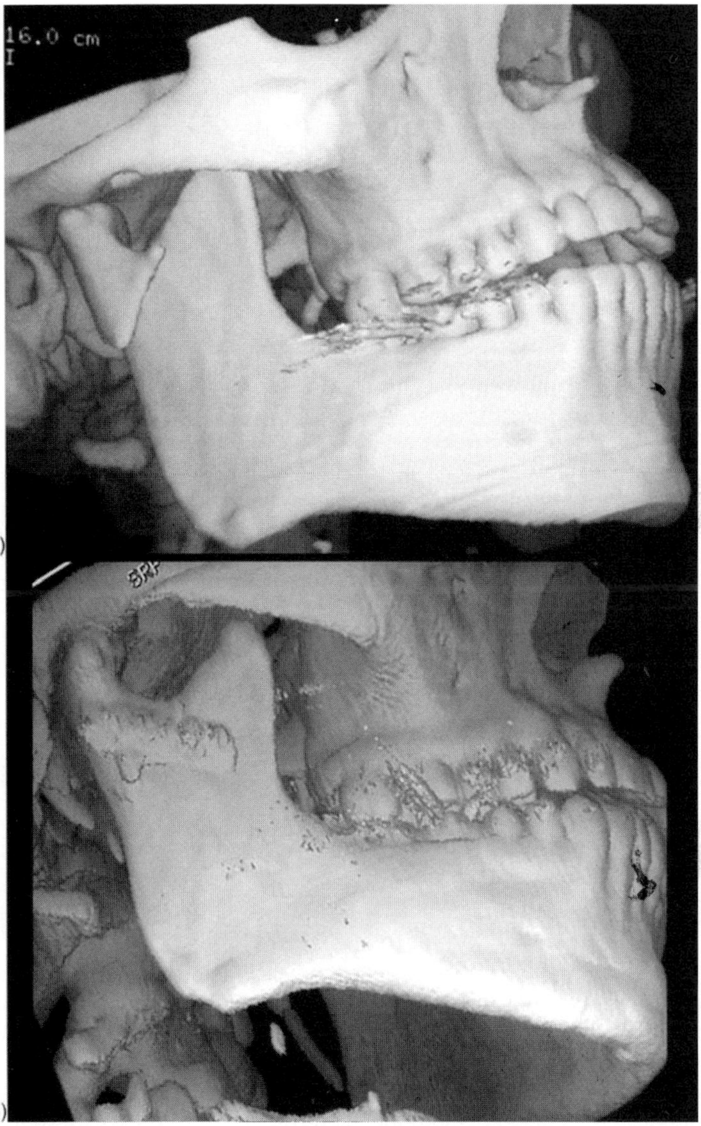

(A)

(B)

Figure 1 Three-dimensional reformatting of the CT scan of a patient's subcondylar fracture allowed the surgeon to predict a relatively straightforward repair in this case of lateral override displacement, which was confirmed on the postoperative CT scan. In medial override displacement the proximal segment would be located medial to the ramus.

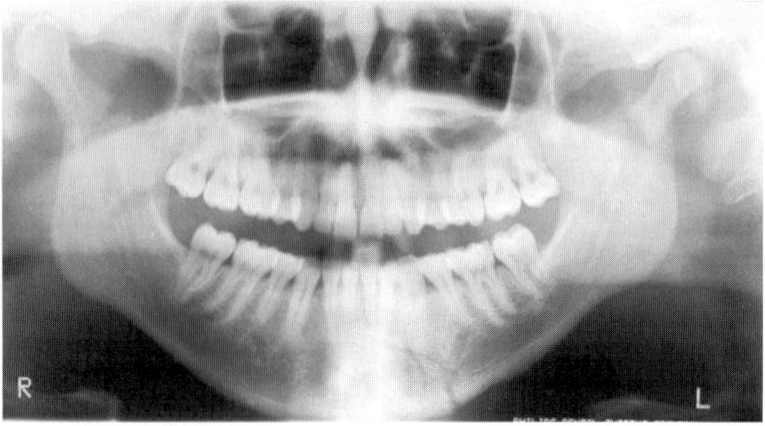

(1a)

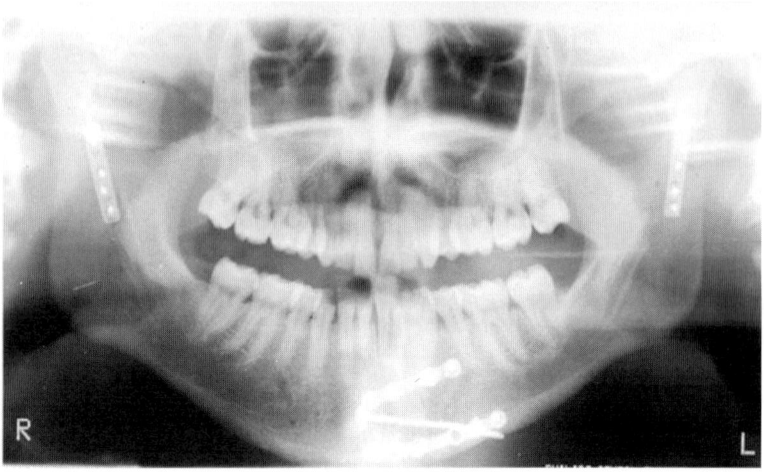

(1b)

Figure 2 Patient who suffered bilateral subcondylar fractures before and after endoscopically assisted open reduction and internal fixation. (1a) Preoperative panoramic radiograph showing bilateral displaced subcondylar fractures. (1b) Postoperative panoramic radiograph. (2a) Preoperative coronal CT scan showing displacement and loss of posterior mandibular height. (2b) Postoperative CT scan showing anatomical restoration of the ramus-condyle unit. (3a) Preoperative frontal view. (3b) Postoperative frontal view. (4a) Preoperative view showing open-bite malocclusion. (4b) Postoperative view showing closure of open-bite. (5a) Preoperative maximal interincisal opening. (5b) Postoperative opening. (6a) Preoperative lateral view showing loss of projection through pogonion. (6b) Postoperative lateral showing restoration of sagittal projection.

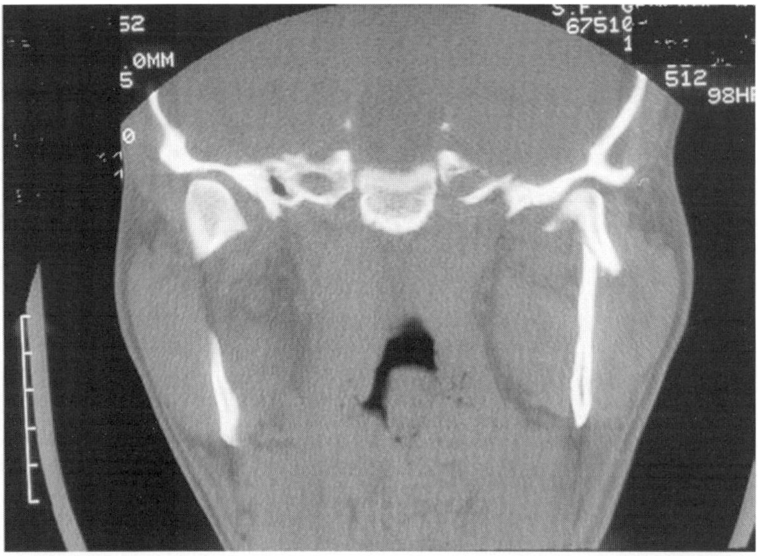

(2a)

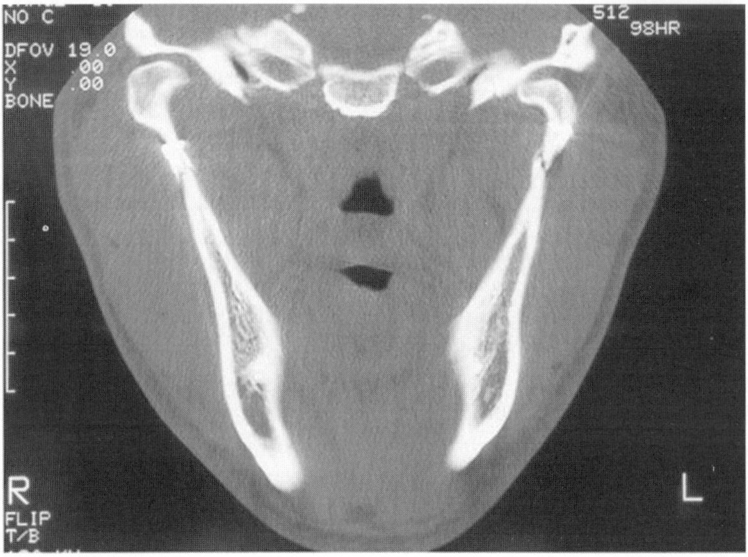

(2b)

Figure 2 (Continued)

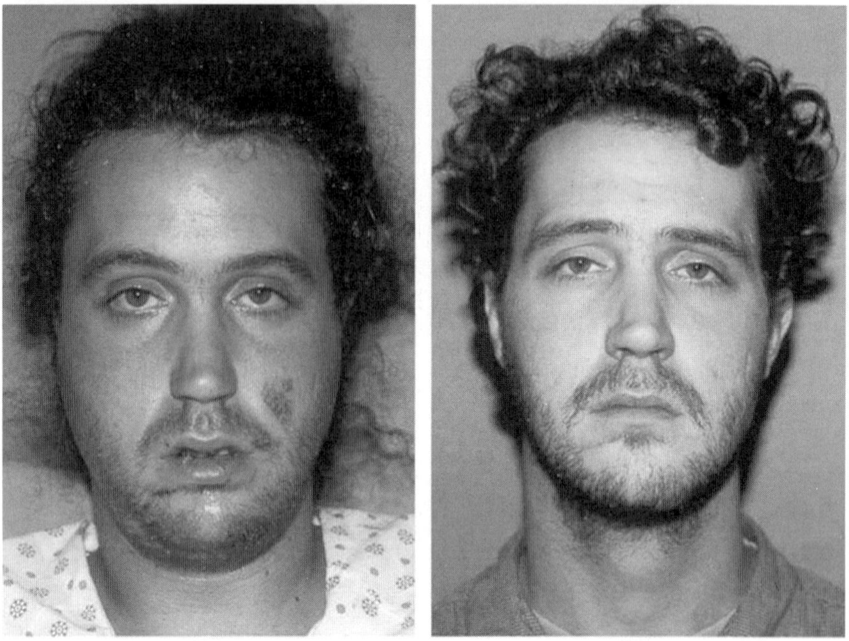

(3a) (3b)

Figure 2 (Continued)

F. Treatment

Initially the patient is fitted with Erich-type arch bars. Any extracondylar fractures are treated with traditional rigid ORIF techniques since intact dentoalveolar arches are essential to the EAORIF technique, and a major goal of the procedure is immediate postoperative function. Local anesthetic with epinephrine is injected for hemostasis along the lateral ramus-condyle unit several minutes before an incision is made with the Bovie cautery. The incision follows the anterior border of the ramus and extends down into the buccal sulcus to the molar region. This incision is similar to that used for the sagittal splitting ramus osteotomy procedure, and an adequate cuff of alveolar mucosa is left below the mucogingival junction to allow easy closure later. Subperiosteal dissection exposes the entire lateral ramus from the sigmoid notch to the inferior border, including the fracture site. The optical cavity is maintained with the aid of the endoscope-mounted retractor and/or the transbuccal sleeve-mounted retractor.

To reduce the fracture, inferior distraction at the fracture site is necessary. This traction may be applied to a screw placed in the lateral surface of

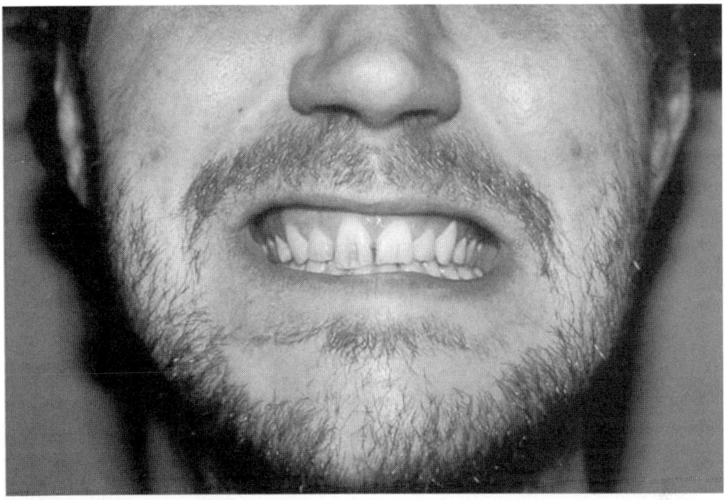

(4a)

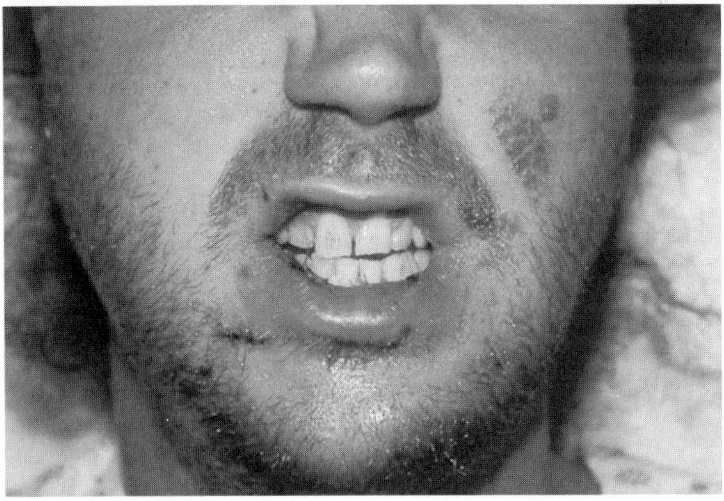

(4b)

Figure 2 (Continued)

the mandibular angle through a 4-mm incision; this incision will be of use also later during reduction maneuvers. Traction is affected through a 26-gauge wire, fed through the sleeve of a large-bore intravenous catheter introduced percutaneously anterior-inferior to the angle, and twisted around the screw. Tight anterior MMF provides the counterforce during distraction maneuvers, and maintains the occlusion in MIP during fixation application later.

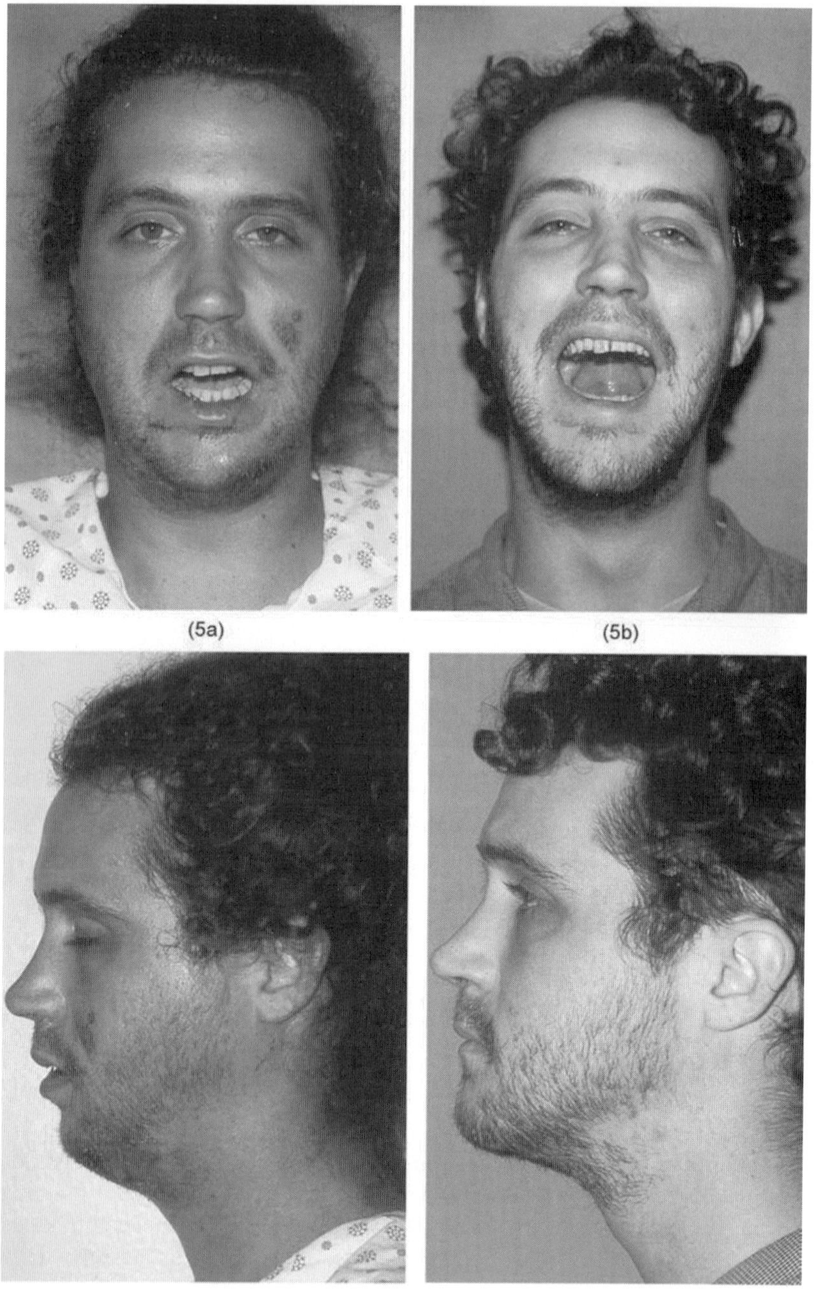

(5a) (5b)

(6a) (6b)

Figure 2 (Continued)

An alternative method of fracture distraction involves placing a small wedge between the ipsilateral molars with the patient in anterior elastic MMF; pressure applied cephalad on the patient's menton by the assistant will effect fracture distraction. Reduction can be tedious and is conducted by the use of endoscope-mounted dissectors and periosteal elevators introduced transorally. A second elevator may be introduced through the incision used for placement of the screw in the mandibular angle, which increases the surgeon's degree of freedom in manipulation. This maneuver can be especially useful in cases of medial override displacement, which are much more demanding to reduce.

Once the fracture is reduced, fixation is carried out using 2-mm miniplates and screws via the transbuccal trocar system. The first plate takes advantage of the thick bicortical bone along the posterior ramus, which is flat enough to take a nonbent plate parallel to the posterior ramal border. If sufficient bone is available, a second plate is placed anterior to the first. The patient is taken out of MMF and the mandible is ranged to ensure that MIP is attainable passively, otherwise the reduction and fixation steps must be done again. The wounds are closed, and if rigid fixation has been achieved the patient is released from MMF at the end of surgery. Gentle guiding elastics may be used to aid in soft-tissue healing during the first postoperative week at the surgeon's discretion. A soft diet is prescribed for 4–6 weeks, and active jaw-opening exercises may commence at 4 weeks. Almost all patients have a maximal interincisal opening of 40–45 mm by the eighth postoperative week (25). A patient example is presented in Figure 2.

III. ZYGOMATIC FRACTURES

A. Rationale

Manson et al. detailed the importance of the horizontal and vertical buttresses of the midface in facial fracture repair (30). Horizontal buttresses may be sagittal or coronal. Gruss et al. have highlighted the central role of the zygomatic arch, a pivotal sagittal buttress, in treatment of complex midfacial fractures and orbitozygomatic injuries (31). The authors feel that adequate reduction of the fractured arch to the stable cranial base is key to reestablishing sagittal projection and facial width. Most isolated arch fractures can be adequately reduced by indirect methods, and maintain adequate reduction without fixation. Furthermore minor redisplacements are often well camouflaged by normal soft-tissue padding. Certain arch fractures demand reduction and rigid fixation. Indirect reduction techniques (Gillies, Keen, etc.) rely on lateral forces to complete the reduction;

therefore, laterally displaced arches are not amenable to these techniques and require ORIF to restore facial width. Posteriorly displaced arches, severe medial displacements, and unstable reductions in patients with thin soft-tissue cover are relatively strong indications for ORIF. Traditional techniques to reduce and stabilize the zygomatic arch rely on use of wide exposure through the coronal incision. Many surgeons and patients feel uncertain about the risk-benefit ratio when comparing the morbidity of a displaced zygomatic arch to that of a coronal approach in anything less than a severe displacement. The long scar of the coronal incision tends to be visible when swimming, in the wind, with short haircuts, and in male-pattern baldness. Temporary and permanent palsies of the temporal branch of the facial nerve are recognized complications with significant morbidity. Alopecia, hypesthesia, dysesthesia, and pruritus may occur.

In an effort to improve the risk-benefit ratio of ORIF procedures for the zygomatic arch, in 1996 Lee et al reported a case of EAORIF of a malar fracture, and then in 1998 Lee et al. conducted a cadaver and clinical study of EAORIF of zygomatic arch fractures (12,32). Kobayashi et al. in 1995 reported use of an endoscope to treat zygomatic fractures with a technique involving use of distant temporal and buccal sulcus incisions, which may produce more difficulty when applying fixation (11). Chen et al. have recently reported a series of patients treated by EAORIF of both the zygomatic arch and the zygomaticofrontal suture under visualization of an endoscope placed through a small temporal incision (33).

B. Surgical Anatomy

The zygomatic arch is a key landmark in restoring facial width and sagittal projection in fractures of the zygomatic complex and high-level midface fractures. The soft-tissue cover of the temporalis muscle cephalad to the arch is composed of five layers: (1) skin, (2) subcutaneous tissue, (3) temporoparietal fascia (superficial temporal fascia), (4) loose areolar tissue (subgaleal fascia), and (5) fascia of the temporalis muscle (deep temporal fascia). The key anatomical structure at risk is the frontal (temporal) branch of the facial nerve. This nerve branch has been the subject of intensive clinical-anatomical study in an attempt to identify the safest plane of dissection to avoid it and to identify various landmarks to predict its course (34). The anatomical variability found in these studies highlights the overriding importance of dissecting in a safe tissue plane to avoid postoperative frontalis muscle palsy. Our method, in agreement with the anatomical study findings of Moss et al. based on their dissections of cadaver heads, is to dissect hard on the temporalis muscle fascia (deep temporal fascia) as a reliable method of avoiding the frontal branch of the facial nerve, which is located on the undersurface of the temporoparietal fascia (35). The temporal fat pad is located between the anterior and posterior leaves of the temporalis muscle fascia (deep temporal fascia). We feel that damage to the blood supply of the fat pad, violation of the overlying fascia, or damage to the fat pad itself may result in atrophy of the pad and temporal hollowing.

C. Indications

Indications for EAORIF of the zygomatic arch depend on patient, surgeon, and fracture variables. The patient's desire to avoid an unaesthetic coronal scar may be strong, especially in balding men and thin-haired women. A surgeon familiar with the anatomy and theory of the technique combined with appropriate training and/or cadaver experience is essential to avoid prolonged operative times and unsatisfactory results. Fracture patterns that may be appropriate for EAORIF include: (1) significant lateral arch displacement, (2) severe medial displacement, (3) comminuted, unstable fractures in patients with thin soft-tissue cover, (4) posteriorly telescoped arch fractures, (5) arch fractures in complex midface injuries that do not require a coronal incision for other reasons.

D. Endoscopic Instrumentation

See Sec. II.E.

E. Technique

Our technique for EAORIF for orbitozygomatic complex fractures utilizes two small cutaneous incisions and an ipsilateral upper-buccal sulcus incision (32). The first incision is made in a pre-auricular crease anterior to the upper helix and extending approximately 2-cm superiorly into the scalp. A second, 1-cm incision is made in a transverse fashion in the lateral orbital region above the canthus, in the thinner eyelid skin. Through the pre-auricular incision a superior dissection is carried out, hard on the temporalis muscle fascia (deep temporal fascia) to create a superior optical cavity. The endoscope and endoscope-mounted retractor are then introduced for visualization of further anterior and inferior dissection. With the optical cavity maintained by the endoscope-mounted retractor it is possible to dissect down to the zygomatic arch staying on the temporalis muscle fascia (deep temporal fascia) and leaving the loose areolar tissue (subgaleal fascia) on the overlying temporaparietal fascia

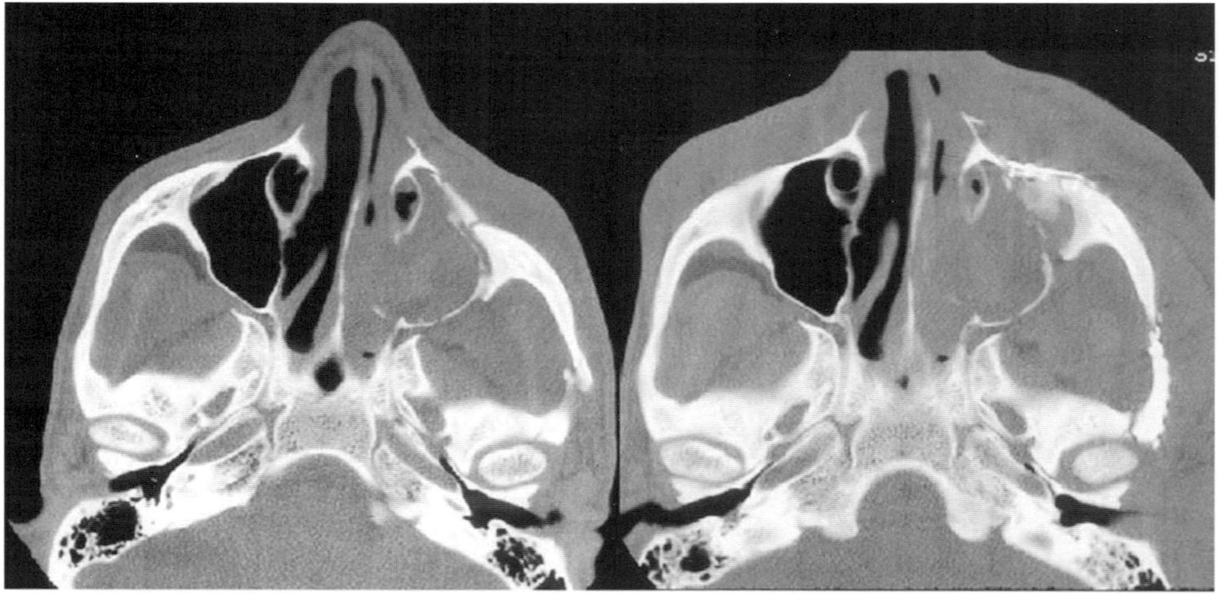

(1)

Figure 3 Patient who suffered a highly displaced left orbitozygomatic-complex fracture who was treated with open reduction and internal fixation, including an endoscopic approach to the zygomatic arch. (1) Pre- and postoperative axial CT scans showing the anatomical restoration of midface projection and width at the malar prominence and arch. (2) Pre- and postoperative frontal views showing restoration of malar prominence and facial width clinically. (3) Pre- and postoperative frontal views showing preservation of frontalis function after endoscopic approach, which had been paretic preoperatively. (4 and 5) Pre- and postoperative lateral and worm's-eye views showing restoration of sagittal malar prominence after anatomical restoration of the zygomatic arch with endoscopic assistance.

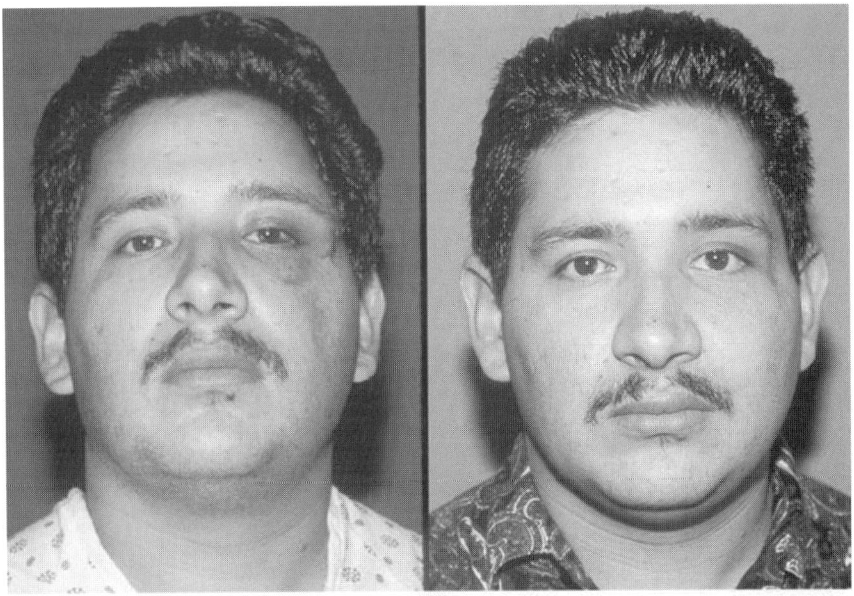

(2)

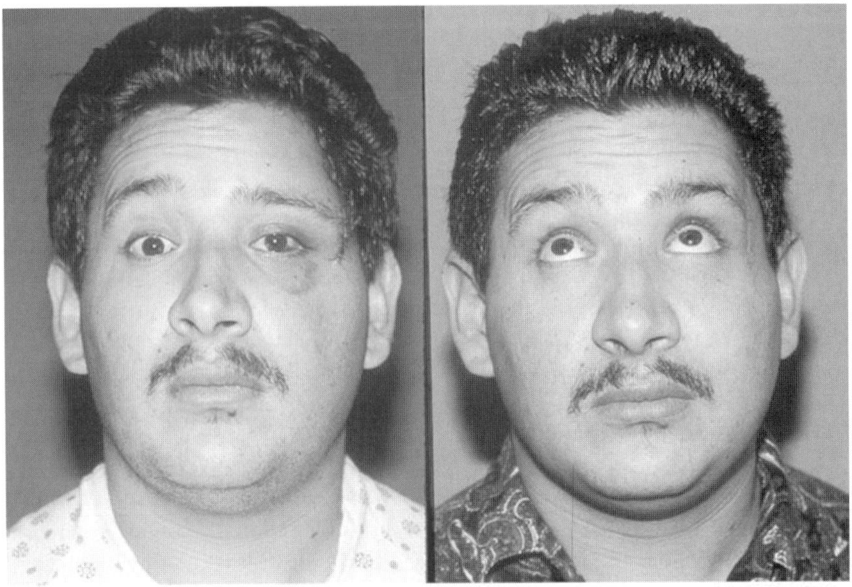

(3)

Figure 3 (Continued)

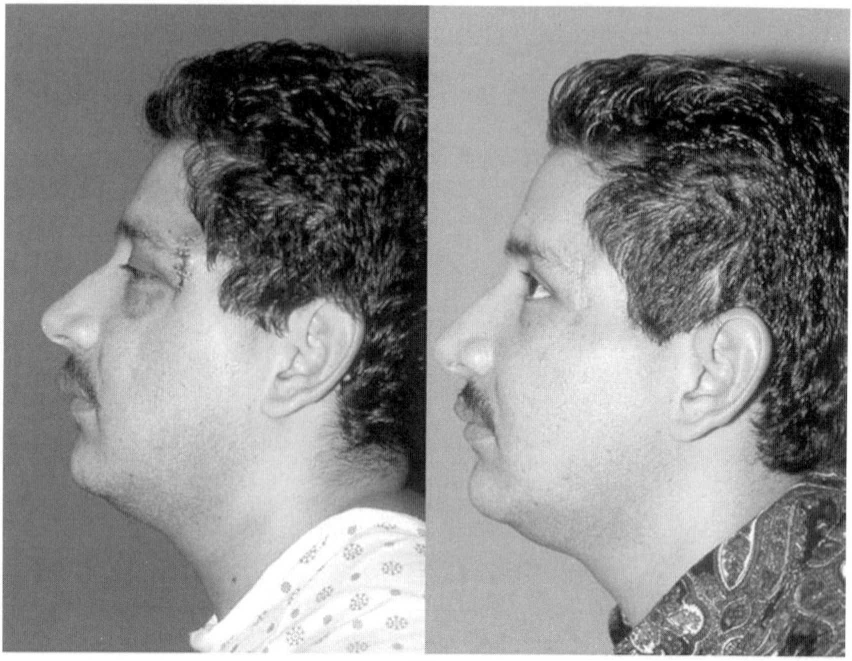

(4)

Figure 3 (Continued)

(superficial temporal fascia), thus leaving the temporal branch of the facial nerve undisturbed without the necessity for direct visualization and protection. The fractured arch is identified without entering the temporal fat pad to avoid postoperative temporal hollowing. The periosteum overlying the arch is incised and the fracture segments exposed subperiosteally. All fracture sites are then visualized while the fractures are reduced. Fracture sites are then sequentially plated. The fractured arch is plated with the aid of a percutaneous trocar system for introduction of drill bits and screws. A patient example is presented in Figure 3.

A series of 15 patients treated by EAORIF of the arch has been reported by Lee et al. (32). Facial width and projection were subjectively restored in all patients, and only one transient (1 week) frontal branch palsy was noted to develop after surgery. Chen et al. later reported a similar approach in 15 patients but dissected between the superficial and deep layers of the temporalis muscle fascia (deep temporal fascia), which may explain the one case of temporal hollowing postoperatively in their series (33).

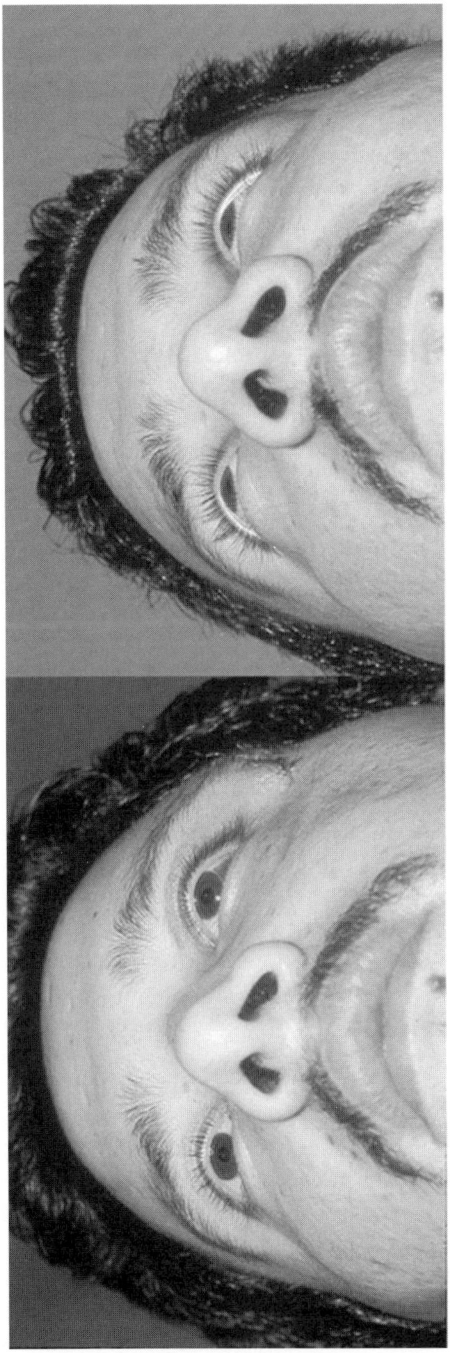

(5)

Figure 3 (Continued)

IV. ORBITAL FRACTURES

Recently interested surgeons have attempted to use the endoscope to advantage in the treatment of isolated orbital fractures. Blowout fractures of the orbital floor and medial orbital walls have been the two main targets of these approaches. Conceptually this approach is attractive. The presence of an adjacent hollow sinus cavity is related to the susceptibility of these unsupported walls to fracture. These same spaces have been exploited as natural optical cavities for both diagnostic and therapeutic aims. In 1997 Saunders et al. studied the utility of transantral endoscopy in diagnosis and treatment of orbital floor fractures in cadavers and clinically (36). They suggest that the endoscope may be useful in: (1) identifying cases of orbital fracture that would benefit from lid approaches for orbital reconstruction, (2) assisting in fracture reduction and identifying the stable posterior ledge for implant placement, and (3) reducing entrapped periorbital tissue caught in trapdoor-type fractures. In 1998 Mohammad et al. performed a cadaver study to assess the feasibility of transantral endoscopically assisted repair of surgically created orbital floor defects (37). The authors were encouraged by their results, although technical difficulties were encountered. A series of nine patients with orbital fractures treated with endoscopically assisted orbital floor reconstruction without lid incisions was reported by Chen and Chen in 2001 (38). Two orbitozygomatic and seven orbital floor fractures were treated with titanium mesh or Medpor implants, with complete correction of enopthalmos in eight patients. Preoperative diplopia resolved postoperatively in two of three patients and improved in the third. No ocular complications resulting from the surgery were reported. Ikeda et al. reported a transnasal endoscope-assisted approach to orbital floor fractures, although they used a balloon catheter to aid in fracture reduction (39). Fears of displacement of fracture fragments into the orbit, causing ocular or optic nerve trauma, are the main drawbacks cited in regard to these techniques.

Fractures of the medial orbital wall have also received the attention of surgical endoscopists. Chen et al. in 1999 reported on a medial transconjunctival endoscopically assisted approach to medial orbital fracture reduction and bone grafting (40). Mun et al. reported on 21 patients treated with a similar medial transconjunctival "slit" incision with endoscopic assistance and calvarial bone grafting; only one patient required revision surgery (41). In 2000 Jin et al. reported on 16 patients treated with a transnasal approach to reduction of medial orbital wall blowout fractures (42). Fourteen patients remained free of enopthalmos while only two required lid approaches subsequently for implant placement to treat residual symptoms. Rhee et al. reported a cadaver study and clinical case of an endonasal endoscope-assisted approach to reduction of the medial orbital wall and implant placement (43). In 2002 Lee et al. reported an additional 16 patients treated by endoscopic endonasal medial orbital fracture reduction with 15 showing complete resolution of symptoms, and only a single case of residual diplopia, which was responsive to prism therapy (44).

In spite of the tempting presence of adjacent, natural optical cavities (sinuses), the acceptance of endoscopic approaches to orbital fractures must be considered carefully. In contrast to condylar and zygomatic arch fractures, where significant scarring is expected from traditional exposures, and where endoscopic approaches may reduce the incidence of functional nerve injury, low-morbidity approaches are available for treatment of isolated orbital injuries. The transconjunctival approach to the orbital floor provides excellent direct binocular visualization of fracture anatomy, for implant placement. It presents a quick and simple dissection with a very low incidence of complications associated more commonly with transcutaneous lid incisions (45). With respect to the medial orbital wall, although endonasal approaches may provide a reduction in morbidity over coronal incisions, the direct exposure of the transcaruncular approach has many advantages. Having long been a preferred low-morbidity approach to medial orbital pathology with ophthalmologists, it may be simpler, easier, allow for more accurate implant placement than endonasal approaches, and requires no special instrumentation or training. This approach may deserve further consideration.

Future experience with each of these approaches by interested surgeons who will examine and report their results will clarify the place of each in the arsenal of the facial fracture surgeon.

V. FRONTAL SINUS FRACTURES

Frontal sinus fractures have traditionally been managed by coronal approaches. Rohrich and Hollier provide excellent reviews of management principles and propose a clinically relevant algorithm in recent articles (46,47). One of the first endoscopic applications to plastic surgery was in the fronto-orbital region for aesthetic brow rejuvenation (6,7). The same endoscopic instrumentation utilized for aesthetic procedures has been employed for the treatment of frontal sinus fractures. All reports thus far have been regarding the treatment of isolated anterior wall fractures. Graham and Spring reported a case of endoscopic repair of an anterior wall frontal sinus fracture in a 13-year-old patient (48). Other reports of frontal sinus fracture repair followed, and focused on the reduced morbidity of the approach resulting from the avoidance of a coronal incision (49–51). Diminished blood loss, minimal scarring, preservation of posterior scalp sensation, and avoidance of alopecia are all reported benefits of the approach. An absolute requirement to endoscopic repair is an absence of indications for sinus obliteration or cranialization. High-resolution computed tomography aids in confirming an intact sinus floor, which suggests an intact nasofrontal duct system; this can be further confirmed at surgery by endoscopic inspection in many cases. If nasofrontal duct involvement or posterior wall displacement indicates a need for sinus obliteration or cranialization, respectively, a coronal approach is used.

VI. CONCLUSION

The principles of wide exposure and anatomical reduction with rigid internal fixation clarified and popularized by Manson and Gruss are the gold standard against which all newly proposed techniques of facial fracture repair must be measured. At the same time we must recognize the morbidities of current approaches and attempt to refine them for the benefit of patients. Endoscopic techniques have revolutionized many operations in the fields of general, thoracic, gynecological, and orthopedic surgery owing to reductions in blood loss, incisional morbidity, and reduced recovery times. The endoscope is a late addition to the plastic surgery armamentarium. The lack of natural optical cavities surrounding facial fracture sites has required innovative thinking and anatomical and clinical study to begin to define a role for this technology in facial trauma. The avoidance of long incisions in this conspicuous area with dense neurovascularity is highly desirable. The principle of wide exposure can still be maintained with endoscopic techniques, while avoiding extensive scarring.

The active participation of surgeons in the development of specialized equipment specific for the craniofacial region is beginning to pay off, as commercially available instrumentation is now becoming available. The process of exposing fracture sites in these cases is often not the most difficult step in the operation; rather it is the application of conventional plate and screw fixation that is most difficult through remote incisions. The use of tissue adhesives and bone cements in facial trauma has been reported, and improvements in these technologies would find many applications for delivery through endoscopic approaches.

Criticisms of endoscopic assistance in facial fracture care include the argument that it is too difficult technically. We would argue that to a large degree the difficulty with the endoscopic approach is in the learning process, and that with experience operative times decrease considerably. With continued technology development, clinical investigation, and the availability of high-quality training, the role of endoscopic assistance in fracture treatment will continue to be defined. This effort is certainly justified if it results in reduced morbidity for patients.

REFERENCES

1. Adams WM. Basic principles of internal wire fixation and internal suspension of facial fractures. Surgery 1942; 12:523.
2. Luhr HG. Stable osteosynthesis in fractures of the lower jaw. Dtsch Zahnaerztl 1968; 23:754.
3. Manson PN et al. Midface fractures: advantages of immediate extended open reduction and bone grafting. Plast Reconstr Surg 1985; 76:1.
4. Gruss JS, Mackinnon SE. Complex maxillary fractures: role of buttress reconstruction and immediate bone grafts. Plast Reconstr Surg 1986; 78:9.
5. Phillips JH et al. Periosteal suspension of the lower eyelid and cheek following subcilliary exposure of facial fractures. Plast Reconstr Surg 1991; 88:145.
6. Core GB et al. Coronal facelift with endoscopic techniques. Plast Surg Forum 1992; 15:227.
7. Vasconez LO et al. Endoscopic techniques in coronal brow lifting. Plast Reconstr Surg 1994; 94:778.
8. Cho BC et al. Free latissimus dorsi muscle transfer using endoscopic technique. Ann Plast Surg 1997; 38:586.
9. Spiegel JH et al. Endoscopic harvest of the gracilis muscle flap. Ann Plast Surg 1998; 41:384.
10. Jacobovicz J, Lee C, Trabulsy PP. Endoscopic repair of mandibular subcondylar fractures. Plast Reconstr Surg 1998; 101:437.
11. Kobayashi S, Sakai Y, Yamada A, Ohmori K. Approaching the zygoma with an endoscope. J Craniofac Surg 1995; 6(6):519.
12. Lee CH, Lee C, Trabulsy PP. Endoscopic-assisted repair of a malar fracture. Ann Plast Surg 1996; 37:178.
13. Hayward JR, Scott RF. Fractures of the mandibular condyle. J Oral Maxillofac Surg 1993; 51:57.
14. Silvennoinen U, Raustia AM, Lindqvist C, Oikarinen K. Occlusal and temporomandibular joint disorders in patients with unilateral condylar fracture: a prospective one-year study. Int J Oral Maxillofac Surg 1998; 27:280.
15. Ellis E III, Palmieri C, Throckmorton G. Further displacement of condylar process fractures after closed treatment. J Oral Maxillofac Surg 1999; 57:1307.
16. Hall MB. Condylar fractures: surgical management. J Oral Maxillofac Surg 1994; 52:1189.
17. Members of the Chalmers J Lyons Club: Fractures of the mandibular condyle: a post-treatment survey of 120 cases. J Oral Surg 1947; 5:45.
18. Zide MF, Kent JN. Indications for open reduction of mandibular condyle fractures. J Oral Maxillofac Surg 1983; 41:89.
19. Walker RV. Condylar fractures: nonsurgical management. J Oral Maxillofac Surg 1994; 52:1185.

20. Ellis E III, McFadden D, Simon P, Throckmorton G. Surgical complications with open treatment of mandibular condylar process fractures. J Oral Maxillofac Surg 2000; 58:950.
21. Worsaae N, Thorn JJ. Surgical versus nonsurgical treatment of unilateral dislocated low subcondylar fractures. J Oral Maxillofac Surg 1994; 52:353.
22. Konstantinovic VS, Dimitrijevic B. Surgical versus conservative treatment of unilateral condylar process fractures. J Oral Maxillofac Surg 1992; 50:349.
23. Takenoshita Y, Ishibashi H, Oka M. Comparison of functional recovery after nonsurgical and surgical treatment of condylar fractures. J Oral Maxillofac Surg 1990; 48:1191.
24. Zide MF, Kent JN. Indications for open reduction of mandibular condyle fractures. J Oral Maxillofacial Surg 1983; 41:89.
25. Lee C, Stiebel M, Young DM. Cranial nerve VII region of the traumatized facial skeleton: optimizing fracture repair with the endoscope. J Trauma 2000; 48:423.
26. Bos RR, Ward Booth RP, de Bont LG. Mandibular condyle fractures: a consensus. Br J Oral Maxillofac Surg 1999; 37:87.
27. Thomson HG, Farmer AW, Lindsay WK. Condylar neck fractures of the mandible in children. Plast Reconstr Surg 1964; 4:452.
28. Leake D, Doykos J, Habal MB, Murray JE. Long-term follow-up of fractures of the mandibular condyle in children. Plast Reconstr Surg 1971; 47:127.
29. Lindahl L, Hollender L. Condylar fractures of the mandible. II. Radiographic study of remodelling processes in the temporomandibular joint. Int J Oral Surg 1977; 6:153.
30. Manson PN et al. Structural pillars of the facial skeleton: an approach to the management of Le Fort fractures. Plast Reconstr Surg. 1980; 66(1):54.
31. Gruss JS et al. The importance of the zygomatic arch in complex midfacial fractures and correction of posttraumatic orbitozygomatic deformities. Plast Reconstr Surg 85(6):878, 1990.
32. Lee Ch et al. A cadaveric and clinical evaluation of endoscopically assisted zygomatic fracture repair. Plast Reconstr Surg 1998; 101:333.
33. Chen CT et al. Application of endoscope in zygomatic fracture repair. Br J Plast Surg 1999; 53:100.
34. Gosain AK et al. The temporal branch of the facial nerve: how reliably can we predict its path? 1997; 99(5):1224.
35. Moss CJ et al. Surgical anatomy of the ligamentous attachments in the temple and periorbital regions. Plast Reconstr Surg 2000; 105(4): 1475.
36. Saunders CJ et al. Transantral endoscopic orbital floor exploration; a cadaver and clinical study. Plast Reconstr Surg 1997; 100(3):575.
37. Mohammad JA et al. Endoscopic exploration of the orbital floor: a technique for transantral grafting of floor blowout fractures. J Craniomaxillofac Trauma 1998; 4(2):16.
38. Chen CT, Chen YR. Endoscopically assisted repair of orbital floor fractures. Plast Reconstr Surg 2001; 108(7):2011.

39. Ikeda K et al. Endoscopic endonasal repair of orbital floor fracture. Arch Otolaryngol Head Neck Surg 1999; 125(1):59.
40. Chen CT et al. Endoscopically assisted reconstruction of orbital medial wall fractures. Plast Reconstr Surg 1999; 103(2):714.
41. Mun GH, et al. Endoscopically assisted transconjunctival approach to medial orbital wall fractures. Ann Plast Surg 2002; 49(4):337–343.
42. Jin HR et al. Endonasal endoscopic reduction of blowout fractures of the medial orbital wall. J Oral Maxillofac Surg 2000; 58(8):847.
43. Rhee JS et al. Intranasal endoscopy-assisted repair of medial orbital wall fractures. Arch Facial Plast Surg 2000; 2(4):269.
44. Lee HM et al. Endoscopic endonasal reconstruction of blowout fractures of the medial orbital walls. Plast Reconstr Surg 2002; 109(3):872.
45. Lorenz HP. Primary and secondary orbital surgery: the transconjunctival approach. Plast Reconstr Surg 1999; 103(4):1124.
46. Rohrich RJ, Hollier LH. Management of frontal sinus fractures: changing concepts. Clin Plast Surg 1992; 19(1):219.
47. Rohrich RJ, Hollier L. The role of the nasofrontal duct in frontal sinus fracture management. J Craniomaxillofac Trauma 1996; 2(4):31.
48. Graham HD III, Spring P. Endoscopic repair of frontal sinus fracture: case report. J Craniomaxillofac Trauma 1996; 2(4):52.
49. Lappert PW, Lee JW. Treatment of an isolated outer table frontal sinus fracture using endoscopic reduction and fixation. Plast Reconstr Surg 1998; 102(5):1642.
50. Forrest CR. Application of endoscope-assisted minimal access techniques in orbitozygomatic complex, orbital floor, and frontal sinus fractures. J Craniomaxillofac Trauma 1999; 5(4):7.
51. Onishi K et al. Endoscopic osteosynthesis for frontal bone fracture. Ann Plast Surg 1998; 40(6):650.

10

Orbital Injuries

Peter J. Taub
New York Medical College, Valhalla, New York

Henry K. Kawamoto, Jr.
UCLA School of Medicine, Los Angeles, California, U.S.A.

I. ANATOMY

A. The Bony Orbit

The orbits form the boundaries between the cranial vault and the lower face. They resemble two recessed pyramids, which house the eyes and their related structures (muscles, vessels, nerves, and lacrimal apparatus). Seven interdigitating bones contribute to create the bony orbit: the frontal bone, the zygoma, the maxilla, the ethmoid bone, the sphenoid bone, the palatine bone, and the lacrimal bone (Fig. 1). The outer rim, which faces the external environment, is composed of only three bones: the frontal bone superiorly, the zygomatic bone inferolaterally, and the maxilla inferomedially. Each bone is covered by periosteum, which is continuous with that lining the skull.

The floor of the orbit is formed mainly by the maxilla with contributions from the zygomatic and palatine bones. It separates the orbital contents from the more caudal maxillary sinus. The shape of the floor is concave anteriorly and convex posteriorly. The inferior orbital fissure runs between the floor and the lateral wall. Through this fissure, the infraorbital nerve (off the maxillary nerve, CN V_2) is transmitted. It runs anteromedially along the floor and exits through the infraorbital foramen in the maxilla.

The roof of the orbit is formed almost entirely from the frontal bone with a portion of the lesser wing of the sphenoid contributing to its posterior aspect. The bones in this region are thin and serve to separate the orbit from

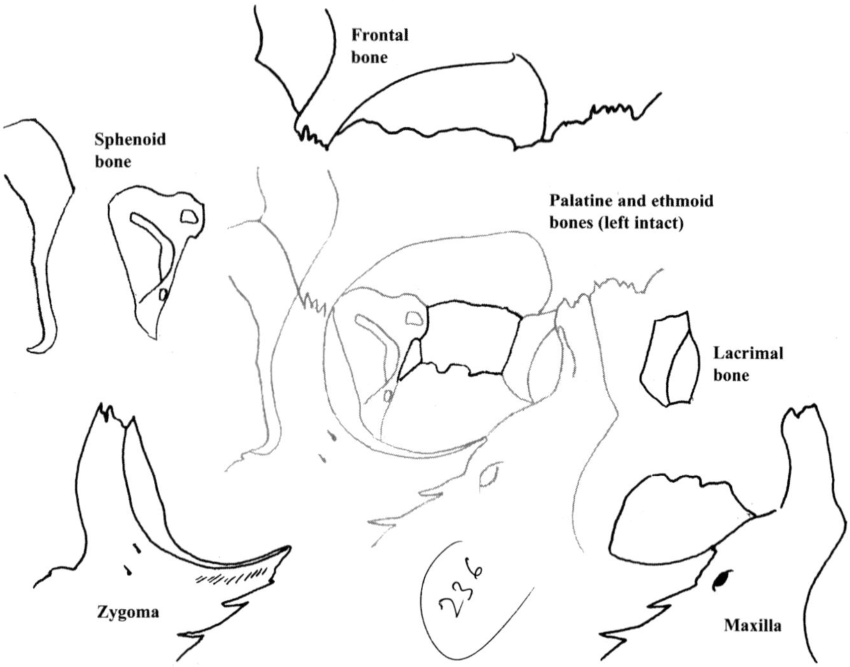

Figure 1 Intact (gray) and exploded (black) orbit demonstrating the positions of the seven bones that comprise the orbit.

the anterior cranial fossa and more medial frontal sinus. The roof is largely concave along its length.

The medial wall is the thinnest portion of the orbit. It is a paper-thin plate formed by four bones: the frontal bone superoanteriorly, the lacrimal bone inferoanteriorly, the sphenoid bone posteriorly, and the lamina papyracea of the ethmoid bone centrally. It separates the orbit from the more medial ethmoidal air cells and midline nasal cavity.

In the anterior portion of the medial wall, a vertical groove houses the lacrimal sac and nasolacrimal duct and is formed anteriorly by the maxilla and posteriorly by the lacrimal bone. The structures in this area are vulnerable to injury when the medial wall is fractured. The nasolacrimal duct terminates in the inferior conchal recess within the nasal cavity.

The lateral wall is the thickest portion of the orbit. It is formed by the frontal process of the zygomatic bone and the greater wing of the sphenoid bone. It separates the orbit from the middle cranial fossa posteriorly and temporal fossa anteriorly. The superior orbital fissure runs between the roof and the lateral wall. It communicates with the middle cranial fossa and is a conduit for several vital structures including: the oculomotor nerve (CN III), the trochlear nerve (CN IV), the abducens nerve (CN VI), branches of the first division of the trigemminal nerve (ophthalmic nerve, CN V_1), and the superior ophthalmic vein.

The apex of the orbit is the posterior termination of the bony orbital pyramid. While the medial walls lie parallel to each other, the lateral walls taper from lateral anteriorly to medial posteriorly. The lateral orbital walls form a 90° angle to one another, while the medial and lateral walls form a 45° angle. The optic canal at the apex of the pyramid transmits the optic nerve (CN II) and ophthalmic artery from the brain. The canal lies approximately 45–55 mm from the outer rim. Safe dissection is possible along most walls of the orbit for a distance of 25–40 mm.

B. Orbital Contents

The supporting structures of the globe include the extraocular muscles, their respective tendons, and the adipose tissue around the muscular cone. The volume of the orbit in the adult is approximately 35 mL. Any change greater than 3.5 mL (10%) is significant enough to produce enophthalmos.

The anterior globe is covered laterally by the sclera, which is a continuation of the dura mater of the central nervous system. A thin layer of bulbous conjunctiva, which is reflected anteriorly to line the superior and inferior fornices and inner lamellae of the eyelids, covers the sclera. Centrally, it abuts the more transparent cornea through which light is transmitted to the retina.

Within the orbit, six muscles move the globe through three axes (sagittal, horizontal, and vertical) and one muscle elevates the upper eyelid (levator palpebrae superioris). The four rectus muscles (superior, inferior, medial, and lateral) all arise from a common tendinous ring that surrounds the optic canal and the junction of the superior and inferior orbital fissures. Each muscle runs as a tangent to the globe inserting just behind the sclerocorneal junction. The medial and lateral recti lie along the same horizontal plane, while the superior and inferior recti lie along the same vertical plane. All are innervated by the oculomotor nerve (CN III), except the superior oblique muscle, which is innervated by the trochlear nerve (CN IV), and the lateral rectus muscle, which is innervated by the abducens nerve (CN VI).

The superior oblique muscle originates from the body of the sphenoid wing superior and medial to the common tendinous ring and inserts into the posterolateral portion of the globe. From its origin, it travels anterior and medial to the superior and medial recti, loops around a fibrocartilagenous structure in the superomedial angle of the orbital wall called the trochlea, and then travels posterior and inferior to insert on the sclera. Contraction of the superior oblique muscle serves to rotate the globe laterally and inferiorly.

The inferior oblique muscle is thinner than the more fusiform superior oblique muscle. It is the only extraocular muscle that does not arise from the common tendinous ring but rather from the anterior floor of the orbit. Thus, it is more prone to injury from inferior-rim fractures and blepharoplasty procedures. It travels posterior and lateral to insert on the sclera.

The levator palpebrae superioris muscle arises from the lesser wing of the sphenoid superior and anterior to the optic canal. It fans out above the upper hemisphere of the globe, becomes aponeurotic at the superior equator, and inserts into the skin and tursil plate of the upper eyelid. Contraction of the muscle elevates the upper eyelid.

The optic nerve (CN II) enters the orbit through the apex of the pyramid. It is surrounded by the common tendinous ring of the extraocular muscles. The ring is pierced in the 7 o'clock position (between the origin of the lateral rectus and the inferior rectus) by the motor nerves supplying the muscles (oculomotor to the medial, superior, and inferior recti and inferior oblique; abducens to the lateral rectus). The nerve itself enters the orbit through the superior orbital fissure. The trochlear nerve enters the orbit slightly more superior and lateral to the ring and supplies the superior oblique muscle.

Adipose tissue within the orbit is either contained within the cone of extraocular muscles or lies outside of it. Posteriorly, most of the fat is intraconal; anteriorly most of the fat is extraconal. In addition, a fine ligamentous system extends throughout the soft tissue of the orbit and serves to interconnect such structures (1). Loss of anterior, extraconal fat results in no significant change in globe position (2). Loss of posterior, intraconal fat, however, can produce clinically significant enophthalmos. The fine ligamentous network alone is incapable of maintaining the full forward position of the globe (3). Posteriorly, the weaker ligamentous support for the fat allows movement of fat from the intraconal position to the extraconal position. With the loss of posterior support, the length of the extraocular muscles can shorten over time and hinder anterior repositioning of the globe. Anteriorly, malposition of the globe allows extraconal fat in the superior aspect of the orbit to fall away from the upper eyelid to produce a characteristic hollowing in the supratarsal area.

C. Normal Orbital Relationships

The globe and orbit must be evaluated in several dimensions, including anteroposterior, lateral-medial, and superoinferior. The projection of the globe in the anteroposterior plane is determined by measuring the distance from the lateral orbital rim to the most anterior surface of the cornea. This is usually performed with a Hertel exophthalmometer. The normal distance in adults ranges from 16 to 18 mm.

The distance between the medial canthal tendons is termed the intercanthal distance (ICD). It measures approximately 28–32 mm in the adult, which roughly equals the palpebral fissure width. The lateral canthus should lie 2–3 mm above the medial canthus, creating a desirable palpebral slant approximately two degrees off the horizontal. The arc of the palpebral fissure usually follows the arc of the eyebrow. The ICD differs from the interorbital distance (IOD), which is the distance between dacryon as measured on posteroanterior cephalogram. Normally, this measures 24–32 mm in males and 22–28 in females. A third measurement is the interpupillary distance (IPD), which is approximately 55–65 mm.

II. EVALUATION AND DIAGNOSIS

A. Evaluation

Evaluation of the patient with periorbital trauma requires a thorough history and physical examination and appropriate radiological studies. In addition, a five-point ocular assessment was recommended by Gossman et al. (4). The five key items are (1) visual acuity, (2) pupillary function, (3) the anterior segment, (4) the posterior segment, and (5) ocular motility (Table 1).

Before visual acuity is tested, a history of the patient's preinjury function must be sought. Testing of near and distant vision should be performed. This can be done with preprinted acuity cards or more readily available package labels. After the initial test, the printed material used should accompany the patient or the chart so that follow-up testing may be performed. If the patient is unable to read any printed material, counting

Table 1 Five-point Ophthalmological Examination, as Proposed by Gossman to Evaluate Ocular Trauma Prior to Formal Ophthalmological Consultation and Surgical Intervention

1. Visual acuity testing	for afferent optic nerve injury
2. Pupillary reactivity testing	for afferent and efferent optic nerve injury
3. Anterior chamber inspection	for corneal laceration and hyphema
4. Posterior chamber inspection	brief demonstration of the red reflex elicited by light reflection off the retina
5. Extraocular muscle function	six fields of the visual axis

fingers and noting the maximum distance at which this can be accomplished should be documented. If the patient is unable to recognize objects such as fingers, the perception of light in all four quadrants should be documented with the contralateral eye occluded. Only when the patient is unable to perceive a bright light (such as from an indirect ophthalmoscope) should vision be declared absent.

Pupillary function should follow visual acuity testing since a very bright light may diminish its reactions. Baseline size, shape, and symmetry of the pupils in normal lighting should be recorded. Ability to accommodate should then be noted in a room with dim lighting. A bright light is focused on one eye and its response noted. Brisk contraction should be recorded as a normal response. The same eye is then retested while the contralateral eye is examined for a response. The light is then shifted and the test repeated on the contralateral eye. Next, the light is alternated between the two eyes while the pupillary response is noted. The first movement of each pupil will be *constriction* followed by slight *dilation* as the light is passed between the eyes. A poor direct reaction may be seen with trauma, glaucoma, iris incarceration, efferent oculomotor nerve injury, massive internal derangement, or optic nerve injury.

A defect in the afferent pathway will result in suboptimal contraction of the pupil with direct stimulation but brisk contraction when the light is shifted to the contralateral eye. This has been termed the "Marcus Gunn" pupil. During the alternating light test, the first pupillary movement noted is *dilation* followed by brisk *contraction* when the light is shifted to the contralateral eye.

Inspection of the anterior segment of the eye is performed by focusing a light slightly anterior and parallel to the plane of the iris and perpendicular to the sagittal plane of the eye. Abnormalities include the appearance of blood in the anterior chamber, alteration in the clarity of the cornea, and asymmetry of the depth of the anterior chamber.

The posterior segment can only be examined with an ophthalmoscope. Acutely, direct inspection may be performed to identify the presence of a red reflex, the absence of retinal folding, the appearance of the macula. When stable, the patient should undergo indirect ophthalmoscopy with pupil dilation by an experienced ophthalmologist.

The three axes of vision should be tested last, after the possibility of globe rupture has been eliminated. As the globe moves through each of the visual axes, any limitation in movement should be sought as this may indicate entrapment and require urgent treatment.

This five-point examination should be performed at the initial examination and repeated during the course of treatment. Loss of vision following fracture reduction is rare (5) but can result from impingement on the optic canal by fracture fragments, bleeding into either the globe or the posterior orbit, central retinal artery occlusion, or edema along the course of the nerve. Postoperative examinations should be carried out as soon as the patient is stable and coherent and serially over the subsequent 48–72 h.

Fractures of the posterior portion of the orbit can involve one or all of the nerves entering through either the optic canal or superior orbital fissure. Injury to all is termed "orbital apex syndrome." The result is inability to move the globe in any direction as well as visual loss. If vision alone is spared, the fracture pattern likely involves the superior orbital fissure and not the optic canal. This is termed "superior orbital fissure syndrome."

B. Diagnosis

Radiological studies to better delineate the nature and location of the injury include plain radiographs, standard and three-dimensional computed tomography (CT), magnetic resonance imaging (MRI), and orbital echography.

The least expensive and most readily available means for imaging orbital injuries is plain radiography. Standard projections include an anterior-posterior (AP) and a lateral projection that show the floor and posterolateral orbital wall. Special projections include the Caldwell view, which better highlights the superior and inferior rims, the medial walls, and the ethmoid and frontal sinuses, and the Waters view, which isolates the orbital roof and floor from surrounding structures. The optic canal can be visualized specifically on basal and oblique projections (6). Plain radiographs, however, have given way to CT as the gold standard.

CT scanning is currently the primary modality for imaging facial fractures, and more specifically, fractures of the orbit (7). While more expensive than plain radiography, its yield is vastly superior. CT scanning readily demonstrates most soft-tissue injuries (8). However, organic matter that becomes lodged in the orbit as a foreign body can be missed or misinterpreted (9). The standard study for facial trauma is 3-mm axial and coronal images without the addition of contrast material. Axial scans should begin at the superior aspect of the frontal sinus and end at the maxillary alveolus. Coronal scans should begin anterior to the nasal pyramid and end posterior to the orbital apex. Thinner, 1.5-mm slices can be obtained if optic nerve injury in the area of the canal is suspected. The data taken from a standard study may then be reformatted to generate a three-dimensional (3-D) image of the craniofacial skeleton. It has been proposed that the 3-D images provide greater spatial information, especially in patients with multiple fracture fragments, but they are not necessary for treatment (10). Plain slices better show the actual amount of displacement.

The drawbacks to CT scanning are the higher cost than plain radiography, higher radiation dose per study (especially if a 3-D reconstruction is requested, which may require up to 100 axial images), and the inability to take true coronal images in the patient with suspected cervical spine injury. Thin-cut CT scan of only the orbit exposes the patient to approximately 0.2–0.3 Gy of radiation, which is similar to a plain orbital series or a standard CT scan of the head.

Spiral CT scanning has been developed as an improvement to conventional techniques. The radiographic beam continuously travels around the patient as the patient is moved through the machine. It provides rapid scanning of a large area with thin slices that may be reformatted into accurate 3-D representations (11). With the more rapid scanning time, motion artifact and radiation exposure are reduced.

Although newer and more sophisticated, MRI remains a secondary study in the imaging of orbital trauma. It is less sensitive in depicting fracture lines and patterns around the orbit. It is, however, more sensitive in showing soft-tissue involvement and more reliably identifies foreign bodies such as wood within the orbit. MRI scanning absolutely is contraindicated in patients with ferromagnetic implants owing to the potential for acute, forceful implant extrusion and severe injury as a result of the study.

Orbital echography should be mentioned in passing but is rarely used as a diagnostic tool in orbital fractures. It is a safe, rapid, and noninvasive means of imaging soft tissues within the orbit (12). It is more reliable for anterior structures that might not be lost in the echoshadow of highly reflective fat and bone. However, it is a poor means for visualizing fracture lines and degrees of misalignment.

III. SURGICAL TREATMENT OF ORBITAL FRACTURES

Several surgical approaches to the orbit can be used alone or in combination, depending on the area of the orbit requiring reconstruction. They include: coronal, brow, lateral upper blepharoplasty, lower blepharoplasty (transcutaneous or transconjunctival with or without lateral canthotomy), and maxillary gingivobuccal sulcus incision (Fig. 2).

A. Orbital Floor

Fractures of the orbital floor were discussed in 1944 by Converse, who was an early advocate of bone grafting in the surgical management of such injuries (13). In 1956, Bordenare provided evidence that muscle and soft-tissue entrapment can occur as a result of orbital floor fractures and

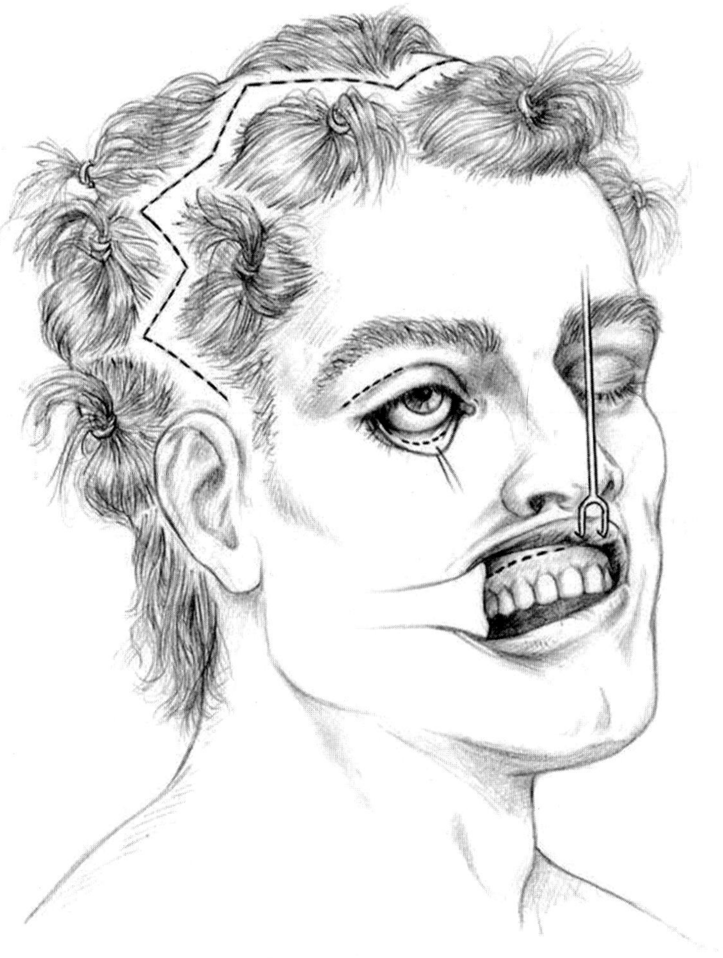

Figure 2 Surgical approaches to orbital fractures.

proposed this as a mechanism for the resultant diplopia seen with such fractures. The term "blowout" fracture was suggested in 1957 when Smith and Regan described fractures of the thin orbital walls. The term was first used to describe those injuries in which the orbital rim remained intact (14). Today, "pure" injuries imply isolated fractures of the floor that spare other components of the orbit. "Impure" injuries involve the floor as well as surrounding structures such as the infraorbital rim, zygoma, and/or maxilla (Fig. 3).

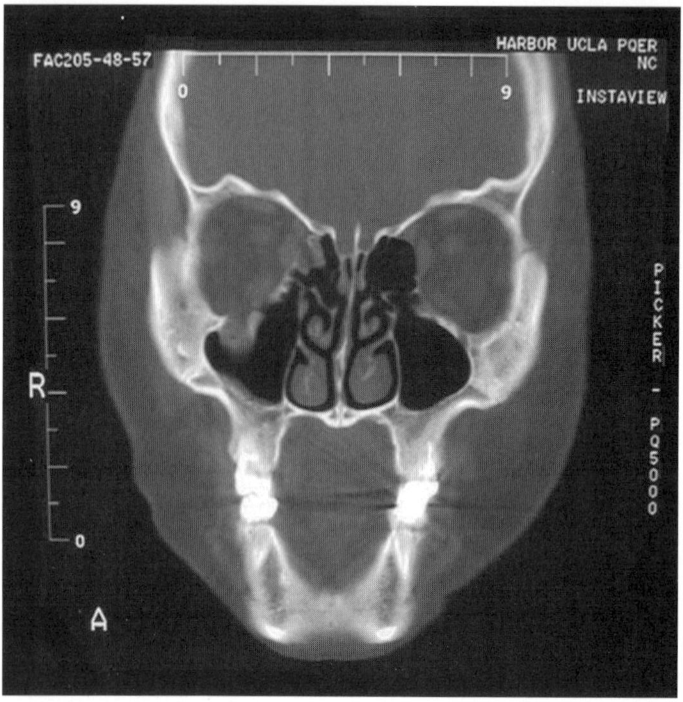

Figure 3 Coronal CT scan image of an orbital floor fracture.

The clinical manifestations of fractures of the orbital floor include signs of trauma, such as edema and ecchymosis, infraorbital nerve injury, from either contusion or disruption, and malposition of the globe. Dystopia refers to altered position of the orbit. Most commonly the globe is inferiorly (hypoglobus) and posteriorly (enophthalmos) displaced owing to the increase in bony orbital volume. The acute swelling of the periorbital tissues often masks the true globe position. Enophthalmos is then unmasked in the postoperative period.

The management of orbital floor fractures has historically been divided into conservative treatment (with delayed intervention for unresolved sequelae) and early surgical intervention. In 1947, Devoe published data supporting conservative management of orbital floor fractures (15). His position was supported by others, including Putterman, who went so far as to recommend that all blowout fractures be followed for 4–6 months before surgical intervention was considered (16). He found that most patients with visually handicapping diplopia resolved with time and none developed enophthalmos that was cosmetically unacceptable. Of note, however, 20% of patients with diplopia continued to have double vision with upward gaze and 20% had enophthalmos that was less than 3 mm. Late treatment was reserved for patients with functionally limiting diplopia and involved strabismus surgery for the diplopia and alloplast implantation for the enophthalmos. With the introduction of improved diagnostic imaging, the indications for surgical intervention are clearer.

Current indications for repair are related to either compromised extraocular muscle function or enophthalmos. Trapping of the inferior rectus muscle into the line of the fracture that prevents full globe retraction on upward gaze is a clear indication for exploration. It is easily tested by asking the patient to look through all six axes of the visual field as well as using forced duction and generation. The anesthetized conjunctiva is grasped in the anterior fornix with forceps and an attempt is made to rotate the globe upward. Inability to do so is termed a positive forced duction test. Then, with the globe in neutral gaze and the inferior rectus grasped, the patient is asked to look down. Shortening of the muscle, such that it retracts out of the forceps, is termed a forced generation. Minimal retraction out of the forceps, on the other hand, implies injury to the muscle with secondary paresis. A positive forced duction test (muscle entrapment) coupled with a negative forced generation test (inadequate retraction) is a definite indication for immediate surgical correction.

Further criteria for acute surgical intervention include enophthalmos of more than 2 mm, extensive soft-tissue herniation into the maxillary sinus, and unresolving diplopia (usually after 10 days of observation). Hawes and Dortzbach in 1983 reported that defects involving over 25% of the fractured orbital floor on CT resulted in enophthalmos (17). Often, however, the degree of enophthalmos is not readily apparent at the time of injury owing to the rapid swelling that accompanies soft-tissue injury. Marginal cases may be monitored for changes in diplopia, extraocular muscle motility, and enophthalmos. In the interim, they can be placed on a rapidly tapering dose of oral corticosteroids for 5–7 days as advocated by Millman et al., who reported faster resolution of diplopia (18).

Reconstruction of pure orbital floor fractures involves identification and reconstruction of the entire floor back to the intact posterior "shelf." Reconstruction of impure fractures additionally must identify and reconstruct the entire inferior orbital rim from stable bone medially. This is vital for avoiding postoperative dystopia and enophthalomos. The position of the globe is an inaccurate means of determining accurate reduction of the fracture because edema can mask a poorly reduced fracture. Thus, anatomical restoration of the skeletal framework is of paramount importance.

Reconstitution of the orbital floor requires a thin spacer to separate and support the orbital contents from the maxillary sinus. Many authors believe that autogenous tissue is superior to alloplastic implants in terms of durability, compatibility, and lower complication rate. Frequently used sources of autogenous bone include the calvarial vault, the rib cage, and the iliac crest. The maxillary antral wall and nasal septum have also been used. In thin individuals, a slight depression of the cheek can be seen if the antral wall is used (Fig. 4).

The list of alloplastic materials placed into the orbit to repair fractures is voluminous. It includes: metal (steel, titanium, Vitallium), Silastic (medical-grade silicone polymer) (19), Teflon (polytetrafluoroethylene, PTFE), polyglactin (Vicryl) (20), porous polyethylene (Medpor) (21), absorbable polydioxanone (22), absorbable polyglycolic acid (Lactosorb) (23), dehydrated human dura mater (24), and banked fascia lata (25). Popularity of these materials relates to their ease of use and absent donor site. Most

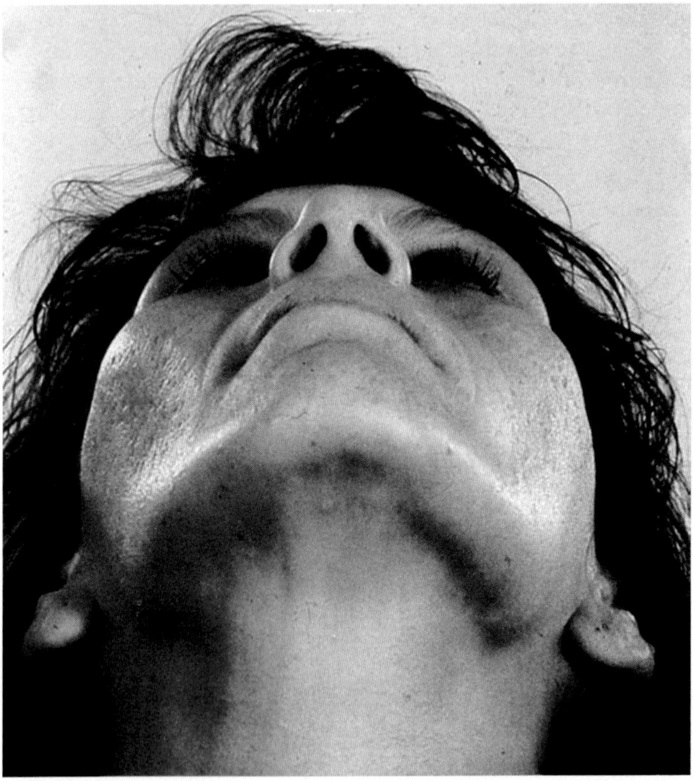

Figure 4 Clinical appearance of collapsed right malar region as a result of a defect in the anterior wall of the maxillary sinus.

come packaged, can be trimmed to fit the recipient defect, and be left forever barring any complications.

Numerous complications have been reported following the use of alloplastic implants for orbital fracture repair. These include: cellulitis, implant extrusion, optic nerve compression, dacrocystitis, hemorrhage (26), and late proptosis (27). Implant extrusion can occur many years after injury (28).

A novel approach to repair of orbital floor fractures recently has been described that utilized transantral endoscopy (29). A 4 mm endoscope introduced via a 1 cm^2 antromy was able to determine fracture size, location, and the presence of entrapped periorbital tissues, as well as assist in fracture reduction.

B. Orbital Roof

Orbital roof fractures account for approximately 5% of facial fractures (30). The superior orbital rim is dense and well supported and, therefore, is fractured only with high-impact trauma (Fig. 5). The more posterior roof is thinner and more prone to injury. While blowout fractures are seen, blowin-type fractures involve the roof more than any portion of the orbit. However, both types of fractures are equally common in this region of the orbit. The levator palpebrae superioris runs beneath a cushion of orbital fat and is frequently contused but rarely incarcerated with this type of injury.

Fracture of the orbital roof is suggested on radiological studies by the presence of pneumocephalus (31). This finding can be noted with penetrating and nonpenetrating injury. The frontal sinus must be examined closely to rule out fractures of the anterior and posterior tables of the sinus. Fractures of the orbital roof that involve displacement of the anterior wall of the frontal sinus require accurate reduction and fixation. Violation of the posterior wall of the sinus may or may not require intervention depending on the extent of dural and neurological injury. The posterior wall is rarely repaired but rather is removed to allow cranialization of the sinus. In this instance, removal of the mucosa and occlusion of the frontonasal ducts with bone graft must be performed to eliminate an ascending route of infection.

C. Medial Wall

Fractures of the medial orbital wall result from direct head-on trauma to the center of the face or orbit. Rarely do fractures in this region produce muscle incarceration requiring surgical intervention (32). In all cases, the integrity of the medial canthal ligament must be ascertained (Fig. 6).

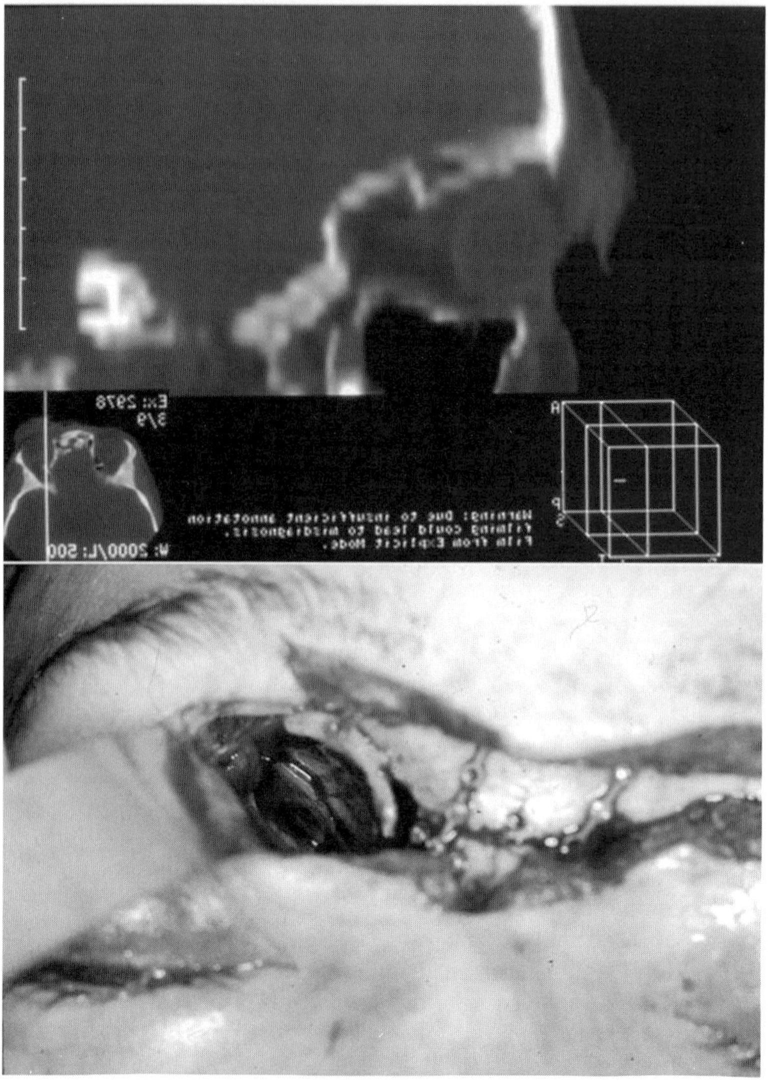

Figure 5 Axial CT scan image and corresponding intraoperative photograph of a patient with an orbital roof fracture.

More anterior fractures in this region may involve the naso-orbito-ethmoid complex (NOE). These fractures may produce shortening and retrusion of the nose, shortening of the palpebral fissure, telecanthus,

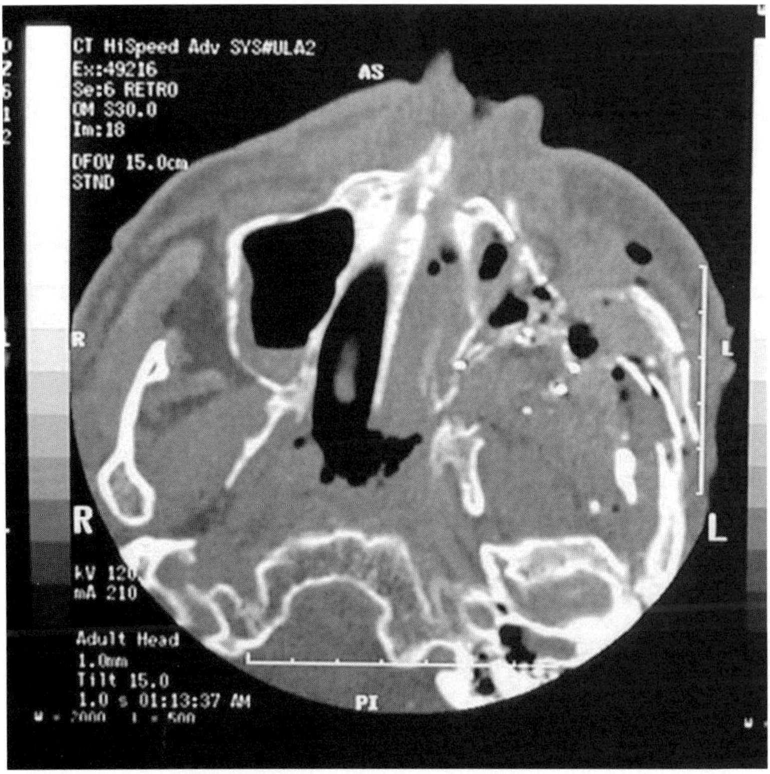

Figure 6 Axial CT scan image of medial orbital wall fracture.

enophthalmos, and ocular dystopia (33). The three patterns of NOE injury are incomplete, complete, and comminuted.

Fractures of the medial or lateral orbital walls can produce hypertelorbitism or telecanthus. Orbital hypertelorism refers to an increase in the distance between the true medial orbital walls as well as lateral displacement of the lateral wall. The severity may be classified into three degrees: 1° (30–34 mm), 2° (34–40 mm), and 3° (>40 mm) (34). Hypertelorism may be seen with certain craniosynostosis syndromes, such as frontonasal dysplasia and Crouzon, but is rare with orbital fractures. Telecanthus, on the other hand, refers to an increase in the distance between the two medial canthi.

Accurate reconstruction in this area is difficult. Treatment must restore projection of the midface and reconstruct the medial canthi. Displaced or mobile NOE fractures require open reduction and internal fixation. This may be accomplished by interfragmentary wiring or plate-and-screw fixation (with or without primary bone grafting). Exposure is obtained via a coronal incision although open lacerations may be utilized. Detachment of the medial canthal tendon is usually only necessary when the fracture extends into the point of insertion. Treatment must also correct any associated nasal deformity. Nasal projection will be lost if bone is lost centrally and not adequately replaced.

D. Lateral Wall

Fractures of the lateral orbital wall are quite common. They can result in either expansion or compression of the orbital volume (Fig. 7). The lateral rectus muscle runs immediately inside the greater wing of the sphenoid and is frequently contused after injury but is rarely incarcerated. Fractures of the lateral wall are often included in those involving the zygomaticomaxillary complex, which is discussed below.

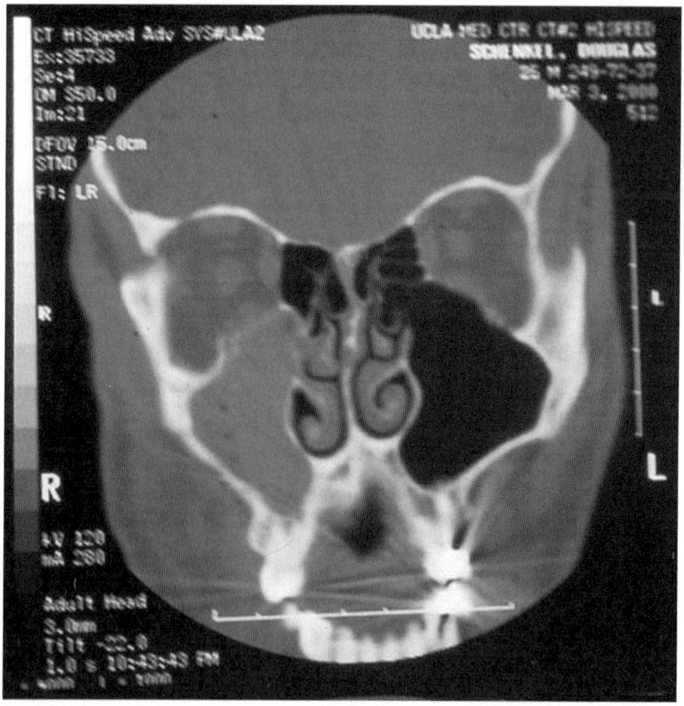

Figure 7 Coronal CT scan image of lateral orbital wall fracture.

E. Zygomaticomaxillary Complex Fractures

Historically, but inaccurately, the term "tripod′ fracture has been used to describe fractures involving the lateral orbital wall and adjacent structures (Fig. 8). A more accurate term is zygomaticomaxillary complex fracture (ZMC). Trauma of relatively low injury may result in fracture patterns that disarticulate the zygoma from the maxilla, frontal bone, temporal bone, and sphenoid bone. Higher-energy injuries result in comminution and rotational deformities.

ZMC fractures are relatively common. They often result from direct trauma as seen with sports-related injury. The injury may produce ecchymosis about the orbit and anesthesia in the distribution of the infraorbital nerve. Resultant depression or deformity of the malar region may not be readily apparent if edema is present.

Accurate reduction of these fractures requires direct inspection of the lateral orbital wall as well as the inferior orbital rim, orbital floor, anterior maxilla, and lateral buttress to identify any rotation. Associated orbital floor defects require additional bone grafting to prevent late enophthalmos.

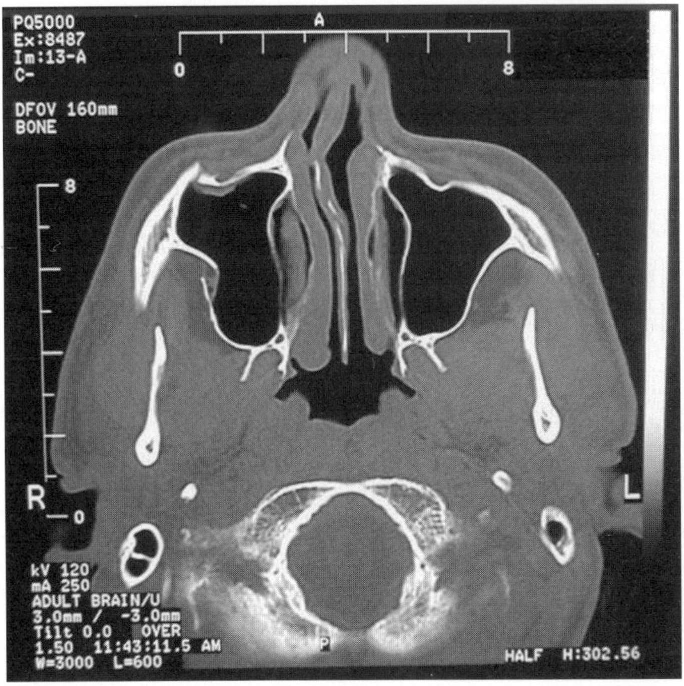

Figure 8 Sagittal CT scan image of a zygomaticomaxillary complex (ZMC) fracture.

F. Pediatric Fractures

In general, minimally or nondisplaced fractures in the pediatric age group may be treated conservatively. Those that are displaced sufficiently, however, will require reduction and fixation. Most often this requires open exposure and treatment follows guidelines similar to those used for adult injuries. The major distinction is the time to healing, which in children requires only 2–3 weeks as opposed to 4–6 weeks in adults.

Orbital fractures in the pediatric population are rare. The orbit does not reach its final form until the age of 8 years, at which time the facial

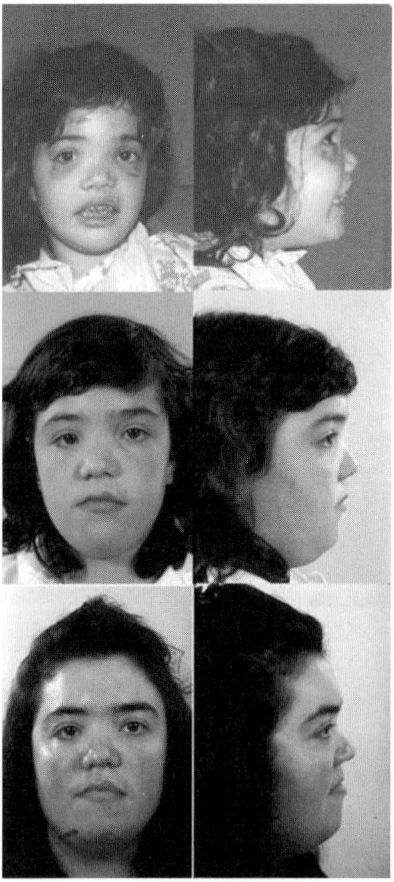

Figure 9 Clinical appearance of retarded bone growth in the adult following fracture as a child.

sinuses are still developing (35). The malleable bones of a child make their orbits less vulnerable to injury. Reports of fractures of the floor in children are sparse (36,37). A series by Posnick et al. revealed that isolated fractures of the floor of the orbit comprise less than 10% of all pediatric orbital fractures (38).

The frontal sinus plays an important role in pediatric roof fractures. In adults, impact to the superior orbital rim creates a force that is transmitted to the frontal sinus and is dissipated to reduce injury to surrounding structures. In children under the age of 7 years, the frontal sinus has not fully developed and these children are more prone to fractures of the roof than are older children with a pneumatized frontal bone (39).

A unique complication of pediatric facial fractures is underdevelopment (Fig. 9). Significant facial fractures have been shown to result in midface hypoplasia as a result of growth arrest (40). Unfortunately, no prospective study has been designed to evaluate the effects of trauma and craniofacial reconstruction in the pediatric population. One retrospective comparison to normal controls showed several changes as a result of childhood trauma. These include decreases in nasal projection, anteroposterior and vertical maxillary size, and upper facial height (41). Possible etiologies include scarring and fibrosis as well as periosteal stripping, which in turn contributes to a decrease in osteogenic potential (42).

IV. SOFT-TISSUE INJURIES

Injury to the orbit not only affects the bony framework but may involve the soft tissues with loss of vision being the most dramatic sequela. Trauma to the orbit results in 40,000 new cases of lost vision each year in the United States, making it the second leading cause of such injury (43). Prospective studies of facial fractures report a rate of approximately 10% (44). The more common injuries to the globe include corneal laceration and hemorrhage into the various chambers of the eye (hyphema, vitreous hemorrhage, retrobulbar hemorrhage, and choroidal rupture). Globe rupture and optic nerve injury are less common but more devastating injuries.

A. Injury to the Globe

Corneal injury is perhaps the most common sequela of ocular injury. Lacerations of the cornea produce photophobia and the sensation of a foreign body within the eye. Minor injuries are difficult to identify in the absence of fluorescein staining. More severe injuries may produce a shadow on the iris when a penlight is directed across the surface. In such instances, intraocular foreign bodies must be ruled out. Peripheral, self-sealing injuries produce almost no visual impairment. Frequently, topical antibiotics are prescribed to prevent secondary infection.

Posttraumatic ocular hemorrhage can occur in any of the various chambers of the eye. The term "hyphema" refers to bleeding into the anterior chamber of the globe. Clinically, this can impair vision initially, but improvement will be noted as the blood settles into the inferior recesses of the chamber. There may be photophobia and dull aching within the globe. Treatment involves prevention of rebleeding by controlling hypertension and maintenance of normal intraocular pressure. The risk of delayed bleeding, which manifests as sudden pain in the improving eye, is greatest within the first 5 days of injury (45). Hemorrhage may also be noted in the posterior chamber and retina, as well as in the postbulbar space causing compression to the surrounding vital structures.

Commotio retinae is seen on ophthalmoscopy as a gray-white opacification of the retina. It is the result of derangement of the outer layers of the retina as occurs with trauma (46). Most frequently, commotio retinae occurs in the temporal quadrants of the retina, but it can also occur around the macula.

Rupture of the globe is perhaps the most dramatic consequence of trauma to the orbit. Like optic neuropathy, this must be excluded prior to fracture reduction or soft-tissue repair. Subtle signs of globe rupture include eyelid perforation, subconjunctival hemorrhage or hyphema, asymmetry of the pupil, and vitreous prolapse. In all cases, a foreign body should be suspect and surgically removed by an experienced ophthalmologic surgeon. In the interim, the globe should be protected from further injury by a metal shield.

Injury to the optic nerve is diagnosed in the relatively normal eye with decreased vision and an afferent pupillary defect. Bone fragments, foreign bodies, blood, or edema can cause direct compression of the nerve along its course. Evaluation includes thin-slice CT scanning to differentiate direct and indirect injury to the optic nerve. Gossman et al. believe that orbital fracture repair should not be undertaken until optic neuropathy has been either ruled out or stabilized (4).

Spontaneous improvement with indirect injury to the optic nerve occurs in 25–30% of cases (47). Direct injury produces less gratifying results. High-dose parenteral steroids may be beneficial in cases of direct and indirect neuropathy. The steroids are maintained until a plateau is reached at which time the dose is tapered.

Surgical approaches to optic neuropathy have included hematoma evacuation alone, fracture reduction alone, nerve sheath fenestration, and decompression (either transcranially or extracranially). Indications for operative decompression include: (1) patients who do not improve after 5–7 days of steroid therapy, (2) condition that worsens on steroids after an initial improvement, (3) those with good vision after impact that then rapidly deteriorates despite steroid treatment, and (4) patients with contraindications to steroid administration. Joseph et al. have reported better than 75% recovery of vision in patients treated with extracranial, transethmoid optic nerve decompression (48).

B. Injury to the Surrounding Structures

Ocular trauma in the vicinity of the medial wall can produce injury to the lacrimal apparatus. Suspicion of such injury warrants careful examination of the wound for transected duct ends and specialized diagnostic studies. Application of fluorescein to the inferior fornix should produce fluorescein in the nasal cavity. In addition, injection of contrast material into the lacrimal sac may highlight the course of the nasolacrimal duct and the presence or absence of injury to the duct. The treatment of such injury should be primary repair if it is easily accomplished. This may be facilitated by intubation of the duct ends with a 0.025-OD silicone catheter. Cases in which the diagnosis is uncertain or the repair difficult may warrant observation alone. In such cases, delayed reconstruction by dacrocystorhinostomy is required in approximately 5–20%.

V. COMPLICATIONS OF REPAIR

Postoperative complications include diplopia, ectropion, and sinusitis. Diplopia is usually due to globe malposition or extraocular muscle imbalance. Ectropion of the lower eyelid is often a sequela of incisions placed in the lower eyelid. Early management involves taping of the eyelid for support and massaging the eyelid to soften the scar tissue.

A. Enophthalmos and Diplopia

In 1889, Lang correctly attributed orbital enlargement to the finding of enophthalmos (49). In 1943, Pfeiffer highlighted several additional causes of enophthalmos, including fat atrophy, soft-tissue fibrosis, neurogenic injury, and posterior and inferior soft-tissue incarceration (50). Today, we realize that posttraumatic enophthalmos is the result of inadequate reduction of orbital fractures that result in changes in the volume of the orbit. More commonly, the volume of the orbit increases and produces posterior and inferior displacement of the globe (enophthalmos and hypoglobus), rather than decreases, producing proptosis (exorbitism). Associated with any change in orbital volume there may be globe malposition and symptoms of diplopia.

The most common cause of posttraumatic enophthalmos is incomplete reduction of fractures involving the orbitozygomatic complex (Fig. 10). The malpositioned zygoma is usually inferior and lateral, producing an increase in the orbital volume. The globe secondarily assumes a dependent position in the orbit, which is too far posterior and too far inferior as compared to the contralateral eye. Careful physical examination will reveal deepening of the supratarsal fold and malposition of the lateral canthus.

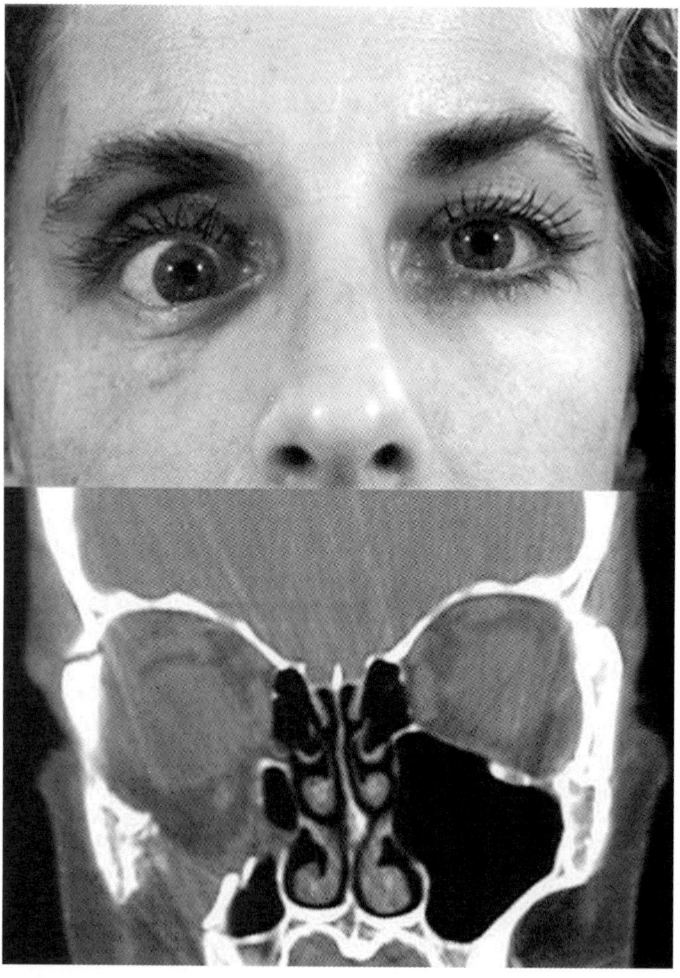

Figure 10 Clinical appearance of posttraumatic enophthalmos and hypoglobus.

Inadequate reduction results usually from failure to explore all components of the fracture. It is incorrect to assume that accurate reduction at the lateral orbital rim and inferior orbital rim will produce an adequate reduction. Rotation of the zygoma upon these two fixed points can still produce malposition of the fracture fragment. It is thus necessary to confirm reduction at least at a third point along the lateral buttress of the maxilla. This is easily achieved via a gingivobuccal sulcus incision and periosteal dissection along the anterior wall of the maxilla and buttress. Checking the alignment of the lateral orbital wall is another safeguard.

The other significant cause of posttraumatic enophthalmos is failure to recognize a concominant medial wall fracture. The bulk of the medial wall lies posterior to the globe so loss of periorbital contents into the ethmoid sinus will cause posterior displacement of the globe. Another minor contribution is the loss of orbital fat.

The most important step in managing postoperative enophthalmos is prevention. Accurate reduction and stable fixation of the fractures at the time of the initial injury will usually prevent posttraumatic enophthalmos. Secondary mild deformity may be corrected with autogenous bone graft (calvarial) to increase the posterior volume of the orbit. Prosthetic components (silicone, metal, or Medpore) also are used.

Severe malposition will manifest with significant cosmetic deformity of the globe. When the displacement of the zygoma is minor, the defects can be camouflaged with autogenous bone grafts or alloplastic material. Greater displacement warrants recreation of the fracture, repositioning of the fragment, and stable fixation with or without the use of autogenous bone grafts. This can be achieved with limited exposure via lateral upper blepharoplasty, transconjunctival, and intraoral incisions (51); however, a coronal approach is recommended unless the surgeon has considerable experience in managing these deformities (52).

The authors prefer to begin the fixation of the repositioned fracture fragment at the frontozygomatic suture with horizontally placed 26-gauge steel wire. Next, miniplates are utilized to stabilize the lateral buttress. Finally, the orbital floor and rim are addressed via the tranconjunctival incision.

REFERENCES

1. Koorneef L. Spatial aspects of the orbital musculo-fibrous tissue in man. Amsterdam: Swets & Zeitlinger, 1977.
2. Manson PN, Clifford CM, Su CT, et al. Mechanisms of global support and postraumatic enophthalmos. I. The anatomy of the ligament sling and and its relation to intramuscular cone orbital fat. Plast Reconstr Surg 1986; 77:193–202.

3. Manson PN, Ruas EJ, Iliff NT. Deep orbital reconstruction for correction of post-traumatic enophthalmos. Clin Plast Surg 1987; 14(1):113–121.
4. Gossman MD, Roberts DM, Barr CC. Ophthalmic aspects of orbital injury: a comprehensive diagnostic and management approach. Clin Plast Surg 1992; 19:71–85.
5. Ord RA. Postoperative retrobulbar hemorrhage and blindness complicating trauma surgery. Am J Oral Surg 1981; 19:202–207.
6. Nugent, R, Rootman J, Robertson W. Applied investigative. In: Rootman J, ed. Diseases of the Orbit. Philadelphia: Lippincott, 1988:35–48.
7. Bair AL, Wells RG, Massaro BM, Linder JS, Lewandowski MF, Harris GJ. Imaging in orbital trauma. Semin Ophthalmol 1994; 9:185–192.
8. Kelly JK, Lazo A, Metes JJ. Radiology of orbital trauma. In: Spoor TC, Nezi FA, eds. Management of Ocular, Orbital, and Adnexal Trauma. New York: Raven Press, 1988:247–269.
9. Roberts CF, Leehy PJ. Intraorbital wood foreign bodies mimicking air at CT. Radiology 1992; 185:507–508.
10. Gillespie JE, Isherwood I, Barker GR, Quayle AA. Three dimensional reformations of computed tomography in the asessment of facial trauma. Clin Radiol 1987; 38:523–526.
11. Lakits A, Steiner E, Scholda C, Kontrus M. Evaluation of intraocular foreign bodies by spiral computed tomography and multiplanar reconstruction. Ophthalmology 1998; 105:307–312.
12. Byrne SF, Green RL. Trauma and periorbital disease. In: Byrne SF, Green RL, eds. Ultrasound of the Eye and Orbit. St. Louis: Mosby-Yearbook, Inc, 1992: 431–461.
13. Converse JM. Two plastic operations for repair of the orbit following severe trauma and extensive comminuted fracture. Arch Ophthalmol 1944; 31:323.
14. Smith B, Regan WF. Blow-out fractures of the orbit: mechanism and correction of internal orbital fracture. Am J Ophthamol 1957; 44:733–739.
15. Devoe AG. Fracture of the orbital floor. Trans Am Ophthalmol Soc 1947; 45:502.
16. Putterman AM, Stevens T, Urist MJ. Nonsurgical management of blow-out fractures of the orbital floor. Am J Ophthalmol 1974; 77:232–239.
17. Hawes MJ, Dortzbach RK. Surgery on orbital floor fractures (influence of time of repair and fracture size). Ophthalmology 1983; 90:1066–1070.
18. Millman AL, Della Rocca RC, Spector S, et al. Steroids and orbital blow-out fractures. Adv Ophthalmol Plast Reconstr Surg 1987; 6:265–268.
19. Mauriello JA Jr, Antonacci R, Mostafavi R. Hinged silicone covered metallic implant for repair of large fractures of internal orbital skeleton. Ophthal Plast Reconstr Surg 1995; 11:59–65.
20. Mauriello JA Jr, Wasserman B, Kraut R. Use of Vicryl (polyglactin-910) mesh implant for repair of orbital floor fracture causing diplopia: a study of 28 patients over 5 years. Ophthal Plast Reconstr Surg 1993; 9:191–195.
21. Rubin PA, Bilyk JR, Shore JW. Orbital reconstruction using porous polyethylene sheets. Ophthalmology 1994; 101:1697–1708.

22. Konito R, Suuronen R, Suuronen O, Paukku P, Konttinen YT, Linqvist. Effectivenes of operative treatment of internal orbital wall fracture with polydioxanone implant. Int J Maxillofac Surg 2001; 30:278–285.
23. Hollier LH, Rogers N, Berzin E, Stal S. Resorbable mesh in the treatment of orbital floor fractures. J Craniofac Surg 2001; 12:242–246.
24. Guerra MF, Perez JS, Rodriguez-Campo FJ, Gias LN. Reconstruction of orbital fractures with dehydrated human dura mater. J Oral Maxillofac Surg 2000; 58:1361–1367.
25. Bedrossian EH Jr. Banked fascia lata as an orbital implant. Ophthal Plast Reconstr Surg 1993; 9:66–70.
26. Rosen CE. Late migration of an orbital implant causing orbital hemorrhage with sudden proptosis and diplopia. Ophthal Plast Reconstr Surg 1996; 12:260–262.
27. Stewart MG, Patrinely JR, Appling WD, Jordan DR. Late proptosis following orbital floor fracture repair. Arch Otolaryngol Head Neck Surg 1995; 121: 649–652.
28. Brown AE, Banks P. Late extrusion of alloplastic orbital floor implants. Br J Oral Maxillofac Surg 1993; 31:154–157.
29. Saunders CJ, Whetzel TP, Stokes RB, Wong, GB, Stevenson TR. Transantral endoscopic orbital floor exploration: a cadaver and clinical study. Plast Reconstr Surg 1997; 100:575–581.
30. Flanagan JC, McLachlan D, Shannon GM. Orbital roof fractures. Ophthalmology 1980; 87:325–329.
31. Hunts HU, Patrinely JR, Holds JB, Anderson RL. Orbital emphysema staging and acute management. Ophthalmology 1994; 101:960–966.
32. Converse JM, Smith B, Woodsmith D. Orbital and naso-orbital fractures. In: Converse JM, ed. Reconstructive Plastic Surgery. Philadelphia: WB Saunders, 1977:748.
33. Markowitz BL, Manson PN, Sargent L, Vander Kolk CA, Yaremchuck M, Glassman D, Crawley WA. Management of the medial canthal tendon in ansoethmoid orbital fractures: the importance of the central fragment in classification and treatment. Plast Reconstr Surg 1991; 87:843–853.
34. Tessier, P. Orbital hypertelorism. I. Scand J Plast Reconstruct Surg 1972; 6:135–155.
35. James D. Maxillofacial injuries in children. In: Rowe NL, Williams JL, ed. Maxillofacial Injuries. Edinburgh: Churchill Livingstone, 1985:538–557.
36. Converse JM, Smith B, Obear MF, Wood-Smith D. Orbital "blow out" fractures: a 10-year survey. Plast Reconstr Surg 1967; 39:20–32.
37. Bartkowski SB, Krzytkowa KM. Blow out fracture of the orbit, diagnostic and therapeutic considerations, and results of ninety patients treated. J Maxillofac Surg 1982; 10:153–164.
38. Posnick JC, Wells M, Pron GE. Pediatric facial fractures: evolving patterns of treatement. J Oral Maxillofac Surg 1993; 51:836–844.
39. Messinger A, Radowski M, Greenwald MJ, Pensler JM. Orbital roof fractures in the pediatric population. Plast Reconstr Surg 1989; 84:213–218.

40. Ousterhout DK, Vargervik K. Maxillary hypoplasia secondary to midfacial trauma in childhood. Plast Reconstr Surg 1977; 80:491–497.
41. Rock WP, Brain DJ. Effects of nasal trauma during childhood upon growth of the nose and midface. Br J Orthodont 1983; 10:38–41.
42. Munro IR. The effect of total maxillary advancement on facial growth. Plast Reconstr Surg 1978; 62:751–758.
43. National Society for the Prevention of Blindness: Fact Sheet. New York, 1980..
44. Jabaley ME, Lerman M, Sander HJ. Ocular injuries in orbital fractures: a review of 119 cases. Plast Reconstr Surg 1975; 56:410–418.
45. Parrish R, Bernadino V Jr. Iridectomy in the surgical management of eight-ball hyphema. Arch Ophthalmol 1982; 100:435–437.
46. Suppereley JO, Quigley HA, Gass JDM. Traumatic retinopathy in primates. Arch Ophthalmol 1978; 96:2267–2273.
47. Wolin MJ, Lavin PJM. Spontaneous visual recovery from traumatic optic neuropathy after blunt head injury. Am J Ophthalmol 1990; 109:430–435.
48. Joseph MP, Lessell S, Rizzo J, Momorse KJ. Extracranial optic nerve decompression for traumatic optic neuropathy. Arch Ophthalmol 1990; 108:1091–1093.
49. Lang W. Traumatic enophthalmos with retention of perfect acuity of vision. Trans Ophthalmol Soc UK 1889; 9:41.
50. Pfeiffer RL. Traumatic enophthalmos. Am J Ophthalmol 1943; 30:718.
51. Longaker MT, Kawamoto HK Jr. Enophthalmos revisted. Clin Plast Surg 1997; 24:531–537..
52. Kawamoto HK Jr. Established post-traumatic enophthalmos. In: Brent BD. ed. Artistry of Reconstruction Plastic Surgery. St. Louis:CV Mosby, 1987: 209–255.

11

Nasal Injuries

Seung-Jun O
Medical University of South Carolina, Charleston, South Carolina, U.S.A.

Seth R. Thaller
University of Miami School of Medicine, Miami, Florida, U.S.A.

I. INTRODUCTION

Nasal fractures are the most commonly encountered form of facial fractures (1). This is due to the central and prominent location of the nasal complex on the face. The nose is often the target of trauma whether it be directed or misdirected energy. In addition, the fragile nature of the nasal skeleton renders it more susceptible than the adjacent facial bones to trauma. The causes of nasal injuries are numerous but can usually be attributed to several etiologies. These include motor vehicle accidents, assaults/altercations, sporting injuries, and accidental trauma to the face. The widespread use of seat belts and air bags has decreased the incidence and severity of nasal injuries. Nevertheless, nasal injuries are still commonplace and their diagnosis and management continues to be a challenge for the treating physicians. The patients who sustain nasal fractures often delay seeking medical attention or fail to do so at all. Often, when patients are seen in the acute setting, they are evaluated and treated by the most junior house officer or a nonspecialist physician. The end result often is misdiagnosis and/or inadequate treatment leading to the undesired long-term sequela of nasal fractures. The focus of this chapter is to review some fundamental concepts in the diagnosis and management of traumatic nasal injuries.

II. ANATOMY

Nasal anatomy can simply be viewed as being comprised of three major components: (1) cover, (2) support, and (3) lining. However, the interaction of these anatomical components during the injury and the subsequent repair is a dynamic process that requires the surgeon to have a thorough understanding of nasal anatomy. The cover is the skin envelope that can be of variable thickness depending on the gender and ethnic origins of the patient. The density of the adnexal structures contributes to the texture of the skin and its ability to mask the underlying structures. Thick skin does not transmit the work done on the framework as much as thin-skin does. The framework is comprised of paired nasal bones and the upper and lower lateral cartilages. The septum, which is comprised of cartilage and bone, intimately interacts with the nasal bones and the cartilages contributing to dorsal support. When the septum is fractured or malpositioned, nasal aesthetics and function are compromised. The lining is composed of the mucosa of the nasal passages as well as the mucoperichondrium that covers the septum. Though often overlooked, injuries to the lining must be noted and accounted for especially when dealing with posttraumatic injuries resulting in a shortened nose.

III. CLASSIFICATION

Numerous classification systems for nasal fractures have been proposed (2–8). In 1929 Gilles described one of the first systems that was based on the vector of the impact that caused the nasal fracture (2). Correlation to the fractures that were sustained was not described limiting the clinical utility of this information. Becker's often-quoted study of 100 patients with nasal fractures is descriptive but its clinical applicability is minimal (3). Stranc and colleagues broadly categorized nasal fractures sustained from either a lateral blow or a frontal impact (4). They further subdivided the frontal-impact injuries into three groups according to the plane of injury. Plane 1 injury involves structure anterior to a line extending from the end of the nasal bones to the anterior nasal spine. Plane 2 injuries are limited to the external nose and do not have orbital involvement. Plane 3 injuries involve the nose as well as orbital and intracranial structures, much akin to a naso-orbito-ethmoid (NOE) fracture. Further discussion describing the clinical finding and management of these fractures is limited. Harrison's retrospective and cadaveric study yielded a four-tiered classification system for patterns of nasal fractures (5). He described a nasal fracture with lateral displacement without sepetal involvement usually the result of a lateral blow. Reduction of the nasal bones resulted in centralization of the septum. He further described fractures with lateral displacement and septal injuries. The pathomechanics of this type of fracture pattern is the result of a septal injury first followed by the bony injury. Treatment should address both the bony and septal injury for optimal results. Fractures of the nasal cap with a concomitant septal injury were the result of a direct frontal blow. Again both the septum and osseous components must be corrected to achieve good results. Severe frontal injuries with comminution and septal fractures should be treated in a similar fashion. Interestingly, Harrison, observed a consistent pattern of septal fracture and displacement. The septal fracture line involves the foot of the cartilaginous septum and passes vertically into the vertical plate of the ethmoid. The configuration is analogous to a reverse "C" and adequate treatment requires resection of both the cartilage and bone to straighten the septum.

Murray and associates reported a study performed in manner similar to Le Fort and midface fractures (6). Weights were dropped on cadaveric heads and the patterns of nasal fractures were described both anatomically and radiographically. Seven broad classifications were elucidated and optimal management often necessitates manipulation of the injured septum. The Haug and Prather classification of nasal fractures derived from a small series of patients includes septal fractures and correction with a closed technique (7). The patterns described are simplified and may limit use of the classification as a descriptive tool.

Pollock categorizes acute nasal injuries according to the "vault" that is injured (8). He divides the nasoseptal complex into the lower, middle, and upper vaults. The lower vault is made up of the alar cartilages and the inferior buttress of the septal cartilage. The injury pattern commonly seen involves a perpendicular caudal septal fracture with displacement or separation of the alar cartilages. Middle-vault injuries involve two predominant patterns of injury. Upward force causes a buckling of the septum due to perpendicular fractures that results in a zigzag fracture configuration. Frontal injuries create fractures in the septum parallel to the nasal floor with possible avulsion of the upper lateral cartilages. The upper vault is comprised of the paired nasal bones and the cartilaginous and bony septum. Patterns of injury range from simple nondisplaced fractures to frank comminution. Pollock describes the septal buttresses and their relationship with his classification of nasal fracture. He goes on to review the Brown-Grus vault compression test as a means to assess the degree of injury of the affected vault and its structural integrity following repair. A comprehensive classification of nasal fractures with widespread clinical applicability is an elusive target. These past reports each offer a descriptive tool to describe patterns of injury and the pathomechanics of their formation (2–8).

IV. ACUTE NASAL INJURIES

Most acute injuries are encountered in the emergency department and are usually the result of some antecedent trauma. A thorough history is the initial step in the management algorithm. The nature and direction of the inciting event should be elicited as well as the appearance of the nose in the preinjury state. Often an identification card can serve as a readily available photograph of the nose prior to the traumatic event. Otherwise, examination of preinjury photos should be viewed prior to operative intervention. As important as the appearance of the nasal deformity, any history of respiratory obstruction or difficulty should be obtained. Preinjury airway obstruction often indicates pre-existing underlying septal or turbinate pathology that may not be corrected with some closed-reduction techniques.

A thorough nasal examination should not preclude a systematic trauma evaluation. The examiner should always be cognizant of concomitant maxillofacial or cervical spine injuries especially in a multiply injured patient. When the patient has rhinorrhea, the presence of a cerebrospinal fluid (CSF) leak should suspected and appropriately diagnosed and treated. External lacerations and nasal deformities such as deviations should be noted. If there has been a delay in seeking medical attention, external deformities are often not readily apparent owing to soft-tissue edema. A comprehensive intranasal examination should be performed with good lighting and a nasal speculum. The use of an endoscope can be very helpful with the intranasal examination especially when evaluating the posterior septum. The use of a vasoconstrictor spray can temporarily reduce the edema and help with the visualization of any mucosal rents, septal perforation, and septal hematomas. Palpation of the framework should be directed for bony stepoff, mobile cartilaginous structures, and crepitus.

V. RADIOLOGY

Several studies have examined the role of plain film radiographs in the evaluation of nasal fractures (9–11). The impact of routinely obtaining x-rays of suspected nasal fractures raises some interesting questions. The interpretation of plain nasal films is fraught with inaccuracies and misdiagnosis. It is not uncommon to miss hairline fractures or interpret vascular markings as fractures. In addition, whether the fracture in question is an acute injury or a healed fracture can be difficult to discern. Nigam and colleagues found a sensitivity of 63.3% and a specificity of 55.7% of detecting nasal fractures with plain radiographs (10). Thus with a significant number of both false positives and false negatives the validity of such studies even in a medicolegal arena is suspect. This should preclude the use of plain nasal films for medicolegal purposes since the interpretation of nasal radiographs is unreliable (11). Finally, the financial burden placed on the facility includes not only the cost of the film and equipment but also the labor of obtaining the film and its interpretation. Therefore, the role of plain radiography in evaluating nasal fractures is of little value and the diagnosis must be made clinically based on a thorough history and physical examination.

Other imaging modalities such as computed tomography (CT) can give excellent information regarding facial fractures including septal fractures. This can be useful, especially when evaluating patients with complex NOE fractures. However, routine use of CT to examine nasal fractures in the absence of other suspected facial bone fractures or intracranial pathology is not indicated and should not be done. Hirai and colleagues reported the use of high-resolution ultrasonography to examine facial fractures including nasal fractures (12). Imaging nasal fractures with ultrasonography, with all its advantages, is an attractive concept. However, its use is limited and has not been validated as an accurate means of examining nasal bone fractures. Therefore, the routine use of radiographic imaging of isolated nasal fractures is not indicated and should be reserved for patients with multiple facial fractures.

VI. TREATMENT OF ACUTE NASAL INJURIES

Once a diagnosis has been made, treatment initially entails stabilization of the acute injury. All external lacerations should be thoroughly cleansed with saline irrigation and repaired. Internal mucosal rents and tears should be identified and, if significant, packed with antibiotio-ointment-impregnated gauze. Untreated mucosal injuries can result in the formation of synechiae or webs that can cause airway obstruction. It is of paramount importance that any septal hematoma be identified and appropriately drained. If a septal hematoma is identified, the hematoma is drained via a hemitransfixion at its most dependent portion with a knife blade. Nasal packing offers some degree of compression and can be placed to reduce recurrence of the hematoma. An undrained septal hematoma can result in pressure necrosis of the cartilaginous septum with resultant scarring and loss of dorsal support. If significant dorsal support is lost, a "saddle nose deformity" may occur.

A. Closed Versus Open Reduction

Nasal bone fractures can be treated by either closed or open techniques. Prior to choosing a method of reduction, the status of the septum must be established. If the septum is fractured and displaced, attempts at closed reduction often result in unsatisfactory results. Closed treatment should be reserved for simple unilaterally displaced nasal fractures without any significantly displaced septal fractures. Results following closed reduction have been examined in some past reports. Crowther and O'Donoghue reported the result of closed reduction of nasal fractures with 85% of the patients satisfied with their nasal appearance (13). A Danish study reported similar favorable long-term results at 3 years following closed reduction of nasal fractures (14). These past reports suggest that in the appropriate patient closed reduction can be an extremely useful modality to treat simple nasal fractures with significant septal pathology.

B. Closed Reduction

The timing of closed reduction for nasal fractures is determined by the stability of the patient and the time elapsed since the injury. Soft-tissue swelling, which can occur 6 h postinjury, generally precludes immediate attempts at reduction if presentation is delayed and should be deferred 4 or 5 days until the resolution of nasal edema. Delayed attempts at reduction should be done before fracture healing occurs, which takes 2–3 weeks. An exception may be the patient with a severe traumatic injury and delayed presentation (up to 4 weeks). Such a patient may benefit from an attempt at osseous reduction with subsequent septorhinoplasty at a later date. Caution must be exercised not to worsen the injury by comminuting the remaining bony segments. The early realignment of the bony components allows for healing in the anatomical position and may obviate the need for major osteotomies and bony respositioning at the time of septorhinoplasty. Attempts at closed reduction can be done in the emergency department or office. However, closed reduction in the operating room with the aid of general anesthesia can be less traumatic for the patient and the surgeon, especially in children or patients with a low threshold for pain.

Proper instrumentation is critical when performing closed reduction of nasal fractures. After the instillation of a local anesthetic and a vasoconstrictor spray, a Boies elevator or scalpel blade handle, with digital counterpressure, is used to reduce a depressed lateral nasal fracture. Impacted lateral fracture segments can be reduced with the aid of Walsham forceps. Closed reduction and manipulation of septal dislocation can be performed with Asch forceps. If a septal dislocation or fracture does not reduce with attempts at closed reduction, septoplasty with submucous resection may be indicated. Temporary nasal packing and external splintage will help maintain reduction and provide protection. Early and frequent monitoring in the office can allow for detection of bony malposition that may be amenable to minor adjustments.

C. Open Reduction

The indications for open reduction of nasal fractures include severe and/or bilateral injury with significant septal involvement. Proper diagnosis and management of septal injuries is fundamental to the correction of these injuries. The distinction between open reduction and open rhinoplasty may be semantic; however, it must be made. The primary goals of open reduction are to restore the preinjury anatomical relationship and airway. Access for open reduction can be done with endonasal incisions, external incisions, traumatic lacerations, or a combination of the aforementioned. Traditional endonasal or closed incisions include intercartilaginous, intracartilaginous, infracartilaginous, and marginal incisions. Open approaches can be done via the transcolumellar, paranasal, and coronal incision. A laceration sustained at the time of injury can also serve as an access portal to perform the reduction. Reduction of fracture segments should be done with the least amount of disruption of the periosteum and mucosa. Fixation can be obtained with miniplates and screws as well as interfragmentary wires. Nasal packing, internal splints, and external splints can provide temporary protection following the operation.

VII. MANAGEMENT OF SEPTAL INJURIES

Treatment of the deviated septum is critical to the success of restoring nasal appearance and function. The nasal septum is intimately associated with the paired nasal bones, upper lateral cartilages, and lower lateral cartilages. Therefore, injuries and deformation of the nasal septum directly affect the appearance and function of the nasal complex. Fry in his classic report further elucidated the potential effects of deforming forces on septal cartilage, which he termed "interlocked stresses" (15). He built upon earlier works of Gibson and Davis on costal cartilages, and stated that septal trauma may cause the release of these deforming forces resulting in septal deviation (16). These past reports suggest that septal injury whether partial or a complete dislocation can result in septal as well as external nasal deformation.

Many techniques have been described to address septal deformities (17–23). Freer described a technique of radical submucous resection including the quadrangular cartilage and vomer-ethmoid complex (17). This approach was modified by Killian, who retained a supporting caudal and dorsal strut (18). The concept of retaining an "L"-shaped strut that provides both dorsal and caudal integrity has been advocated by others (19). Techniques for septoplasty were described by Cottle to treat the deflected septum (20). Numerous modifications have since been described and offer some degree of success in treating the deviated septum. Gruber and Lesavoy describe an interesting method of septal repositioning utilizing a nasal speculum to fracture the bony septum and the turbinates (21). Techniques employing complete septal removal with extracorporeal modifications and replacement have also been described to treat severe septal deviations (22,23).

The approach to septal injury is directed toward the degree and location of the pathology and does not rely on one method of correction. Open approaches allow for easier visualization of the anatomy. In addition, the less experienced surgeon may find this approach more reproducible and comfortable. However, Killian incisions can be used to address simple septal injuries and should provide more than adequate exposure. The use of hydrodissection by the instillation of local anesthetic in the subchondral plane markedly lessens the difficulty of the subperichondral dissection. Reduction of the dislocated septum to the vomerine groove and judicious submucous resection are operative principles that must be adhered to. The presence of a bony spur at the base of the septum should be resected. Spreader grafts placed between the upper lateral cartilages and nasal septum can correct misalignment and airway obstruction. Internal splints (Doyle) as well as through-and-through mattress sutures with plain gut on a Keith needle may obviate the need for nasal packing.

Correction of the deviated septum following nasal injury is fundamental to the restoration of nasal appearance and function. The treatment of acute nasal injuries should follow the reparative ladder. Simple injuries without significant septal injury may require only closed reduction, whereas complex injuries may necessitate formal septorhinoplasty. Management algorithms should provide a systematic means of diagnosing and treating acute injuries. However, they should not replace common sense and sound clinical judgment.

VIII. LATE POSTTRAUMATIC DEFORMITY

Untreated or improperly treated nasal injuries can lead to some of the most challenging and difficult secondary deformities even for the most experienced surgeons. These deformities include: the twisted nose, the saddle nose deformity, and the short nose. Posttraumatic nasal deformities do not adhere to classification schemes, but present with facets of multiple deformities.

A. Twisted or Crooked Nose

Classically, the twisted nose, can be defined as a deviation of the nasal complex form the midline when viewed from the AP plane. The pathology of the underlying structure translates to the external appearance of the nose. The key component of the twisted nose is the fractured nasal septum and often involves both the cartilaginous and bony septum. The intimate relationship of the nasal support structures (i.e., the nasal bones, septum, and cartilages) has a causal relationship when one or all of them are injured. Therefore, injuries to the septum result in distortion of the attached nasal bones and upper lateral cartilages.

Many different techniques have been described to straighten the twisted nose. Simply put, these approaches have been a restorative model with anatomical reconstruction with or without camouflage techniques. Reconstructive techniques are based on attempts at restoration of normal septal and bony anatomy and usually entail some form of septoplasty with osseous repositioning (24–27). Gunter and Rohrich emphasize the importance of septal reconstruction in their management of a deviated nose (25). Their techniques are based on the following principles: (1) complete mobilization of all deviated structures, (2) maintenance of as much mucoperichondrial attachment as possible, (3) maintenance or restoration of septal support, and (4) precisely planned osteotomies. They limit their bilateral mucoperichondrial dissection to areas of submucous resection and otherwise perform it in a unilateral fashion on the remaining portion of the septum. Other techniques described include: swinging-door septal flaps, used to straighten caudal deflection; septal release with internal splints, used to correct dorsal L-strut angulations; and suture stabilization of fractured L struts.

Byrd and associates describe their techniques that entail release of the deforming forces by releasing the lower lateral cartilage from the upper lateral cartilage at the adherent scroll area (26). Further mobilization of the septum is initially done sharply and completed with an elevator to extensively mobilize the septum. Release of the upper lateral cartilages from the septum provides the exposure to perform quadrangular cartilage resection. They advocate the use of "Mustarde"-type suture to straighten cartilage convexities. Spreader extension grafts are placed on the concave side and batten grafts are placed on the convex side of the dorsal septum to further straighten the L strut. In a report by Courtiss, he correctly points out that septal cartilage has incredible memory and the septal deflection can recur with time. He further asserts that inferior turbinate hypertrophy must be corrected at the time of surgery to optimize airway patency (24). Although the concept of anatomical reconstruction of the injured components sounds attractive, it is fraught with less than ideal results even with the most properly designed and executed operation. Overmanipulation or handling of the dorsal septum can result in weakening of an already damaged septum and can lead to dorsal collapse. Therefore, dorsal septal structural integrity must be preserved as much as possible or reinforced with grafts.

Other authors advocate the use of camouflage techniques with onlay graft to mask deformities (28–30). Traditional septoplasty techniques and osteotomies are performed to achieve general alignment and restore the airway. According to McKinney, recurrent deviation and a smaller-appearing nose can occur postoperatively (28). He describes a technique using onlay grafts with septal cartilage to correct dorsal- and middle-vault deficiencies. Similarly, Gilbert describes a technique of overlay grafting of lateral wall concavities with both autogenous tissues and nonautogenous implant materials (29). Constantian's technique focuses on restoring balance between the nasal dorsum and base with a combination of resection and augmentation (30). He minimizes dorsal resection and manipulation to preserve dorsal septal integrity and adds graft to conceal the residual deformity. The addition of radix grafts further reduces the amount of dorsal reduction, thereby preserving dorsal support. Tip grafts, lateral wall grafts, and spreader grafts are also used to restore a balanced appearance.

B. Saddle Nose Deformity

Loss of the dorsal nasal concavity is characteristic of saddle nose deformity. Though there are numerous etiologies for this deformity, posttraumatic causes are the result of loss of dorsal support. This dorsal concavity is usually the result of damage to both the cartilaginous and bony support secondary to the traumatic insult. Unrecognized septal hematomas can result in pressure necrosis of the cartilaginous septum and lead to a saddle nose deformity. It is not uncommon for nasal shortening to occur with a saddle nose deformity; however, the classic saddle nose deformity does not involve tip malposition. When tip rotation and increased nasolabial angle occur with a saddle nose deformity this is known as a porcine deformity.

Treatment has been primarily focused on augmenting the nasal dorsum. Both closed and open approaches are utilized to augment the nasal dorsum. If a complex defect requires extensile exposure, an open approach may facilitate the operation and is advocated by some authors (31,32). Through the years a plethora of material has been tried including nonautogenous materials (gold, ivory, leather, titanium, homograft cartilage, and bone) and are mentioned for historical purposes (33). Newer materials have also been tried including silicone, Supramid mesh, Mersilene mesh, Proplast, and Gore-Tex. The use of Gore-Tex has increased in popularity and it is commonly used to augment nasal deficiencies (34–36). The use of autologous tissues has been primarily focused on soft tissue, cartilage, and bone. Soft-tissue fillers, including fat, dermis, and SMAS, have all been used but are plagued with problems such as lack of structural support and propensity for resorption (36). Cartilage grafts from the auricle, septum, and rib have

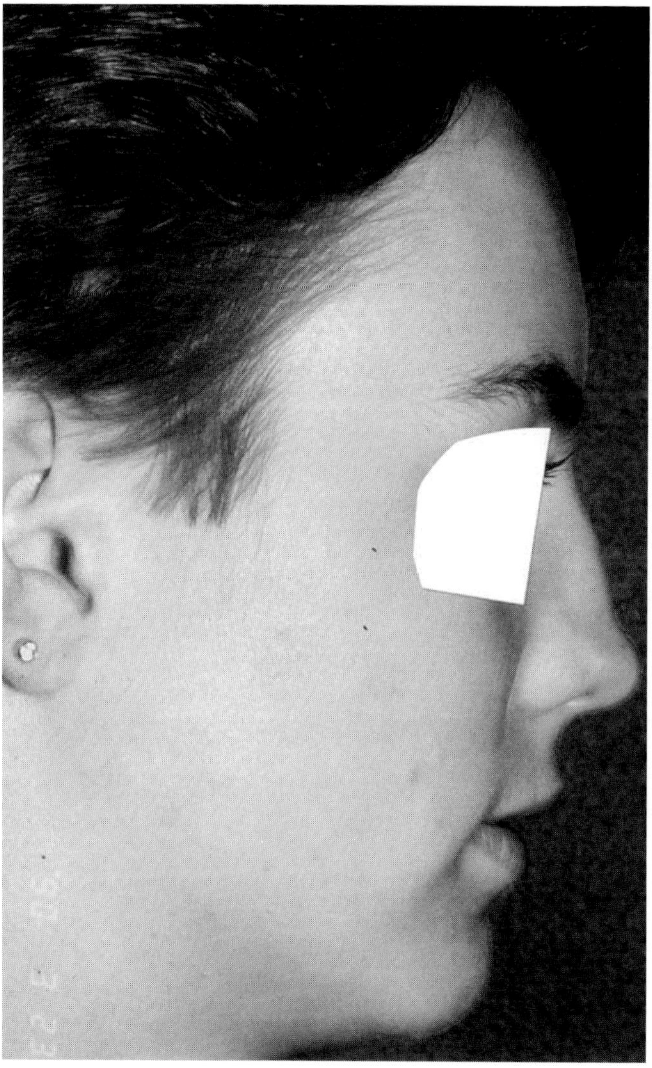

Figure 1

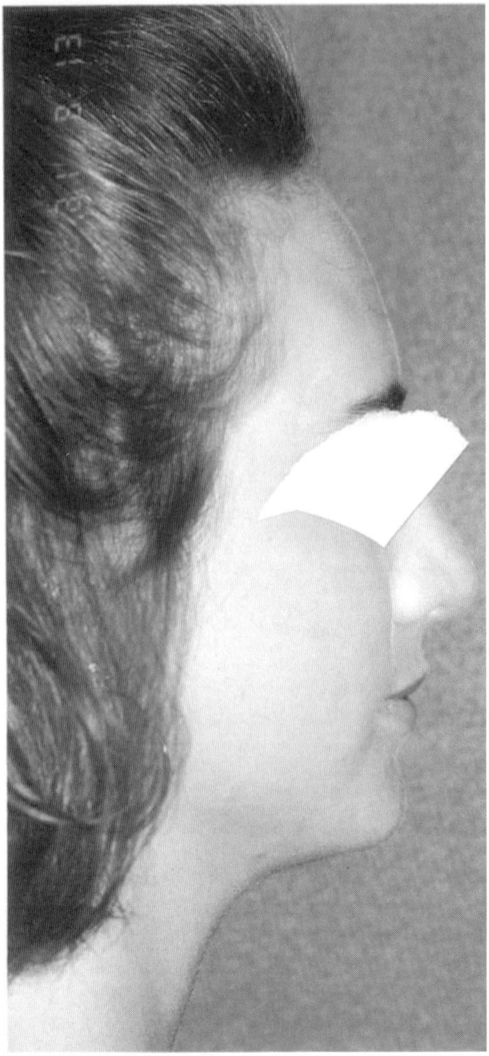

Figure 2

also been used and are championed by some authors (37–39). Auricular and septal cartilage may be appropriate for smaller defects but may not suffice for significant depressions that can be corrected with costal cartilage (Figs. 1,2). The primary concern with cartilage grafts centers around their propensity to warp or deform over time (16,40). To address this issue, Furlan recommends the usage of the anterior free extremities of the eighth and

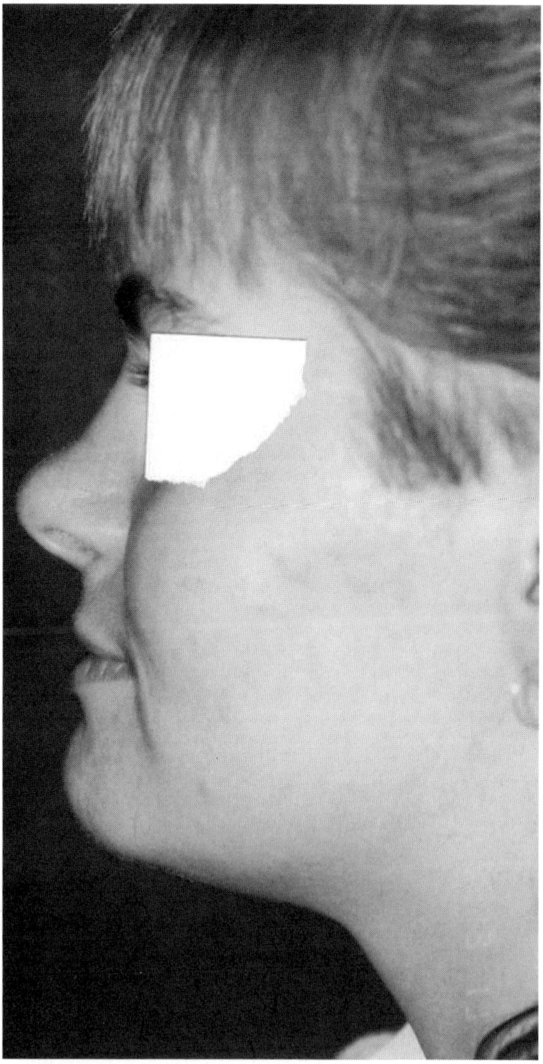

Figure 3

ninth ribs with an intact perichondrium (41). Others have used bone graft from various locations including tibia (42), iliac crest (40), rib (43), and calvarium (44) to correct the saddle nose deformity (Figs. 3,4,5). Calvarial bone grafts, which are readily obtainable from the same operative site and demonstrate less resorption than endochondral bone (45), have become

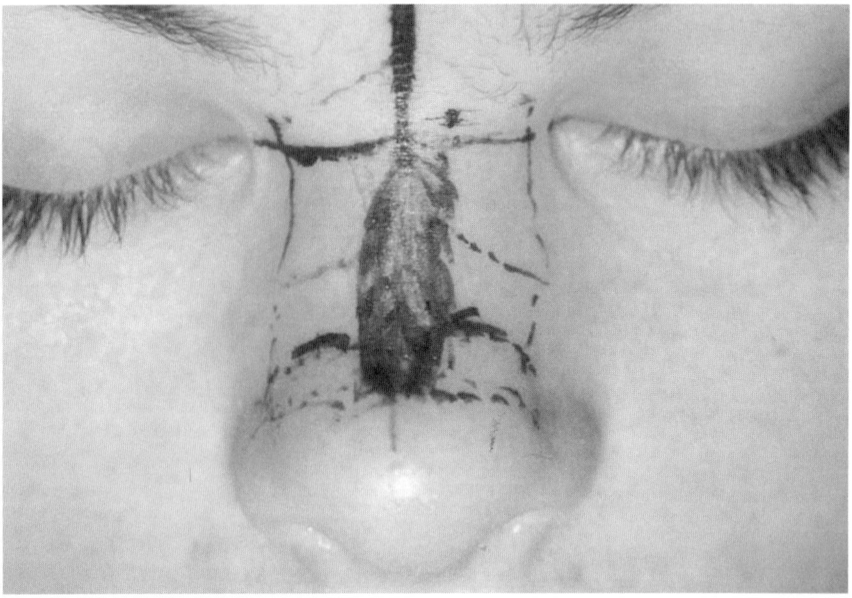

Figure 4

the donor site of choice for bone grafting. The debate over calvarial bone graft and costal cartilage may not have a clear winner. Both have been effectively used to correct saddle nose deformities and have well-known advantages and disadvantages. The surgeon should base his choice of augmentation material on his/her comfort level with the graft and ability to obtain the graft.

C. The Short Nose

As was started earlier, nasal shortening often occurs with a saddle nose deformity. The "short nose" is characterized by decreased nasal length with a deprojected and overrated tip. This deformity manifests with a decreased distance from the nasion to the tip-defining point on the frontal view and an increased nasolabial angle on the lateral view. The cause of a short nose is often multifactorial and can result from loss of dorsal support as with a saddle nose deformity, as well as weakening or loss of lower lateral cartilage support. The significant contribution of circatrial changes to the skin envelope and mucosal lining must also be taken into consideration in post-traumatic nasal shortening.

Many treatments of the foreshortened nose have been described and entail methods of nasal lengthening and tip derotation (46–51). Gunter's method of nasal lengthening involves derotating the tip complex by wide undermining of the skin, complete mobilization and detachment of lower lateral cartilages, and a compensatory caudal dorsal

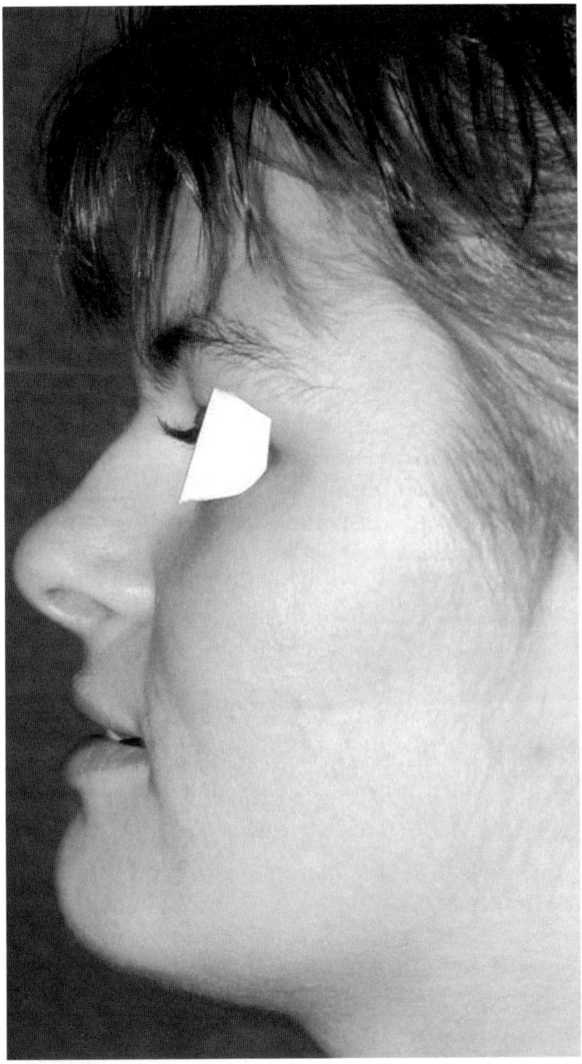

Figure 5

reduction (46). When necessary, tip grafts are used to augment tip projection and add to the illusion of nasal lengthening. Kamer extended nasal length by the insertion of composite auricular grafts to the septum that have been incised in a staggered fashion to release the septocolumellar unit (47). However, tip derotation and support are not specifically addressed. Giammanco employed a staged approach by extending the caudal septum with an anterocaudally based composite septal graft (48). Intercartilaginous deficits were addressed with composite auricular graft interposed between the lower lateral and upper lateral cartilages on the mucosal side. The second stage entailed the placement of dorsal graft with septal cartilage and bone for augmentation.

Gruber's procedure involved several key elements: (1) complete mobilization and release of skin envelope and cartilages, (2) staggered bilateral releasing incisions of the septal mucoperichondrium, and (3) batten grafts to extend nasal length (49). Tip grafts, tip suture techniques, and interpositional composite grafts were added when the need for additional length was encountered. Dyer's method, with the addition of columellar strut graft to extended spreader grafts that control tip placement, is aptly named dynamic adjustable rotation tip tensioning (DAART) (36). Naficy and Baker's "flying buttress graft" is similar but further describes the use of radix graft as well as intercartilaginous interposition grafts (50). Wolfe's application of craniofacial techniques employs major osteotomies with bone grafts as well as lining replacement for the treatment of markedly foreshortened noses (51). This departure from the traditional techniques described was applied in both congenital and posttraumatic noses. Treatment of the short nose is one of the most difficult maladies to correct, if not *the* most difficult. The numerous reports in the literature attest to this and should be kept in mind when approaching these late posttraumatic deformities.

IX. SEPTAL PERFORATIONS

Septal perforations have a wide spectrum of presentation from minor irritations to airway obstruction. The clinical significance is dependent on the size and location of the perforation, with large anterior perforation exhibiting more symptomatology. Posttraumatic causes include direct injury or an unrecognized septal hematoma. Treatment of septal perforations can be technically demanding owing to the trilayer nature with bilateral mucoperichondrium with interposing cartilage. Reconstructive aims should be recreation of the trilayer septum in a tension-free manner. Techniques employing local mucosal flap with an intervening grafts have been described (52,53). Romo described the repair of large perforations (>2 cm) with a staged approach using flaps raised from expanded nasal floor mucosa (54). Regional flaps of pericranium (55) and labial buccal mucosa (56) have also been described. When surgical repair is not feasible or desired, the use of prosthetic buttons or obturators has been described (57,58).

X. NASAL INJURIES IN CHILDREN

Nasal fractures are the most commonly seen facial fracture in children (59). The seemingly trivial nature of the injury often results in delayed presentation or no treatment at all. The principles of management of acute nasal injuries apply to both adults and children. Prompt recognition and treatment are critical to successful outcomes because children exhibit rapid fracture healing. In addition, procedures in younger children (<16 years) should be performed in the operating room with appropriate anesthesia and instrumentation. The optimal method, be it open or closed reduction, for the treatment of nasal fractures in children remains controversial. Some authors advocate closed-reduction techniques with satisfactory results (60,61), whereas others have reported good results with open reduction (62,63). The debate centers around the effects of nasal surgery on future nasal growth. Experimental and clinical studies have examined the effects of nasal surgery on nasal growth with no apparent resolution (60,61,64–72). Furthermore, it is unclear whether the surgical procedure, the traumatic insult, or a combination of the two affects nasal growth. All things considered, treatment of children with nasal fractures should not deviate significantly from the care of the adult patient when clear operative indications exist. These include septal hematoma/abscess, significant airway obstruction, and gross external nasal deformity. Otherwise, a conservative approach of closed reduction for obvious deformities with formal corrective septorhinoplasty following nasal growth is a reasonable approach.

XI. CONCLUSION

Nasal trauma is commonplace and can result in a wide range of injuries. The spectrum of pathology can range from an acute nasal fracture to a complex posttraumatic deformity. Systematic and detailed history and physical examination must be performed on every patient to arrive at a correct diagnosis. Once the diagnosis is made, knowledge of nasal anatomy is fundamental in the treatment of these patients. The approach and techniques that are used are numerous but must adhere to the basic surgical principles of nasal surgery. The end results of a carefully planned and executed surgery are restoration of airway function as well as nasal aesthetics.

REFERENCES

1. Martinez SA. Nasal fractures: What to do for a successful outcome. Postgrad Med 1987; 82:71.
2. Gilles HD, Kilner T. The treatment of the broken nose. Lancet 1929; 1:147.
3. Becker OJ. Nasal fractures: analysis of 100 cases. Arch Otolaryngol 1948; 48:344.
4. Stranc MF, Robertson GA. Classification if injuries to the nasal skeleton. Ann Plast Surg 1979; 2:468.
5. Harrison DH. Nasal injuries: their pathogenesis and treatment. Br J Plast Surg 1979; 32:57.
6. Murray JAM, Maran AGD, Busuttil A, Vaughn G. A pathologic classification of nasal fractures. Injury 1986; 7:338.
7. Haug RH, Prather JL. The closed reduction of nasal fractures: an evaluation of Two techniques. J Oral Maxillofac Surg 1991; 49:1288.
8. Pollock RA. Nasal trauma: pathomechanics and surgical management of acute injuries. Clin Plast Surg 1992; 19:133.
9. DeLacey G, Wignall BK, Hussain S, Reidy JR. The radiology of nasal injuries: problems of interpretation and clinical relevance. Br J Radiol 1977; 50:412.
10. Nigam A, Goni A, Benjamin A, Dasgupta AR. The value of radiographs in the management of the fractured nose. Arch Emer Med 1993; 10:292.
11. Ilum P. Legal aspects of nasal fractures. Rhinology 1991; 29:263.
12. Hirai T, Manders EK, Nagamoto K, Saggers GC. Ultrasonic observation of facial bone fractures: report of cases. J Oral Maxillofac Surg 1996; 54:776+.
13. Crowther JA, O'Donoghue GM. The broken nose: Dose familiarity breed contempt? Ann R Coll Surg Edin 1987; 69:259.
14. Illum P. Long-term results after treatment of nasal fractures. J Laryngol Otol 1986; 100:273.
15. Fry HJH. Nasal skeletal trauma and the interlocked stresses of the nasal septal cartilages. Br J Plast Surg 1967; 22:146.
16. Gibson T, Davis WB. The distortion of autogenous cartilage grafts: its cause and prevention. Br J Plast Surg 1958; 10:257.
17. Freer O. The correction of the nasal septum with a minimum of traumatism. JAMA 1902; 38:636.
18. Killian G. The submucous window resection of the nasal septum. Ann Rhinol Laryngol 1905; 14:363.
19. Dingman RO, Natvig P. The deviated nose. Clin Plast Surg 1977; 4:145.
20. Cottle MH. Modified nasal septum operations. Eye Ear Nose Throat Mon 1950; 29:480.
21. Gruber R, Lesavoy M. Closed septal osteotomy. Ann Plast Surg 1998; 40:283.
22. Briant TDR, Middleton WG. The management of severe nasal septal deformities. J Otolaryngol 1985; 14(2):120.
23. Gubuisch W. The extracorporeal septumplasty: a technique to correct difficult nasal deformities. Plast Reconstr Surg 1995; 91:229.

24. Courtiss EH. Septorhinoplasty of the traumatically deformed nose. Ann Plast Surg 1978; 1:443.
25. Gunter JP, Rohrich RJ. Management of the deviated nose: the importance of septal reconstruction. Clin Plast Surg 1988; 15:43.
26. Byrd SH, Salomon J, Flood J. Correction of a crooked nose. Plast Reconstr Surg 1998; 102:2148.
27. Ramirez OM, Pozner JN. The severely twisted nose: treatment by separation of its components and internal cartilage splinting. Clin Plast Sur 1996; 23:327.
28. McKinney P, Shively R. Straightening the twisted nose. Plast Reconstr Surg 1979; 64:176.
29. Gilberts SE. Overlay grafting for lateral wall nasal concavities. Otolaryngol Head Neck Surg 1998; 119:385.
30. Constantitian MB. An algorithm for correcting the asymmetrical nose. Plast Reconstr Surg 1989; 83:801.
31. Johnson CM, Toriumi DM. Open structure rhinoplasty. Philadelphia: WB Saunders, 1990.
32. Adamson PA. The over-resected dorsum. Facial Plast Surg Clin North Am 1995; 3:407.
33. Lupo G. The history of aesthetic rhinoplasty: special emphasis on the saddle nose. Aesth Plast Surg 1997; 21:309.
34. Waldman SR. Gore-Tex for augmentation of the nasal dorsum: a preliminary report. Ann Plast Surg 1991; 26:520.
35. Owsley TG, Taylor CO. The use of Gore-Tex for nasal augmentation: a retrospective analysis of 106 patients. Plast Reconstr Surg 1994; 94:241.
36. Dyer WK, Beaty MM, Prabhat A. Architectural deficiencies of the nose. Otolaryngol Clin North Am 1999; 32:89.
37. Horton CE, Mathews MS. Nasal reconstruction with autologous rib cartilage: a 43 year follow-up. Plast Reconstr Surg 1992; 89:131.
38. Ortiz Monasterio, Olmedo A, Oscov LO. The use of cartilage grafts in primary aesthetic rhinoplasty. Plast Reconstr Surg 1981; 67:597.
39. Sheen JH. Tip grafts: A 20 year retrospective. Plast Reconstr Surg 1993; 91:48.
40. Wheeler E, Kawamoto H, Zarem H. Bone grafts for nasal reconstruction. Plast Reconstr Surg 1982; 69:9.
41. Furlan S. Correction of saddle nose deformity by costal cartilage-a technique. Ann Plast Surg 1982; 9:32.
42. Farina R, Cury E, Ackel IA. Saddle and boxer's nose. Aesth Plast Surg 1983; 7:171.
43. Gerow FJ, Stal S, Spira M. The totem pole rib graft reconstruction of the nose. Ann Plast Surg 1983; 11:273.
44. Stuzin JM, Kawamoto HK. Saddle nose deformity. Clin Plast Surg 1988; 15:83.
45. Hardesty RA, Marsh JL. Craniofacial onlay bone grafting. Plast Reconstr Surg 1990; 85:5.
46. Gunter JP, Rohrich RJ. Lengthening the aesthetically short nose. Plast Reconstr Surg 1989; 83:793.
47. Kamer FM. Lengthening the short nose. Ann Plast Surg 1980; 4:281.

48. Giammanco PF. Lengthening the congenitally short nose. Arch Otolaryngol Head neck Surg 1987; 113:1113.
49. Gruber RP. The short nose. Clin Plast Surg 1996; 23:297.
50. Naficy S, Baker SB. Lengthening the short nose. Arch Otolaryngol Head Neck Surg 1998; 124:809.
51. Wolfe SA. Lengthening the nose: a lesson from craniofacial surgery applied to posttraumatic and congenital deformities. Plast Reconstr Surg 1994; 94:78.
52. Kridel RWH. Septal perforation repair. Otolaryngol Clin North Am 1999; 32:695.
53. Fairbanks DNF. Closure of nasal septal perforation. Arch Otolaryngol Head Neck Surg 1980; 106:509.
54. Romo T 3rd, Scalfani AP, Falk AN, Toeffel PH: A graduated approach to repair of nasal septal perforations. Plast reconstr Surg 103:66, 1999.
55. Paloma V, Samper A, Cervera-Paz FJ. Surgical technique for reconstruction of the nasal septum: the pericranial flap. Head Neck 2000; 22:90.
56. Tipton JB. Closure of large septal perforations with labial-buccal flap. Plast Reconstr Surg 1970; 46:514.
57. Eliacher I, Mastros NP. Improved nasal septal prosthetic button. Otolaryngol Head Neck Surg 1995; 112:347.
58. Facer GW, Kern EB. Nasal septal perforations: use of silastic button in 108 patients. Rhinology 1979; 17:115.
59. Anderson PI. Fractures of the facial skeleton in children. Injury 1995; 26:47.
60. Dommerby H, Tos M. Nasal fractures in children-long term results. ORL J Otolayrngol Relat Spec 1985; 47:272.
61. Chmielik M, Gutkowska J, Kossowska E, Praglowska B. Reduction of nasal fractures in children. Int J Pediatr Otolaryngol 1986; 11:1.
62. Moran WB Jr. Nasal trauma in children. Otolaryngol Clin North Am 10:95, 1977.
63. Pirsig W. Clinical aspects of the fractured growing nose. Rhinology 1983; 27:107.
64. Wexler MR, Sarnat BG. Rabbit snout growth. Arch Otolaryngol 1961; 74:305.
65. Sarnat BG, Wexler MR. Growth of the face and jaw after resection of the septal cartilage in rabbits. Am J Anat 1966; 118:755.
66. Bernstein L. Early submucous resection of nasal septal cartilage: a pilot study in canine pups. Arch Otolaryngol Head Neck Surg 1973; 97:273.
67. Freng A. Mid-facial sagittal growth following resection of the nasal septum-vomer: a roentgencephalometric study in the domestic cat. Acta Otolaryngol 1981; 92:363.
68. Verwoerd CDA, Urbanus NAM, Nijdam DC. The effects of septal surgery on the growth of nose and maxilla. Rhinology 1979; 17:53.
69. Huizing EH. Septum surgery in children: indications, surgical technique and long term results. Rhinology 1979; 27:91.
70. Ortiz-Monasterio F, Olmedo A. Corrective rhinoplasty before puberty; a long term follow-up. Plast Reconstr Surg 1981; 68:381.
71. Grymer LF, Gutierrez C, Stoksted P. Nasal fractures in children: influence on the development of the nose. J Laryngol Otol 1985; 99:735.
72. El-Hakim H, Crysdale WS, Abdollel M, Farkas LG. A study of antropoometric measures before and after external septoplasty in children. Arch Otolaryngol Head Neck Surg 2001; 127:1362.

12

The Management of Naso-orbital-ethmoid Fractures and Avoidance of Untoward Sequelae

Paul Manson
Baltimore, Maryland, U.S.A.

I. INTRODUCTION

Naso-orbital-ethmoid (NOE) fractures are inherently complex and challenging to repair, reflecting the intricate nature of the relevant anatomy and the necessarily exquisite attention to detail required for optimal surgical intervention. To restore the preinjury appearance, we must attain meticulous reduction of these fractures and stable, durable internal fixation in a timely fashion. The soft tissue and the bone must be considered. Posttraumatic deformities are profound and problematic, and may be persistent after ill-performed or delayed surgical procedures. Further we have little ability to effectively resolve these secondarily despite our ever-expanding armamentarium of surgical techniques.

II. ANATOMY

The NOE region is the watershed of the central midface, as the point of confluence between the nose, cranium, paranasal sinuses, inferior midface, and bony orbits. The junctions of no fewer than nine bones are involved in this area—the bilateral nasal bones, maxillae, ethmoids, and lacrimals. as well as the frontal bone.

The orbit is composed of seven bones in its entirety. Superiorly, the frontal bone constitutes the orbital roof. The vertical portion gives rise to the slightly convex, projected forehead, while serving as the encasement of the frontal sinus and the anterior wall of the anterior cranial fossa. A horizontal component of the frontal bone forms the supraorbital rims, the main horizontal buttress of the upper face. Between the supraorbital ridges, the frontal bone becomes the galabella and then projects caudally to articulate with the paired nasal bones and maxillae. The nasofrontal ducts are located centrally along the posterior floor of the frontal sinus and are sometimes vulnerable to disruption and obstruction with trauma to the NOE area.

The lacrimal and ethmoid bones comprise the eggshell-like medial orbital wall, also known as the lamina papyracea. These bones are not only important in their anatomical location as the medial limit of the bony orbit, but also serve to contain, transmit, and attach important anatomical structures. Concomitant injuries to these structures are seen with NOE fractures. The lacrimal sac is located within a depression of the lacrimal bone between the anterior and posterior lacrimal crests. The anterior crest represents the junction of the frontal process of the maxilla with the lacrimal bone. Coursing inferiorly from the lacrimal sac and occupying an excavated, narrow cavity within the medial maxilla is the nasolacrimal duct. The nasolacrimal system terminates in the inferior meatus, just beneath the inferior turbinate. Two neurovascular foramina are intimately associated with the medial orbital wall. The anterior ethmoidal artery and nasociliary nerve emerge from the anterior ethmoid foramen, encountered in the frontoethmoid suture line approximately 24 mm posterior to the anterior lacrimal crest at the level of the cribiform plate. Continuing deeper into the orbit, the posterior ethmoid foramen, transmitting the artery and nerve of the same name, is located 36 mm past the anterior crest. Most important, the optic foramen and nerve are found at a distance of 4–7 mm from the posterior arterial branch within the lesser sphenoid wing. Skeletal disruption of this region may produce traumatic shearing of these structures, leading to orbital hematoma and/or blindness.

The medial canthal tendon is the critical soft-tissue structure within the NOE region. Recognized as the fibrous condensation of the pretarsal, preseptal, and orbital orbicularis oculi muscle, it stretches medially to surround the lacrimal gland and insert onto the anterior and posterior lacrimal crests. A portion of the tendon extends horizontally onto the nasal bone medial to the eyelid commissure and lacrimal sac. Functionally, the medial canthal tendon provides support to the globe as an integral component of an enveloping sling system consisting of the tarsal plates, Lockwoods and Whitnails ligaments. The posterior limb also functions to keep the lids tangentially applied to the globe. NOE fractures are characterized by isolation and instability of a central bony fragment to which the medial cathal tendon is attached. Lateral displacement of the fragment results in shortening of the eyelids and a laxity along the entire suspensory sling of the globe and lower eyelid. Consequently, NOE fractures are associated with telecanthus, central globe displacement, and reduction of the length of the palpebral aperture. Avulsion of the tendon from the lacrimal bone is rare; there usually remains a sizable fragment onto which the tendon remains inserted. Precise reduction of this unstable canthal-bearing fragment with medial repositioning, followed by internal fixation, provides the most acceptable aesthetic and functional outcomes for this difficult problem.

The interorbital space represents that area between the medial orbital walls and caudal to the central anterior cranial fossa, inferior to the cribiform plate. The ethmoid bone is the cornerstone of this area. The perpendicular plate of the ethmoid partitions the nasal cavity into left and right cavities. Extension of this midline structure for a variable distance intracranially is termed the crista galli. Bisecting the perpendicular plate in a horizontal orientation is the cribiform plate, through which the delicate second-order neurons of the olfactory nerve pass via bony fenestrations. Posteriorly, the space is bounded by the anterior face of the sphenoid (rostum). Contained within these boundaries is the honeycomb-like labyrinth of the anterior and posteior ethmoidal air cells. These air-filled spaces (approximately 12–15 per side in an adult, with a total average volume of 14–15 mL) consist of eggshell-thin bone segments blanketed by a thin, well-vascularized mucoperiosteum. Drainage of these sinuses is to the middle meatus for the anterior cell grouping and to the superior meatus for the cells located posterior to the ground lamella, the thickened wall of bone separating the groups. Significant traumatic forces applied/translated to this area result in obliteration of the normal sinus architecture, with pulverization of the labyrinth and creation of a common cavity filled with blood, bony spicules, and mucosal debris.

III. DIAGNOSIS

A. Physical Examination

The presentation of a patient with a history of an impact to the facies from an automobile accident, a fall from a height, or an object with great mass or velocity should raise the suspicion of an NOE complex fracture. Initial evaluation of the blunt, multisystem trauma patient should follow the principles set forward elsewhere, with prompt attention to airway control, ventilatory assessment and assistance, and hemodynamic evaluation. Associated cervical spine and intracranial injuries are common with central midface trauma and should always be suspected in this injury pattern.

Consultation for facial fracture evaluation and treatment should begin with visual inspection. Patients presenting with significant bony facial trauma usually exhibit facial edema, the extent of which corresponds to the severity of injury. Panfacial fractures associated with NOE fractures result in generalized facial edema, while isolated NOE fractures display more localized edema over the nasal, periorbital, and glabellar regions. Periocular ecchymoses are usually present. A spectacle hematoma displays a sharp demarcation at the rim of the orbit and is produced by a fracture within the orbital cavity. There is broadening and flattening of the nasal root area. Retrodisplacement of the nasal complex occurs with comminution of the underlying ethmodial complex and results in loss of nasal projection and height. The nose loses bridge support (palpation) and has an acute columella-lip angle with palpable loss of caudal septal support. Also apparent upon examination will be the development of epitcanthal folds, obscuring the relatively sharp medial canthal angles. Lateralization of the medial canthi is noted, with a compensatory increase in intercanthal distance (traumatic telecanthus) and decrease in palpebral fissure length. The preinjury intercanthal distance generally equals the palpebral fissure length. The pronounced facial edema present, which tends to worsen over 48 hours after the traumatic event, may exaggerate the characteristic widening and flattening of the nasal dorsum, while simultaneously blunting the perception of telecanthus. Lacerations are noted and gently explored for foreign material or bone spicules. Lacerations overlying the medial canthus may indicate complete dislocation of the tendon from the lacrimal crests and damage or transection of the lacrimal system.

Formal ophthalmological evaluation is mandatory. Prior to this, a basic ocular examination should be completed. Because of severe edema, retraction of the eyelids may be extremely difficult. Careful use of two long cotton-tipped applicators placed on the upper- and lower-lid edges followed by gentle pressure and distraction superiorly and inferiorly facilitates direct observation of the globes. Water-bag edema of the conjuctiva (chemosis) and subconjuctival edema and hematoma are nearly universal findings in the setting of NOE fractures. Pupillary response, gross visual acuity, extra-ocular muscle motion, and the presence of diplopia should be assessed. Often, the patient demonstrates a severely decreased level of consciousness or is unable to fully participate in this part of the evaluation, but pupillary response to light may still be assessed.

Tactile examination of the NOE area follows visualization. Gentle pressure with a single digit on the nasal tip and dorsum demonstrates a lack of bony and cartilaginous support, with little force required to collapse the nose. Because of the extent of comminution seen with these fractures, crepitance and mass movement of the entire nasal complex are appreciated on palpation utilizing the thumb and index finger. Laxity of the medial canthal tendon is assessed by the Furnas traction test. While the attachment of the tendon is palpated medially, the lower eyelid is gently stretched laterally. Tactile resistance to increasing lateral traction is recognized as "bowstringing." This finding indicates an intact medial canthal tendon insertion. In the setting of a grossly comminuted NOE fracture, these is loss of tension with this test and bony fragment movement may be perceived. Bimanual examination utilizing a Kelly clamp inserted intranasally is important for diagnosis and for operative decision making. This maneuver is performed by first estimating the position of the medial canthal tendon by surface anatomical landmarks, and then introducing a blunt clamp into the nasal cavity. Careful advancement of the clamp superiorly, just until there is contact of the intranasal portion of the medial orbital rim bearing the medial canthal tendon by the clamp tip, is performed. The examiner's contralateral index finger is simultaneously placed externally over the tendon insertion. Gentle rocking movements allow a determination of bony stability. Mobility of the canthus-bearing bone not only confirms the pathology, but also provides indication for operative intervention. A lack of mobility implies that there is tight periosteal adherence of the bony fragments, impaction of the fracture, or no true NOE fracture at all. These stable fractures can be managed nonoperatively, provided there is no dislocation of the central fragment.

Anterior rhinoscopy utilizing a nasal speculum and portable light source is also mandatory. Blood and debris should be gently removed with bayonet forceps and proximal suctioning with a Frazier tip. The mucosa is noted to be edematous and congested. The septum may be obviously fractures, with overlying laceration of the mucosa or hematoma development. Septal perforation is common. Clear cerebrospinal fluid (CSF) may emanate from the nares, indicative of a disruption of the cranial base. Acutely, this is mixed with blood and difficult to confirm.

B. Radiology

Radiographic evaluation with high-quality CT scanning is invaluable. Plain-film radiography has been replaced by more modern techniques and now plays no role in diagnosis or treatment planning. The severe nature of the head trauma present in patients where NOE fractures are suspected, a CT scan with axial and coronal images both for evaluation of intracranial injury and visualization of the nose and orbits must be performed by the time plastic surgical consultation is obtained. If necessary a preliminary axial cut soft tissue window CT can yield important information prior to the performance of a dedicated facial CT. Importantly, no contrast is administered for either the head or facial CT. Frequent concomitant intracranial injuries include subarachnoid hemorrhage, parenchymal contusions (frontal and temporal lobes), and extradural or parenchymal hematoma formation. For evaluation of the craniomaxillofacial skeleton, the bone windowed scans are the most elucidating. All sinuses are identified and assessed for opacification, which may indicate fracture of the surrounding walls. The pterygoid plates are examined for fractures, which would provide the basis for diagnosis of a Le Fort fracture. The cribriform plate and orbital floor are not optimally visualized on axial sections, as these are axially oriented structures. Radiographic evidence of NOE complex fractures includes opacification of the ethmoid air cells with loss of bony sepation within the sinuses, comminution of the medial orbital walls with loss of sharp definition of the medial orbital limits, nasal and septal fractures, and air bubbles within the ocular globe. It is worth noting that NOE complex fractures may be either unilateral or bilateral. Simultaneous fractures of the nasal radix/glabella area inferior orbital rim, pyriform aperature, orbital floor and medial orbital wall confirm the diagnosis radiologically.

IV. CLASSIFICATION OF FRACTURE PATTERNS

Fractures of the NOE complex are usually the result of direct frontal-impact blunt trauma but may occur as an extention of high Le Fort II or III fractures. Rather than a single fracture in a single location, the NOE complex fracture necessarily entails fractures at multiple locations. Specifically, fractures are identified at the junction of the nasal bone and maxilla, the junction of the frontal bone and frontal process of the maxilla, the medial orbital wall (the ethmoid and lacrimal bones), and the infraorbital rim extending through the nasomaxillary buttress at the piriform aperture. Within this field of fractures, the medial canthal tendon-bearing bone is isolated as a large or comminuted fragment. This principle forms the basis of fracture pattern classification.

NOE complex fractures may exist as unilateral or bilateral fractures. The fracture may be isolated within the central midface or may extend to involve the lateral maxilla, the lateral orbit, or the frontal sinus. Three types of fractures have been described according to Manson and Markowitz, with the canthal-bearing bone fragment being the point of differentiation.

Type I fractures are characterized by isolation of a large canthal-bearing segment along the fracture lines outlined above. No comminution is present. Type I fractures may be either unilateral or bilateral. The most subtle fractures observed are displaced only inferiorly at the inferior orbital rim and pyriform aperature, and are hinged (greenstick) superiorly. In this fracture telecanthus does not occur, but the palpebral fissure is lengthened by medial displacement of the canthal ligament. A relatively moderate amount of applied blunt force is responsible for this injury, and there is the potential in this setting for incomplete fractures at the inferior orbital rim and the frontal bone–maxilla junction that retain periosteal integrity. A special case under the type I designation is the bilateral, complete NOE complex fracture, also known as the monoblock NOE fracture. In this situation, the entire NOE region is isolated from the remainder of the midface, but maintains continuity across the midline. True traumatic telecanthus is not a feature in the monoblock NOE fracture, as the medial canthal tendon via transnasal canthopexy is not undertaken.

In contrast to type I fractures, type II injuries are characterized by comminution of the central fragment outside the medial canthal insertion. The canthal-bearing segment if sizable can be effectively manipulated during repair. Reduction of the fragment medially is followed by fixation with microplates and screws. A transnasal wire reduction of this fragment provides the most stable anatomic reduction.

The distinguishing feature of type III fractures is the more extensive comminution, which extends into the medial canthal tendon insertion. Instead of the tendon being attached to a bone fragment of meaningful size, it is continuous with little more than a bony spicules. Repair necessarily includes bone graft replacement of the tendon insertions for stabilization of the tendon. Rarely, the medial canthal tendon is completely avulsed from its insertion.

V. OPERATIVE TREATMENT

Successful surgical management of these complex fractures depends upon accurate identification of the extent of injury and timely operative intervention. Recognition of the type of fracture is the cornerstone of surgical treatment planning, as the techniques employed are based on the extent and location of injury. Preoperative CT scans may differentiate between type I, II and III fracture patterns, but direct observation of the condition of the central fragment in the operating room ultimately determines the means of repair. Because this injury produces profound facial deformities that are difficult, if not impossible, to resolve on satisfactorily a secondary basis, prompt initial meticulous repair is of paramount importance.

13

Management of Acute Injuries to the Frontal Sinus and Management of Untoward Sequelae

Danny J. Enepekides and Paul J. Donald
University of California, Davis Medical Center, Sacramento, California, U.S.A.

I. INTRODUCTION

Fracture of the frontal sinus requires considerable force, owing to the density, thickness, and arched configuration of its anterior wall. When compared to the rest of the maxillofacial skeleton, fracture of the frontal sinus necessitates greater force. Therefore, isolated frontal sinus fracture due to blunt trauma is rare. The majority of cases are associated with other midface fractures and are often accompanied by intracranial injuries.

Frontal sinus fractures are most often the consequence of blunt trauma. With the implementation of seat belt laws and improved automobile safety, the incidence of severe maxillofacial trauma associated with motor vehicle accidents (MVA) has decreased. However, MVA remains the leading cause of frontal sinus fracture. Penetrating trauma, as a consequence of violent crime with firearms, unfortunately, also remains a relatively common mechanism of injury.

II. ANATOMY OF THE FRONTAL SINUS

Embryologically, the frontal sinus develops either as an expansion of anterior frontoethmoidal air cells into the frontal bone or from superior extension of the frontal recess, the most anterosuperior portion of the infundibulum of the middle meatus (1). The sinus is absent at birth and usually begins its development by 3 years of age. It continues to enlarge into adolescence. The frontal sinus reaches its maximal size by the age of 16–18 years in boys and 12–14 years in girls (2).

The volume of the frontal sinus varies tremendously and has implications with respect to trauma. Well-aerated sinuses require significantly less force to fracture than smaller, more contracted ones. When present, the average frontal sinus measures 28 mm in height, 27 mm in width, and 17 mm in depth. Complete aplasia of the sinus is seen in 15% of Caucasians and in 35% of people of other ethnicity (4). Unilateral aplasia is rare, seen in only 3–4% of the population (5). The sinus is usually divided into two halves by an intersinus septum. Supernumerary septa may be present but are often incomplete.

As shown in Figure 1, the frontal sinus is pyramidal in shape. The base of the pyramid forms its floor. The convex anterior wall of the frontal sinus is formed by thick, dense bone. Its arched configuration distributes forces of impact efficiently across the brow and frontal bone. By comparison, the posterior wall is much thinner and transgressed by bridging veins to the intracranial cavity. It is far more susceptible to fracture. Laterally, the sinus extends over the orbits. Here, the floor of the sinus contributes to the

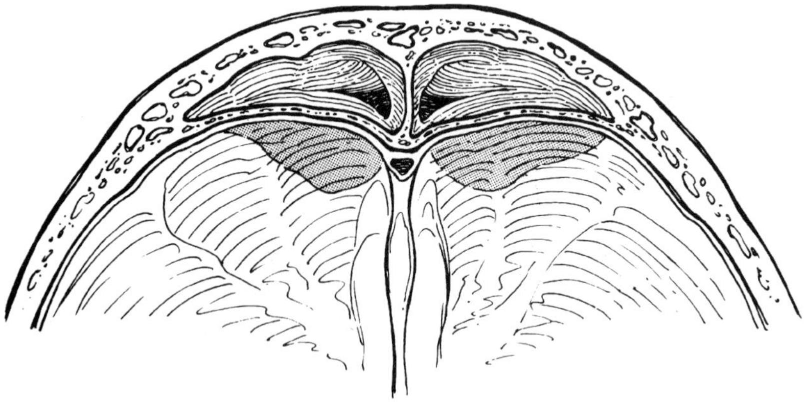

Figure 1 Schematic of the frontal sinus in the axial plane. Note the thick convex anterior wall of the sinus and its much thinner posterior wall. (From Ref. 32.)

medial orbital roofs. The central portion of the frontal sinus floor forms the roof of the nasal cavity anterior to the cribriform plate. Posteriorly, the sinus may extend, deep to the floor of the anterior cranial fossa, to the lesser wing of the sphenoid. Such significant posterior extension makes complete removal of sinus mucosa during obliteration procedures difficult.

The falx cerebri takes origin from the crista galli and is densely adherent to a small spine on the intracranial surface of the frontal sinus' posterior table. As a consequence, fractures of the posterior wall often result in dural tears. The frontal vein, origin of the superior sagittal sinus, enters the cranium through the foramen cecum just anterior to the crista galli. Injury to the superior sagittal sinus is serious. Ligation of the sinus posterior to the coronal suture line usually results in quadriplegia and death due to severe cerebral edema. The proximal third of the superior sagittal sinus may be ligated with some risk (Fig. 2).

The route of drainage of the frontal sinus into the nasal cavity is variable and dependent on its embryological origin. As already mentioned, the sinus

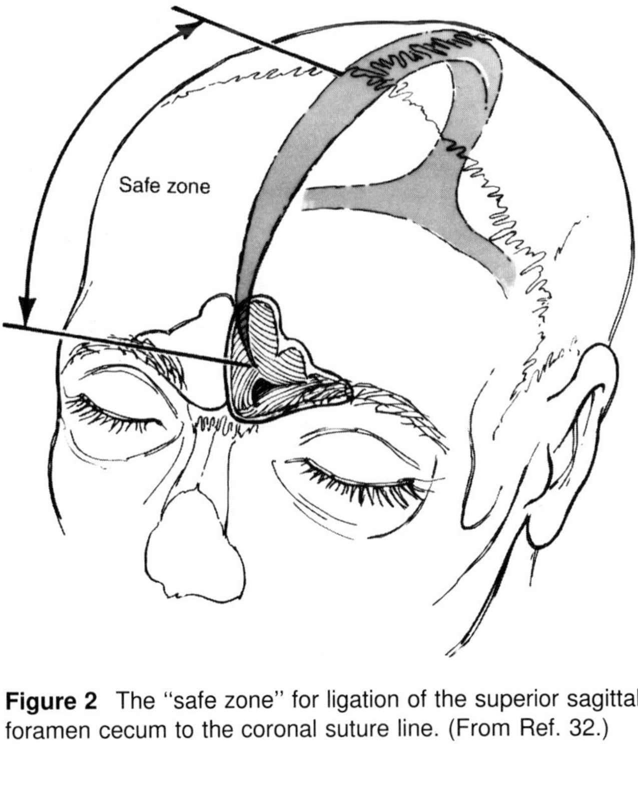

Figure 2 The "safe zone" for ligation of the superior sagittal sinus extends from foramen cecum to the coronal suture line. (From Ref. 32.)

may originate as a cephalad expansion of the frontal recess. In this situation, present in roughly 25% of the population, the sinus drains into the anterosuperior portion of the middle meatus through a true sinus ostium. Otherwise, the sinus drains through a nasofrontal duct (Fig. 3). The duct is often surrounded by anterior ethmoid air cells commonly referred to as frontoethmoid cells. It opens into the anterosuperior portion of the infundibulum (4).

The blood supply to the frontal sinus is primarily from the internal carotid system via the supraorbital branch of the ophthalmic artery. The anterior ethmoid artery may also contribute. Venous drainage occurs through the anterior facial, angular, and superior ophthalmic veins, which communicate with the cavernous sinus. Alternate routes of venous drainage, first documented by Mosher and Judd in 1933, are valveless transosseous channels passing through the foramina of Breschet in the posterior table of the sinus (6). These venous channels pass directly into the subarachnoid space and serve as potential routes of spread for infection. Sensory innervation of the frontal sinus is by way of the supraorbital and supratrochlear nerves, branches of the ophthalmic division of the trigeminal nerve.

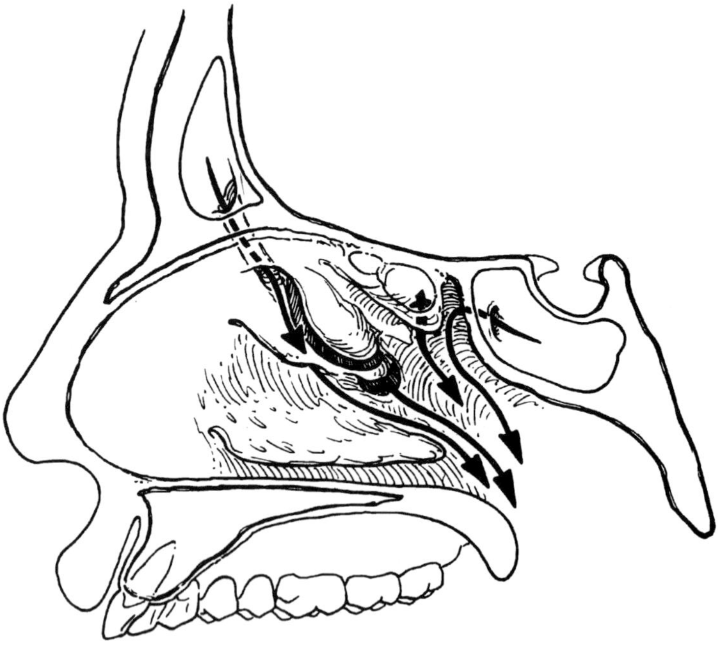

Figure 3 Drainage routes of the paranasal sinuses. The nasofrontal duct drains the frontal sinus into the superior portion of the infundibulum. (From Ref. 32.)

III. PATHOPHYSIOLOGY OF FRONTAL SINUS MUCOSA

To avoid the formation of frontal mucoceles and their untoward sequalae, a basic understanding of the pathophysiological response to trauma of the frontal sinus mucosa is required. Unlike the lining of the other paranasal sinuses, the mucosa of the frontal sinus tends to form cysts in resposne to trauma. As opposed to the previously held notion that mucocele formation implied nasofrontal duct injury and obstruction, the work by Lotta and Schall (7), Schenck (8), and the senior author (9) has shown that injury to the frontal mucosa in and of itself can lead to cyst formation. There is a dense fibrous response to trauma in the submucosa that accompanies these mucosal cysts. In addition, a brisk inflammatory infiltrate ensues and the normally ciliated epithelial cells either lose their cilia or their cilia become immotile in the acidic environment. The cysts subsequently accumulate fluid that results in their expansion. The associated bone loss is the result of either bone erosion from pressure or activation of osteoclasts at the periphery of the cyst. The majority of mucoceles form as a result of nasofrontal duct injury and obstruction. In these cases a true cyst does not form. Rather, mucous becomes inspissated within the obstructed sinus eventually resulting in bone erosion, usually along the paths of least resistance into the anterior cranial fossa, medial orbital roof, or nasal cavity. However, when mucosa becomes traumatized or trapped within a fracture line, mucosal cysts will form and eventually lead to clinically apparent mucoceles. This may occur despite the presence of a patent nasofrontal duct.

For these reasons, careful assessment of the nasofrontal duct and removal of all trapped or traumatized mucosa is paramount. However, the frontal sinus mucosa is tenacious. This characteristic is due in part to the variable anatomy of the sinus with its nooks and crannies that can be difficult to see and access and also to the microanatomy of the sinus. The foramina of Breschet, as already mentioned, are located in the posterior table of the sinus. The transosseous venous channels that pass trough the foramina have been shown by Donald to be accompanied by imbricating tongues of sinus mucosa (9). These microscopic projections of mucosa may serve as a nidus for mucocele formation if not completely removed during obliteration procedures.

IV. CLINICAL PRESENTATION AND EVALUATION

Of all facial bones, the frontal requires the greatest force to fracture. Between 800 and 1600 pounds of force are needed to result in frontal bone fracture. This is significant when compared to the 500–900 pounds of force required for mandibular fracture (10). Given its strength, it is not surprising that the majority of frontal sinus fractures are accompanied by other maxillofacial injuries. This was highlighted in a series of 72 frontal sinus fractures seen at University of California, Davis Medical Center between 1974 and 1986. As expected, MVA was the leading cause of injury, accounting for 71% of cases. However, 69% of patients had at least one other craniofacial fracture (11).

Patients suffering injuries to the frontal sinus are often victims of polytrauma. Given the tremendous forces invovled, cervical spine injury must be ruled out in all cases. Many present with altered levels of consciousness or other serious injuries requiring immediate attention. Unless it is obvious, it is easy to overlook frontal sinus fracture during the initial trauma evaluation. Certain findings should increase suspicion of frontal sinus injury. Forehead swelling, unless patients are examined immediately after the insult, is an invariable finding. Often lacerations are present over the sinus. In cases of compound anterior table fracture, bone fragments may be seen within the laceration. A palpable stepoff is a helpful diagnostic clue. Unfortunately, in many cases, this finding is obscured by subgaleal hematoma. Epistaxis, commonly associated with frontal sinus fracture, is most often due to accompanying midface injury. It is extremely important to look for cerebrospinal fluid (CSF) rhinorrhea in all cases of suspected frontal sinus fracture. When present, it is indicative of serious posterior table injury with violation of the dura and possible direct trauma to the frontal lobe of the brain. In severe cases of through-and-through fracture involving both walls of the sinus, brain matter may be seen through an overlying laceration.

Periods of unconsciousness often accompany fractures of the frontal sinus. Many patients will demonstrate signs of concussion including amnesia and headache. Hyposmia and anosmia are also common complaints. This may be the result of cribriform fractures or nasal vault edema and obstruction. Another important mechanism is shearing of the olfactory nerves from the olfactory bulbs as a consequence of kinetic energy transfer to the intracranial space. Hypesthesia of the forehead and scalp is indicative of injury to the supraorbital and supratrochlear neurovascular bundles. When it is present, it is helpful to determine if the sensory deficit is only evident above the laceration. In such cases it may be assumed that the neurovascular injury occurred at the site of laceration. In contrast, when the entire forehead is numb the nerves have usually been injured at the brow within the supraorbital foramen or notch. In either case, careful and clear preoperative documentation of all sensory deficits is mandatory.

Isolated nasofrontal duct injury is very difficult to diagnose and requires a high index of suspicion. In fact, this injury most often manifests as a mucocele or mucopyocele many months after the trauma. A persistent air-fluid level in the frontal sinus 10 or more days after the injury suggests the diagnosis. This nonspecific finding may simply be due to frontoethmoid mucosal edema. In fact, many polytraumatized patients will have indwelling nasogastic and nasotracheal tubes that alone could obstruct the frontal sinus.

Definitive diagnosis of frontal sinus fracture requires diagnostic imaging. In the past, plain films of the facial skeleton were relied upon to demonstrate these injuries. The facial series and Caldwell view in particular could reveal fracture lines and opacification of the sinus. The European fifth view, a hyperextended submentovertex projection, was used to evaluate the posterior table of the frontal sinus. These studies have now become obsolete and replaced by high-resolution computed tomography (CT). CT is currently the gold standard for imaging of craniofacial trauma (Fig. 4a–c). Adequate evaluation of frontal sinus fractures requires both axial and coronal fine-cut (1–2 mm) images through the sinus. Often true coronal images cannot be obtained owing to cervical spine precautions. In such

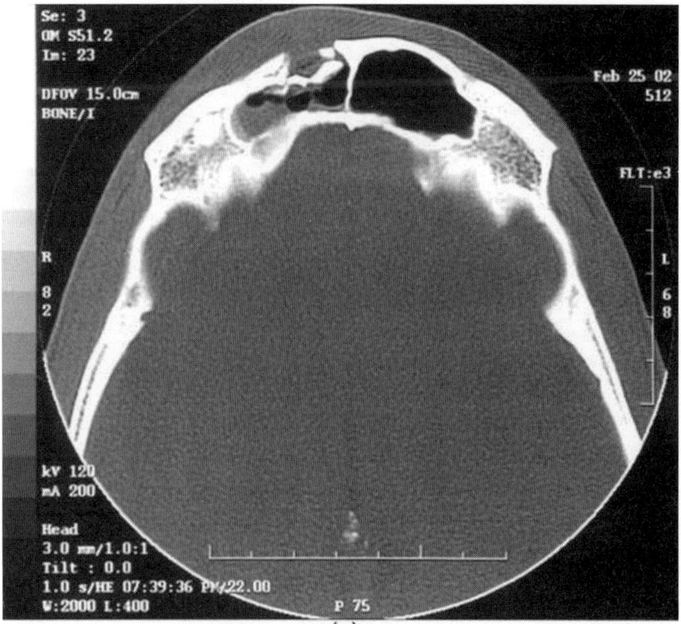

(a)

Figure 4 CT scan of frontal sinus fractures. (a) Axial image of a depressed anterior wall fracture. (b) Coronal image of a depressed anterior wall fracture. The depressed bone fragments can be seen within the sinus interior. (c) Axial image of a nondisplaced anterior and posterior wall frontal sinus fracture.

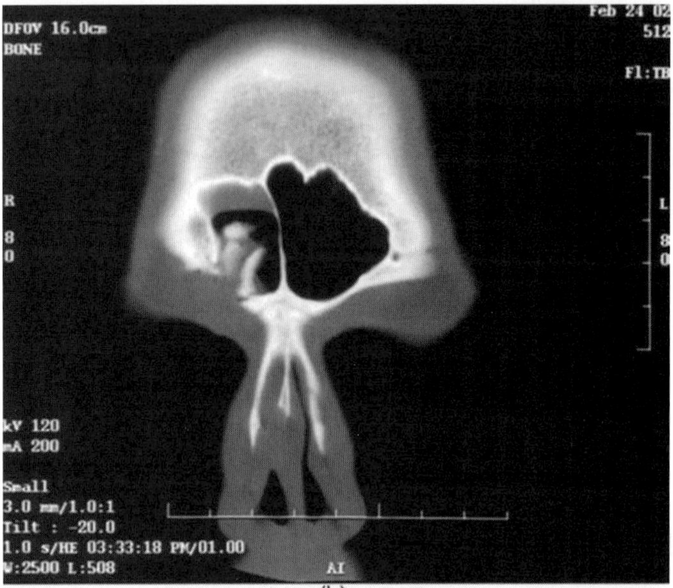

(b)

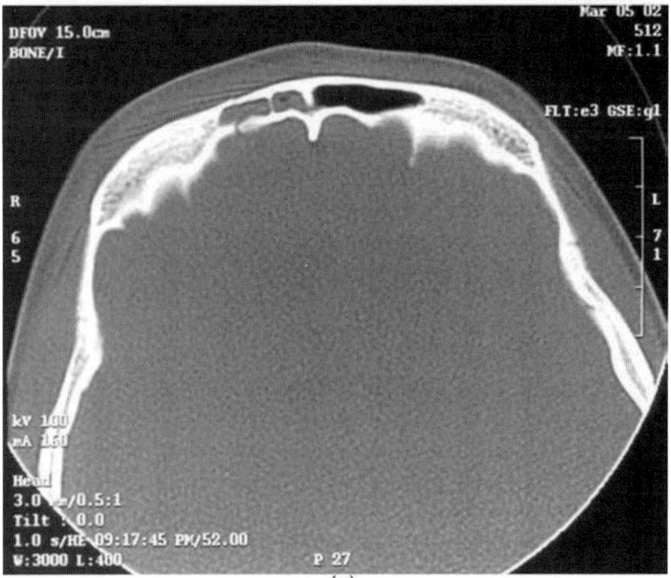

(c)

Figure 4 *(continued)*

cases, coronal reconstructions from fine-cut axial images may substitute. CT scan very accurately defines fractures of the anterior wall of the sinus. The bone of the posterior table of the sinus may be extremely thin. As a consequence, certain posterior table fractures can be difficult to diagnose despite high-resolution CT scan. This is particularly true for linear nondisplaced fractures. Coronal images are also helpful in evaluating the sinus floor and nasofrontal ducts. Magnetic resonance imaging (MRI) serves primarily as an adjunct to CT scan. It is particularly helpful when intracranial injury is suspected.

V. CLASSIFICATION OF FRONTAL SINUS FRACTURES

The classification scheme proposed for fractures of the frontal sinus is anatomically based on the structures involved by the injury. This classification system not only strandardizes reporting but also helps guide treatment.

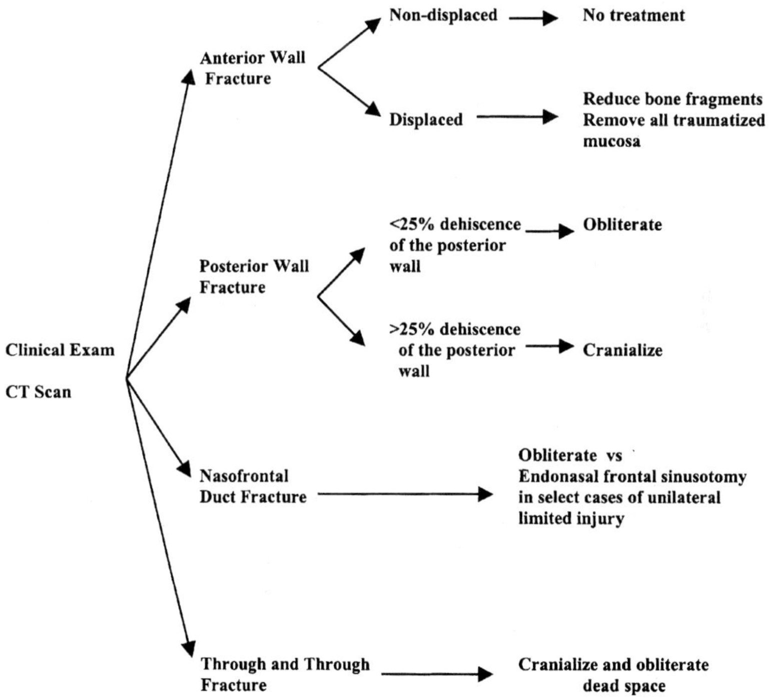

Figure 5 Treatment algorithm for fractures of the frontal sinus.

The categories include anterior wall, posterior wall, nasofrontal duct, and through-and-through fractures. Through-and-through fractures are those that transgress both walls of the sinus and violate the anterior cranial fossa. Further subclassification of the fracture type should include linear, depressed, comminuted, or compound. Injuries of the posterior wall should also be classified according to the presence or absence of CSF leak.

The treatment algorithm for fractures of the frontal sinus (Fig. 5) requires that every fracture be categorized according to this system. As will be shown, the treatment of these injuries is rather straightforward when the extent of the trauma is accurately defined. The appropriate approach, avoidance of late complications, and postoperative cosmetic result all depend on accurate diagnosis of fracture type and location. This necessitates careful intraoperative examination of the sinus interior and surrounding structures.

VI. MANAGEMENT

A. Anterior Wall Fractures

Anterior wall fractures of the frontal sinus are the most frequent fracture subtype encountered. Isolated linear nondisplaced fractures do not require intervention (Fig. 6). These injuries do not typically result in cosmetic deformity. In addition, mucosal entrapment within the fracture line is uncommon and, therefore, posttraumatic mucocele is an infrequent occurrence. On the other hand, all depressed or comminuted fractures should be explored surgically. Patients with such injuries usually have nonpalpable stepoffs at intial evaluation. As previously mentioned, this is due tu subgaleal hematoma and edema. However, if left untreated, these injuries will result in obvious unsightly depressions of the forehead. More important, all of these fractures result in mucosal trauma and entrapment (Fig. 7). Unless the traumatized mucosa is removed, posttraumatic mucoceles are likely.

The surgical approach to the sinus largely depends on the extent of the fracture. When compound, the laceration may be used to access the fracture (Fig. 8). In such cases, the laceration often needs to be extended into a preexisting forehead rhytid to provide adequate exposure. Otherwise the fracture must be accessed through an infrabrow, midforehead, or bicoronal incision (Fig. 9). The choice of incision is largely dependent on the patient's hairline. The bicoronal incision is used most frequently owing to its acceptable cosmetic appearance and the excellent exposure it affords. The incision is made approximately 2 cm behind the hairline. It may be extended inferiorly into the preauricular skin crease if exposure of the zygoma and glabella are required. The skin is elevated in a subgaleal plane to the level of the superior orbital rims. To avoid injury to the frontal division of the

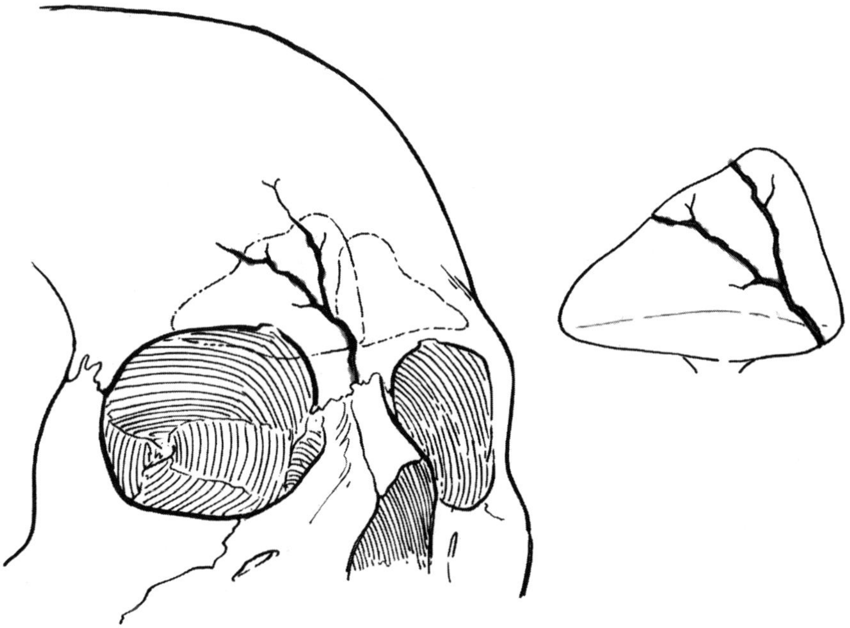

Figure 6 Linear nondisplaced anterior wall frontal sinus fracture. (From Ref. 32.)

facial nerve, it is important to raise the scalp flap deep to the superficial layer of the temporalis fascia. Alternatively, when the patient lacks a well-developed hairline, an infrabrow or midforehead incision can be used. In most instances these incisions result in less satisfactory cosmesis and decreased exposure as compared to the bicoronal incision. The infrabrow incision is made immediately below the eyebrows, beveling the blade to avoid loss of hair follicles and a more conspicuous scar. Whenever possible, the two lateral limbs of the incision are connected across the glabella in a preexisting horizontal skin crease. The midbrow incision may be preferable when deep forehead rhytids are present that help camouflage the scar. Both of these incisions result in limited exposure and should be avoided when the frontal sinus is of considerable size.

Once exposed, the depressed bone fragments should be elevated with a bone hook (Fig. 10). It is not uncommon for the displaced bone fragments to prolapse into the sinus interior (Fig. 11). The interior of the sinus, especially the posterior wall and the nasofrontal ducts, should always be examined carefully. When the fracture is of considerable size, this is easily

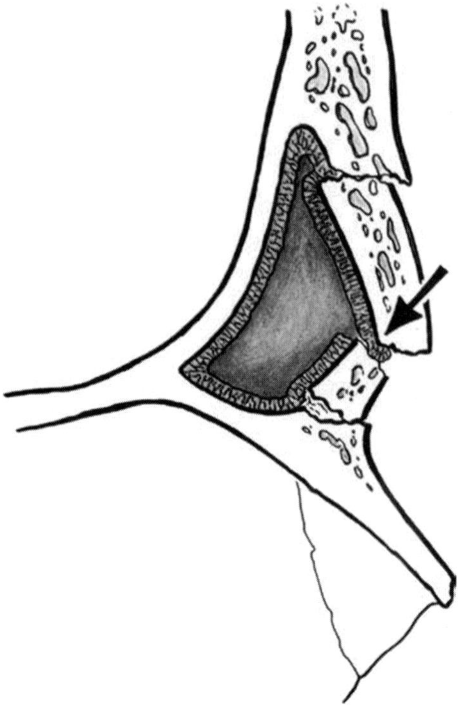

Figure 7 Schematic of a depressed anterior frontal sinus wall fracture. The arrow points out an area of mucosal entrapment between bone fragments. (From Ref. 32.)

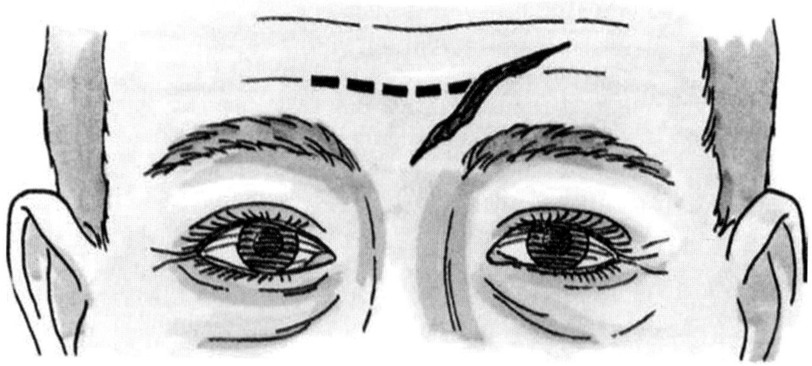

Figure 8 Extension of a laceration into a pre-existing forehead rhytid may provide adequate exposure of compound fractures of the frontal sinus. (From Ref. 32.)

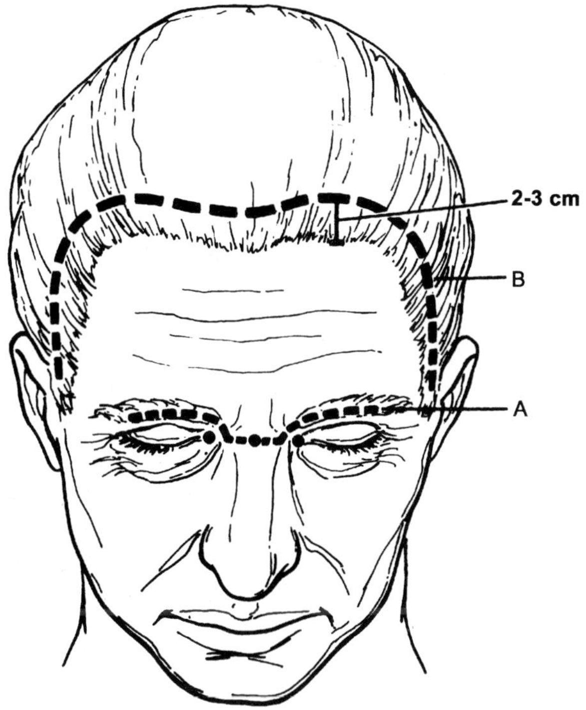

Figure 9 Incisions used for exposure of the frontal sinus. (A) The infrabrow incision. (B) The coronal incision. (From Ref. 32.)

accomplished. A 0° and 30° endoscope may prove useful when examination of the sinus is made difficult by a smaller anterior wall defect.Instilling methylene blue into the sinus and observing its egress into the nasal passages helps confirm patency of the nasofrontal ducts. In the absence of more extensive injury, all bone fragments should be elevated. In severely comminuted fractures, it is possible to lose bone fragments when irrigating wounds or by aspirating them with injudicious use of suction. The mucosa on the inner surface of all bone fragments should be removed carefully and the bone burred down with a drill (Fig. 12). One might consider removing only a circumferential rim of mucosa when the fragment is of considerable size. It is still necessary to drill down the exposed bone on the inner surface of these fragments to prevent mucosal trapping and mucocele formation (Fig 13). The bone fragments should be carefully reduced and fixed in position with titanium miniplates or, in cases of severe comminution, 26- or 28-gauge wire

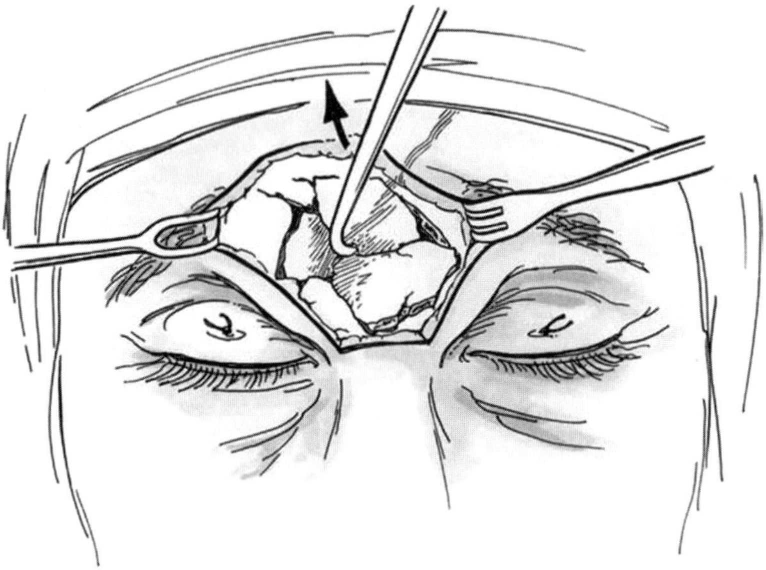

Figure 10 Comminuted fracture of the anterior wall exposed through an infrabrow incision. A hook is used to carefully elevate the displaced bone fragments. (From Ref. 32.)

(Fig 14). Every attempt should be made to avoid areas of missing bone. Small gaps, 1 cm or less, may be left open but it should be realized that this might result in visible depressions as edema subsides. This is especially true in thin-skinned individuals. It is preferable to replace missing bone. This may be achieved with calvarial bone graft. Outer-table calvarial grafts are easily harvested at the time of fracture repair, especially when the bicoronal incision is used. Alternatively, titanium mesh, alone or in conjunction with hydroxyapetite bone cement, may be used (12).

Controversy exists regarding the management of rare compound anterior wall fractures in which large segments of bone are missing. There are two schools of thought. The missing bone may be replaced with titanium mesh and the scalp lacerations meticulously closed. In most instances the sinus should be obliterated with fat following removal of all sinus mucosa and plugging of the nasofrontal ducts. Whenever possible, the titanium mesh should be covered by a vascularized pericranial flap. Hydroxyapatite cement should be avoided in these cases given the significant risk of infection. Alternatively, these complicated fractures can be managed by Reidel ablation. This involves removal of the remaining anterior sinus wall, all of the sinus mucosa, obliteration of the nasofrontal ducts, and closure of the

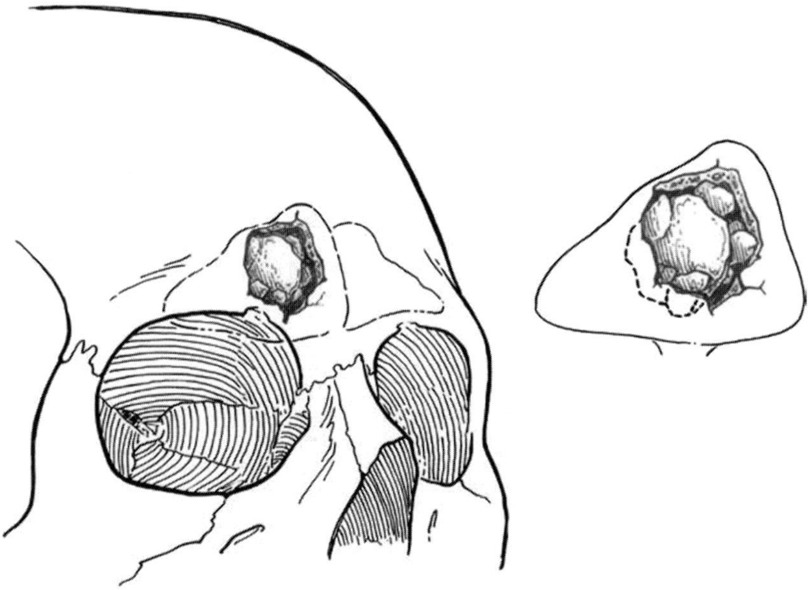

Figure 11 Comminuted fracture of the anterior wall with prolapse of bone fragments into the sinus interior. (From Ref. 32.)

skin over the posterior sinus wall. This procedure results in significant cosmetic deformity requiring secondary reconstruction. It should be reserved for those cases involving delayed treatment and significant contamination of the wound.

B. Posterior Wall Fracture

Posterior wall fractures (Fig. 15) have great potential to result in serious late sequelae when improperly treated. Controversy still surrounds the appropriate management of the linear nondisplaced posterior wall fracture. Despite careful follow-up, untreated fractures often result in mucocele formation and serious intracranial infectious complications. As previously mentioned, the frontal dura is tightly adherent to the posterior wall of the frontal sinus. Even small linear fractures may result in dural tears. The consequences of a missed dural tear may prove disastrous. Furthermore, despite fine-cut CT, it is often difficult to demonstrate slight fracture displacement. For these reasons, we feel strongly that all posterior wall fractures should be explored.

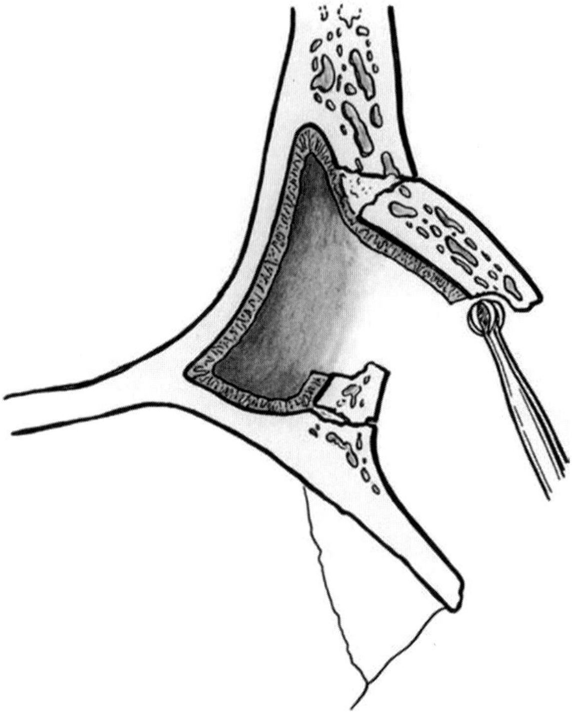

Figure 12 Approximately 2 mm of bone and all trapped mucosa is removed from the margins of all bone fragments. (From Ref. 32.)

Unless one is dealing with a through-and-through fracture, exposure of the posterior wall of the frontal sinus requires an osteoplastic flap of its anterior wall. A bicoronal incision is recommended. The scalp is raised to the level of the superior orbital rims and nasion. The anterior wall of the sinus must be osteotomized and opened without violating the intracranial space. This requires an accurate template of the frontal sinus' location and extent. A 6-ft penny Caldwell radiograph is traditionally used. A cutout of the frontal sinus and superior orbital rims is prepared from the radiograph and sterilized. It is important to include the superior orbital rims so that they may be used a landmark to ensure proper placement of the template. The outline of the sinus is then transferred to the frontal bone with methylene blue. The pericranium is incised and a cutting burr is used to outline the location of the sinus. When reconstruction requires a vascularized pericranial flap, the pericranium should be carefully elevated and protected

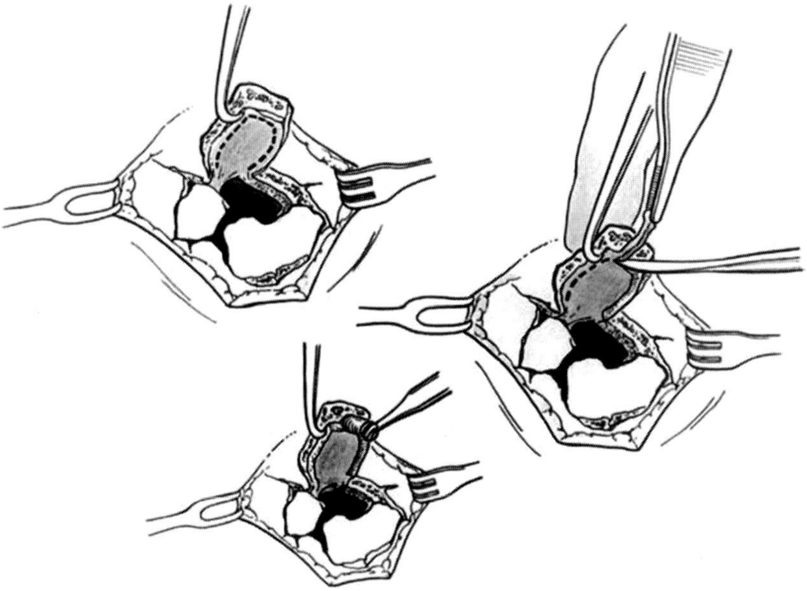

Figure 13 Bone and mucosa are removed from the margins of larger fragments. (From Ref. 32.)

prior to marking and osteotomizing of the bone. The osteotomy is made with a Stryker saw or with a cutting drill bit. It is important to angulate the cutting instrument toward the interior of the sinus (Fig. 16). An osteotome or saw is used to cut the thick bone at the brow and nasion. Finally, the intersinus septum is osteotomized. with gentle upward pressure the anterior wall of the frontal sinus is fractured as a single fragment (Fig. 17). When the intersinus septum is being cut, care must be taken to avoid injury to the sinus floor and nasofrontal ducts. Directing the osteotomy toward the superior aspect of the nasion, in effect fracturing the septum obliquely and leaving the inferior portion intact, achieves this.

Traditionally, the 6-ft penny Caldwell radiograph has been used to locate the frontal sinus for osteoplastic flap procedures. Alternate methods are available that may be used alone or in conjunction with the penny Caldwell x-ray to help confirm its position. An endoscope may be inserted through a small trephine in the anterior wall of the frontal sinus. The operating theater's lights are then turned down and the sinus is nicely transilluminated. This allows excellent visualization of the sinus' location. When available, image-guided navigational systems precisely locate the

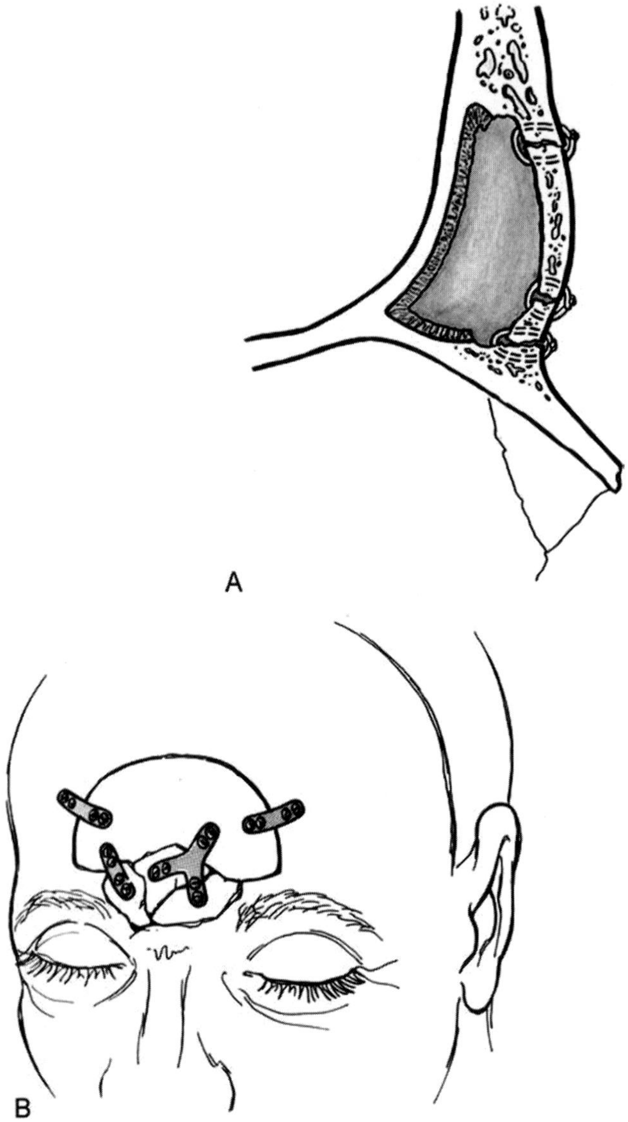

Figure 14 Fixation of bone fragments by (A) wire osteosynthesis or (B) miniplate rigid fixation. (From Ref. 32.)

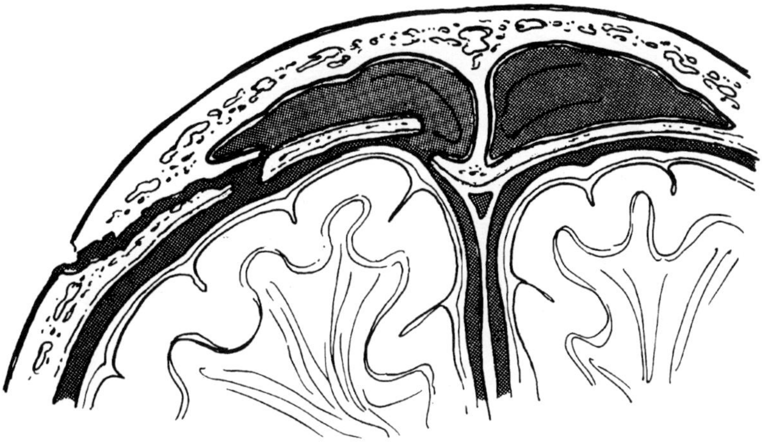

Figure 15 Displaced posterior wall fracture. (From Ref. 32.)

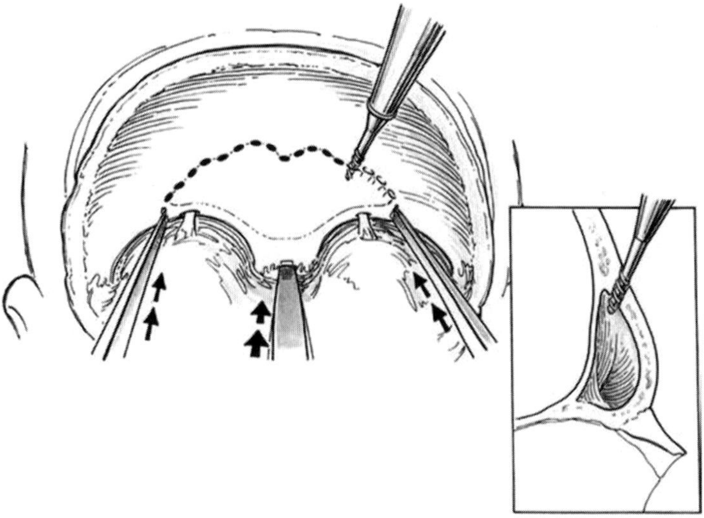

Figure 16 Osteoplastic flap procedure. The outline of the sinus is carefully marked with a template and then perforated with a cutting drill bit. It is important to angulate the drill into the sinus interior (inset) to avoid accidental intracranial injury. The lateral brows and glabella may require osteotomy to facilitate mobilization of the anterior wall of the sinus. (From Ref. 32.)

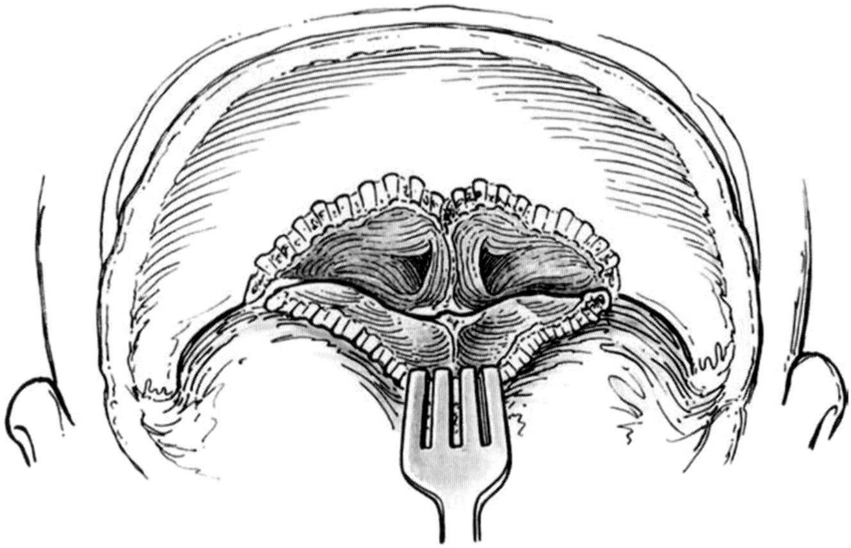

Figure 17 Completed osteoplastic flap. (From Ref. 32.)

sinus. These systems require specialized instrumentation and experience but may prove invaluable in certain situations.

Once open, the posterior wall of the sinus is carefully examined. The posterior wall mucosa is elevated to expose the fracture, In cases of nondisplaced fractures without CSF leak the sinus mucosa is completely removed. Removing all mucosal remnants requires drilling away a 1–2-mm layer of bone. The nasofrontal ducts are then plugged with free temporalis muscle grafts and the sinus interior is obliterated with abdominal fat. The fat is harvested through a left-lower-quadrant incision. The bony anterior wall is then plated back into position. Late complications are avoided by meticulous and complete removal of the sinus mucosa.

If a CSF leak or depressed fracture is encountered, the bone fragments must be elevated carefully and the dura examined. As illustrated in Figure 18, small dural lacerations are repaired with simple interrupted dural sutures. A watertight closure is necessary. The repair should be augmented with a fascial graft (Fig. 19). Neurosurgical consultation is required when the dural injury is more complex or when there appears to be an injury to the frontal lobe or superior sagittal sinus. Complex dural lacerations require duraplasty with temporalis fascia, fascia lata, or lyophilized dura. The repair is reinforced with a second layer of fascia tucked under the margins of the bony defect and may be augmented with

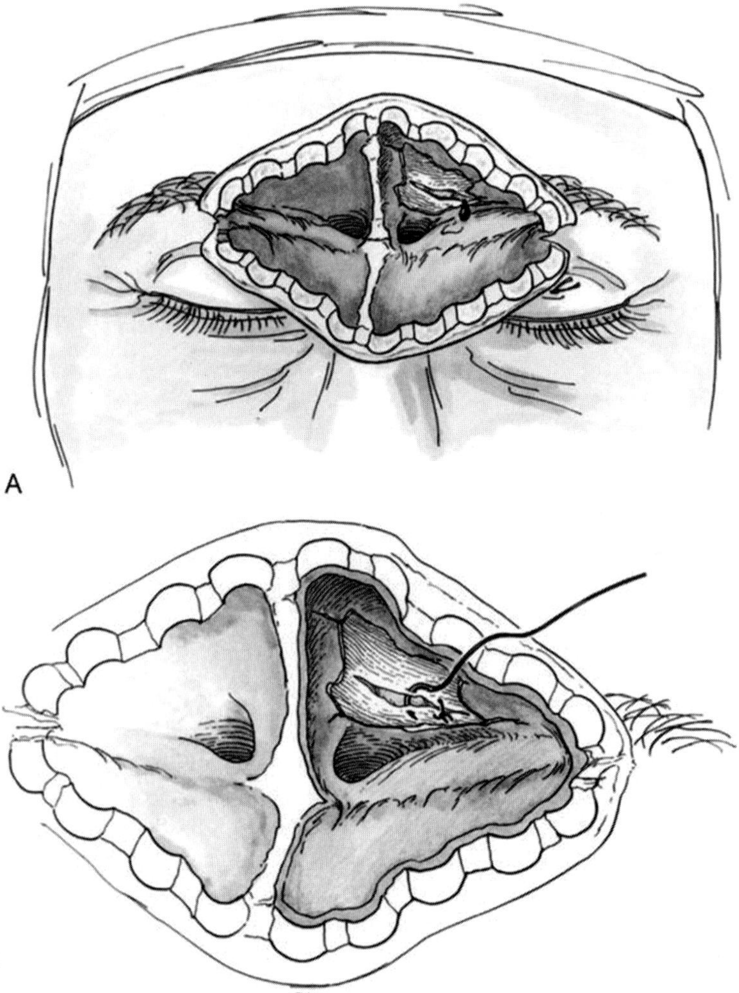

Figure 18 Dural tear and CSF leak exposed. The dural tear is repaired with simple interrupted dural sutures. (From Ref. 32.)

fibrin glue. All displaced bone fragments are then reduced and the sinus obliterated. Unfortunately, loose fragments of bone must be removed. If there is a significant dehiscence in the posterior wall, obliteration is ill advised. As shown by Donald and Ettin, fat obliteration in the presence of significant posterior wall bone loss often leads to fat graft absorption with subsequent re-epithelialization and mucocele formation (13).

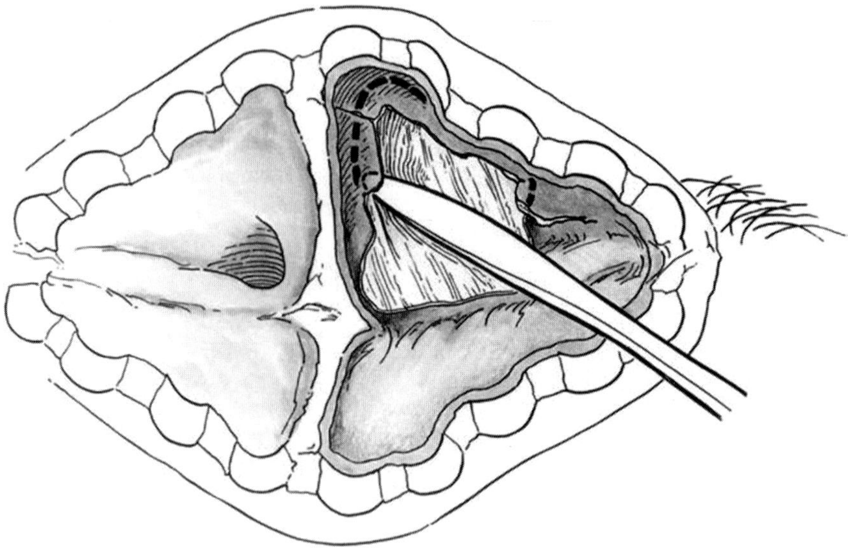

Figure 19 The dural repair should be augmented with a fascial graft that is tucked underneath the margins of the posterior wall bony defect. (From Ref. 32.)

Whenever a small dehiscence exists, consideration should be given to obliteration of the sinus with a vascularized pericranial flap. If greater 25% of the posterior wall is missing, the sinus should be cranialized (14). This involves complete removal of all sinus mucosa as previously described and resection of the remaining posterior wall. The frontal lobes of the brain are allowed to prolapse into the dead space previously occupied by the sinus. It is extremely important to plug the nasofrontal ducts to prevent ascending infection. This is accomplished with temporalis muscle grafts and may be augmented with pericranium. The anterior wall of the sinus is then plated back into position. The procedure is outlined in Figure 20.

C. Nasofrontal Duct Fracutre

Isolated fracture of the nasofrontal duct duct are rare injuries that, as previously mentioned, are hard to diagnose (Fig. 21). In fact, most isolated injuries manifest themselves as late infectious complications secondary to mucopyocele formation. The majority of nasofrontal duct injuries occur in conjunction with other frontal sinus fractures and, as such, are diagnosed at the time of surgical exploration. Isolated injury is suggested by frontal sinus obstruction that persists for more than 10 days. Coronal CT scan may confirm the diagnosis. However, mucosal injuries and nondisplaced fractures are difficult to see radiographically. Instilling methylene blue into

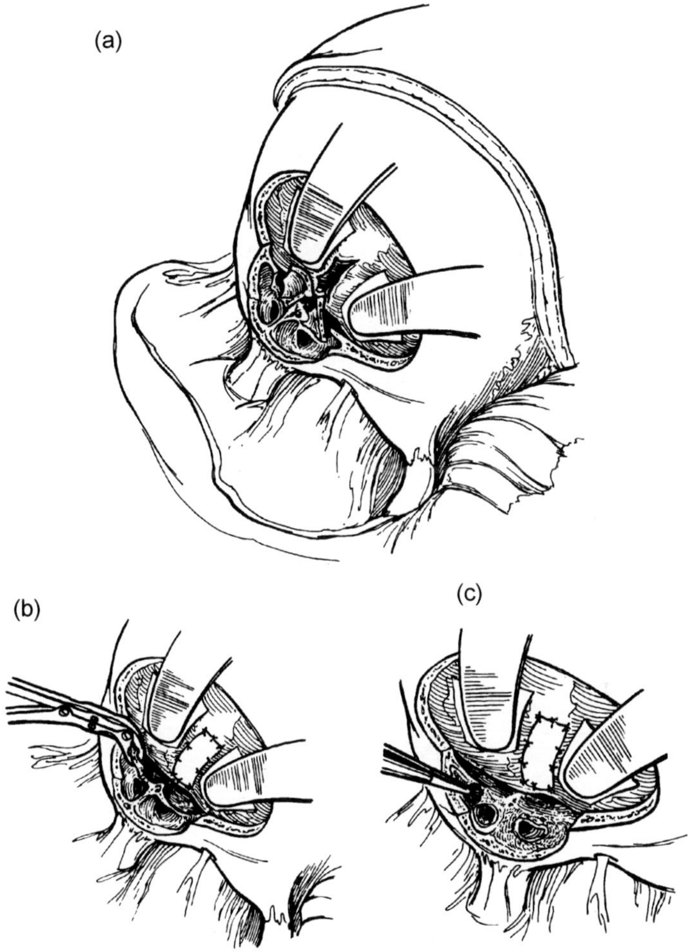

Figure 20 Cranialization procedure. (a) Following osteoplastic flap and frontal craniotomy, the posterior wall fragments are removed and any dural defects are repaired. (b) The remaining posterior wall is resected to the level of the sinus floor. (c) All sinus mucosa and a 2-mm rim of bone are removed. (d) Temporalis muscle plugs are used to obliterate the nasofrontal ducts bilaterally. (e) The frontal lobes are then allowed to expand and fill the defect. (f) The craniotomy and anterior frontal sinus wall are then fixed into position using wire or miniplates. (From Ref. 32.)

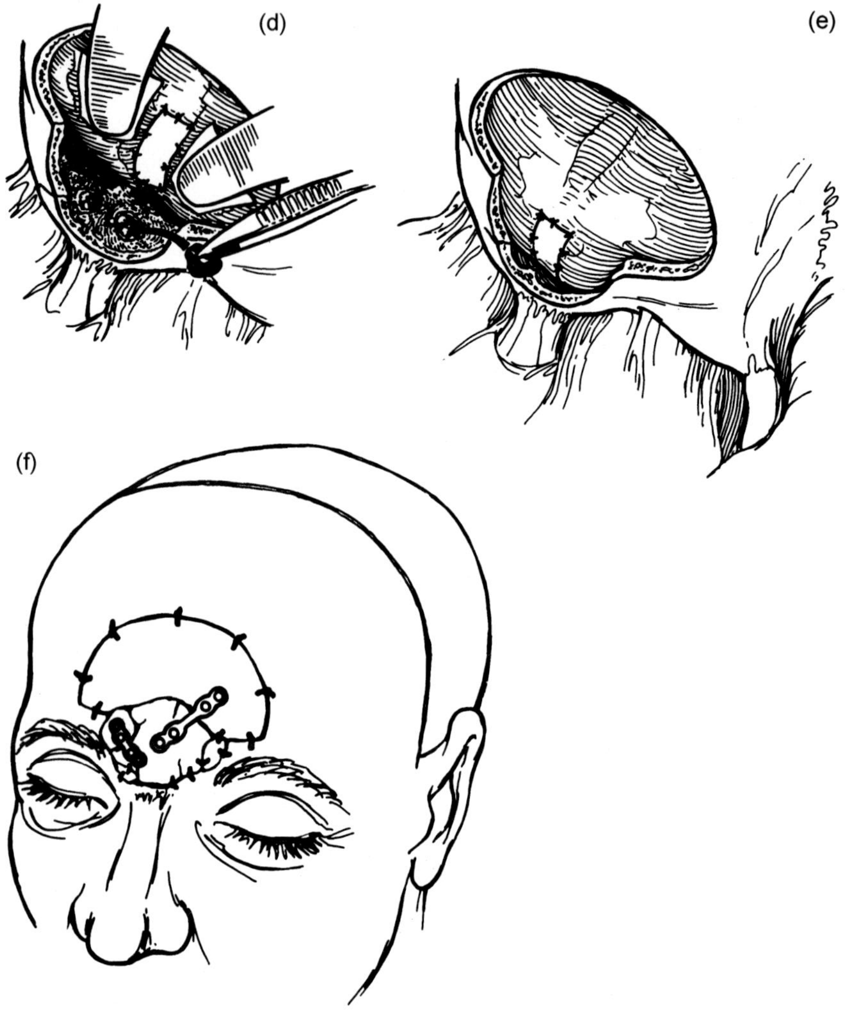

Figure 20 (*continued*)

the sinus via a trephine and observing its egress into the nasal cavity may demonstrate patency of the ducts. If obstructed, drainage of the sinus must be re-established. If this is not possible, the sinus should be obliterated. Occasionally, a unilateral injury may result in unilateral frontal sinusitis. In these situations, endoscopic frontal sinusotomy may be therapeutic and effectively treat the obstruction. Otherwise, the intersinus septurn may be taken down through a trephine, allowing drainage of infection through

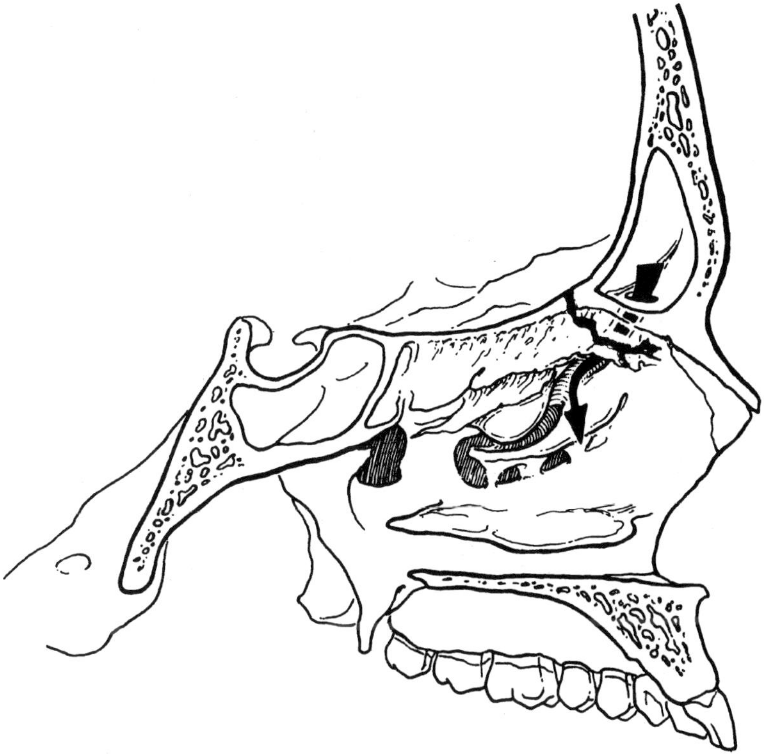

Figure 21 Fracture of the cribriform plate extending through the nasofrontal duct. (From Ref. 32.)

the normal contralateral nasofrontal duct. The normal ciliary beat pattern within the sinus is circular with secretions being carried up the intersinus septum and then along the roof and floor of the sinus prior to reaching the nasofrontal duct (Fig. 22). Simply taking down the intersinus septum, therefore, is an ineffective means of permanently draining an obstructed side of the sinus. However, in cases of acute infection the cilia are dysfunctional and gravity is relied upon for drainage. This is only a temporizing measure to allow treatment of the infection prior to definitive management of the sinus.

The Management of the isolated nasofrontal duct injury remains controversial. The vast majority of fractures require frontal sinus ablation. However, in the rare case of limited unilateral injury one may consider functional preservation of the sinus. Open procedures designed to drain the frontal sinus, including the Lynch and Sewall-Boyden frontoethmoidectomy,

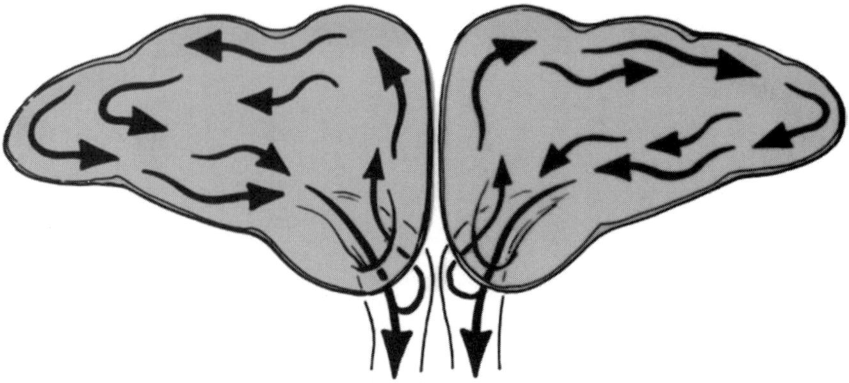

Figure 22 Normal circular flow of the frontal sinus mucosal blanket. (From Ref. 32.)

Lothrop procedure, and variations thereof, were previously considered the gold standard. These have been largely replaced by endoscopic sinus surgery. Endoscopic frontal sinusotomy may be appropriate when dealing with unilateral nasofrontal duct obstruction manifesting as posttraumatic unilateral frontal sinusitis, especially when coronal CT scan fails to show a significant bony abnormality (15). The procedure is demanding and requires experience in sinus endoscopy, specialized instrumentation, and an in-depth appreciation for paranasal sinus and anterior skull base anatomy. A detailed description of these techniques may be found elsewhere and is beyond the scope of this chapter (16).

D. Through-and-Through Fractures

Through and through fractures and devastating injuries. These fractures result in severe trauma to both walls of the frontal sinus and often to the contents of the anterior cranial fossa (Fig. 23). More often than not these fractures are compound and obvious CSF leak or cerebral injury is present at initial evaluation. Almost half of these cases result in death at the scene of the accident or shortly thereafter. The management of these injuries is complex and requires a team approach (17). Immediate neurosurgical intervention is necessary to stop hemorrhage from torn cortical veins or injury to the superior sagittal sinus. The devitalized brain is debrided and the dura is repaired. The type of dural repair depends on the extent of injury but often requires grafting with temporalis fascia, fascia lata, or lyophilized dura. Significant cerebral edema may ensure as a consequence

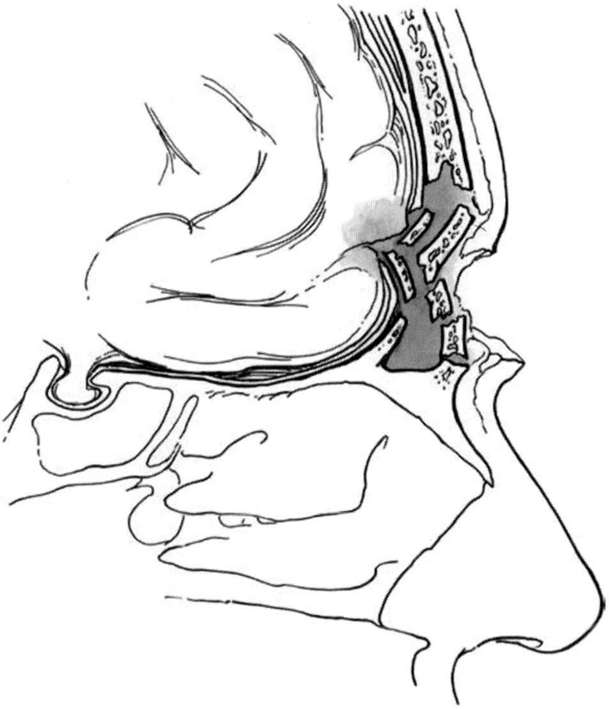

Figure 23 Through-and-through fracture of the frontal sinus with dural and cerebral injury. (From Ref. 32.)

of the cortical injury. Intravenous mannitol, hyperventilation, and an intraventicular drain may be required to help decrease intracranial pressure.

Management of the severely traumatized frontal sinus is complex. Large portions of the anterior will may be missing or contaminated. Fortunately, the work of Nadell and Kline has established the safety of using iodine-proviodine-cleansed bone fragments for anterior wall reconstruction (18). Whenever possible, the periosteum should be preserved. Further complicating matters are the large forehead lacerations or avulsions that often accompany these fractures. Owing to its rich vascular supply, the forehead is resistant to wound infection and necrosis. Therefore, all lacerations should be conservatively debrided and meticulously closed in layers. The sinus itself should be cranialized. A craniotomy is often needed to adequately treat the intracranial injuries. The posterior wall of the sinus should be removed completely, saving as much bone as possible for anterior wall reconstruction. As discussed, the mucosal lining of the sinus must be

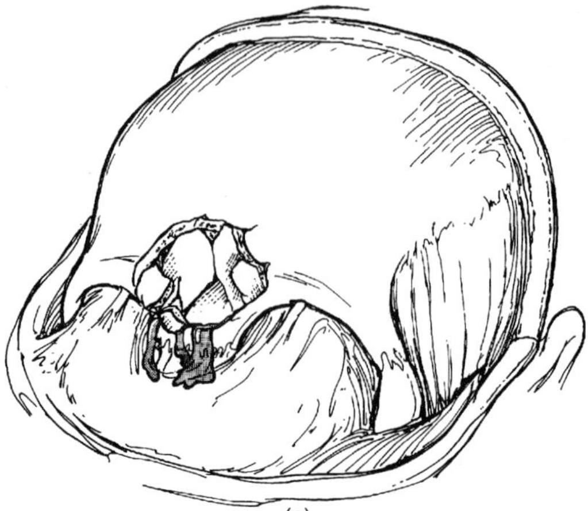

(a)

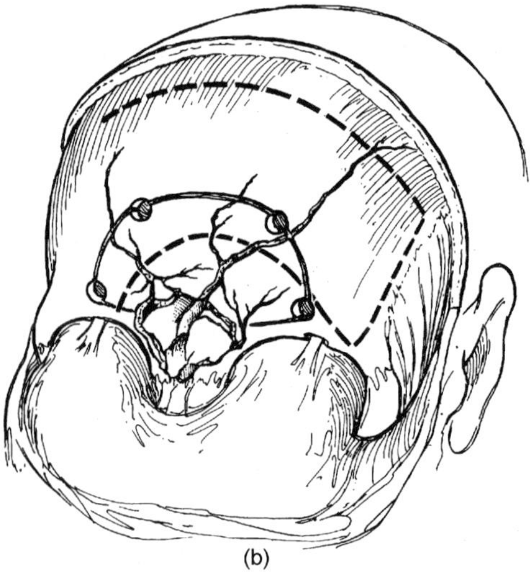

(b)

Figure 24 (a) Through-and-through fracture with obvious CSF leak. (b) The pericranial flap is elevated as outlined, based on the right supraorbital vessels in this case. A frontal craniotomy is then performed. (c) Duraplasty is performed and the dead space is obliterated with abdominal fat following cranialization. (d) An additional rim of bone (dotted line) is removed from the lateral frontal bone ipsilateral to the pedicle of the pericranial flap. This prevents strangulation of the pericranial flap once the frontal bone flap is replaced. (e) The pericranial flap is then tucked into the frontal defect. The flap should be long enough to envelop as much of the fat graft as possible. (f) The frontal craniotomy flap is replaced and the anterior wall of the sinus reduced. (From Ref. 32.)

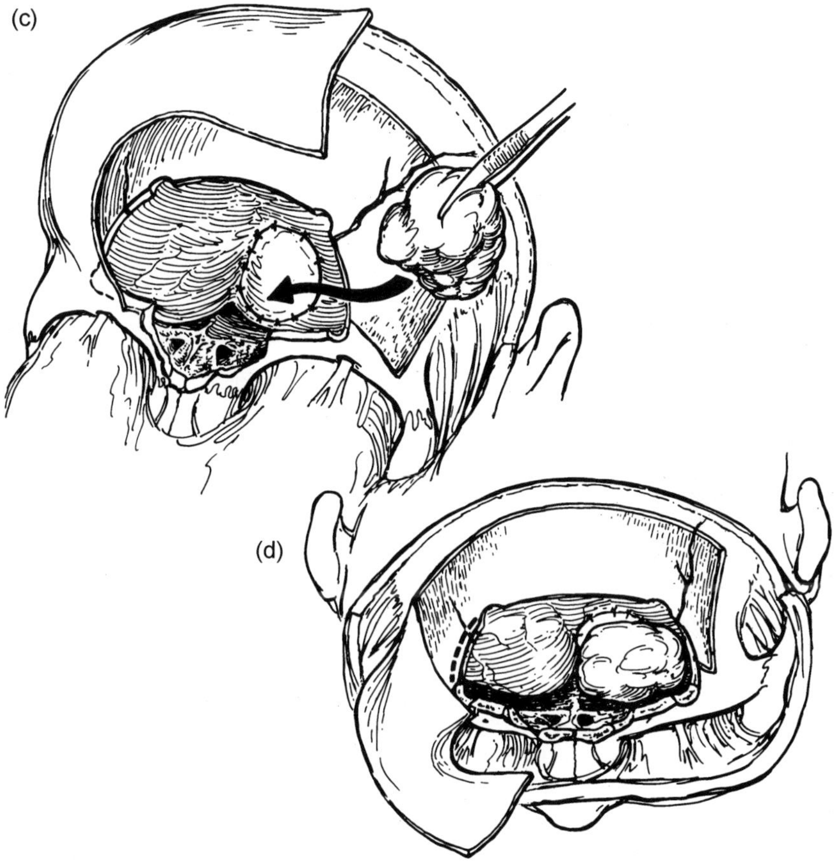

Figure 24 (*continued*)

completely removed and the nasofrontal ducts must be obliterated. The frontal lobes are then allowed to prolapse into the dead space previously occupied by the sinus. Given the extent of frontal lobe edema often encountered, the extra intracranial space is welcomed. However, when dead space persists every attempt should be made to obliterate it. As the authors have highlighted elsewhere, failure to obliterate intracranial dead space in anterior cranial base surgery predisposes to infectious complications (19).

Free fat grafts often absorb when placed against dura, especially when large duraplasties have been performed. In this situation it is recommended to use a vascularized pericranial flap and fat, as illustrated in Figure 24. The pericranium not only improves vascular supply for the fat graft but also

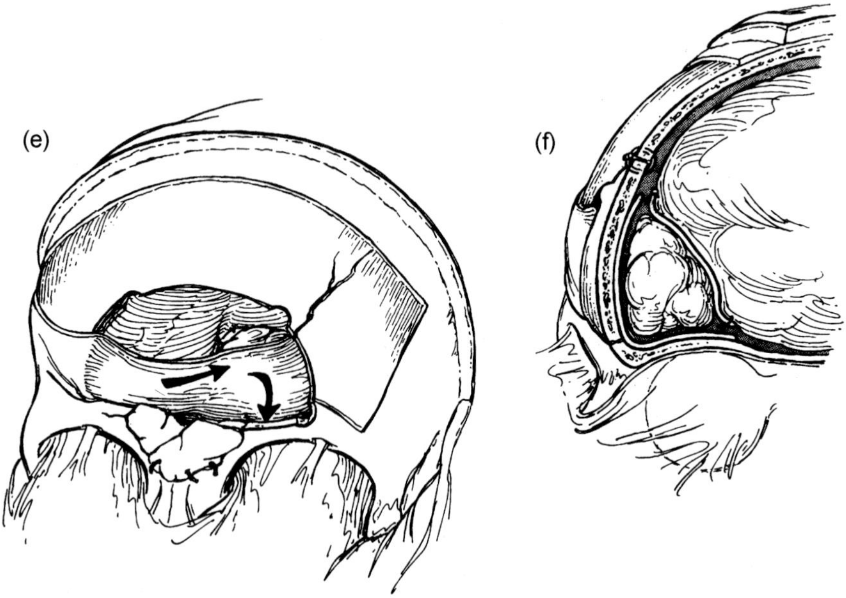

Figure 24 (*continued*)

augments the obliteration of the nasofrontal ducts. The flap should be harvested as a single long sheet of uninjured pericranium based, whenever possible, on both supraorbital pedicles. It should be tucked underneath the frontal lobes and either sutured or glued into position. When length permits, it is helpful to fold it back onto itself sandwiching the fat graft between two layers of vascularized tissue. The anterior wall of the sinus should be reconstructed. This usually requires bone grafts from either the posterior wall of the sinus or the calvarium's outer table. Alternatively, titanium mesh may be used to cover the exposed dura and recontour the forehead. In the past, such extensive injuries were not reconstructed. The sinus was completely removed and the skin was draped over the frontal lobe dura. Not only did this result in a dramatic cosmetic deformity requiring delayed reconstruction, it also placed the brain at substantial risk of injury.

VII. COMPLICATIONS OF FRONTAL SINUS TRAUMA

Many patients with frontal sinus fracture present with serious injuries that require acute care. Although it is rewarding to restore health, function, and cosmesis to these patients, it is imperative to understand that the majority of complications due to frontal sinus trauma manifest months after the injury. Therefore, all patients should be followed carefully. Aside from mucocele, all sequelae are infectious in origin. They may be divided into intracranial and extracranial complications. Fortunately, the bacteriology of these infections is similar to that seen with chronic frontal sinusitis. The most common pathogens include *Staphylococcus aureus*, anaerobic streptococci, *S. epidermidis*, *Streptococcus pneumoniae*, *β-hemolytic streptococci*, *Hemophilus influenzae*, and *Bacteroides melaninogenicus* (20). The management of these complications is both medical and surgical. The choice of antibiotic should be guided by culture results. Obviously, all abscess collections should be drained. The timing and type of surgical intervention required are dependent on the nature and severity of the complication.

A. Extracranial Complications

1. Mucocele

The propensity of the frontal sinus mucosa to form cysts in response to trauma makes mucocele formation a relatively common sequela of fracture. As previously stressed, appropriate management of the nasofrontal ducts and complete removal of all traumatized mucosa help minimize their occurrence. Although, not themselves infectious complications, mucoceles, by virtue of their propensity to erode bone and become infected, periscope patients to all of the serious extracranial and intracranial infectious sequelae of frontal sinus trauma. As the mucocele enlarges, it erodes bone along the paths of least resistance. Typically this results in erosion of the medial orbital roof and floor of the frontal sinus (Fig. 25). Clinically, this manifests as downward and lateral displacement of the globe. In addition, mucoceles may become intracranial owing to erosion of the thin posterior sinus wall. In these cases, the lining of the mucocele may be adherent to dura. Given its thickness, complete erosion through the anterior wall of the frontal sinus is uncommon. This may occur, however, when areas of dehiscence are not repaired. As mucoceles enlarge, they fill with proteinaceous fluid. This creates an ideal medium for bacterial superinfection and mucopyocele formation. Once infected, these cysts rapidly expand, causing pain, swelling, and signs of localized infection. If not effectively decompressed, mucopyoceles may lead to infections of surrounding structures, most notably of the intracranial space and orbit. Mucopyoceles must be drained surgically, often via frontal sinus trephination, and treated with appropriate antibiotics prior to definitive management of the offending mucocele.

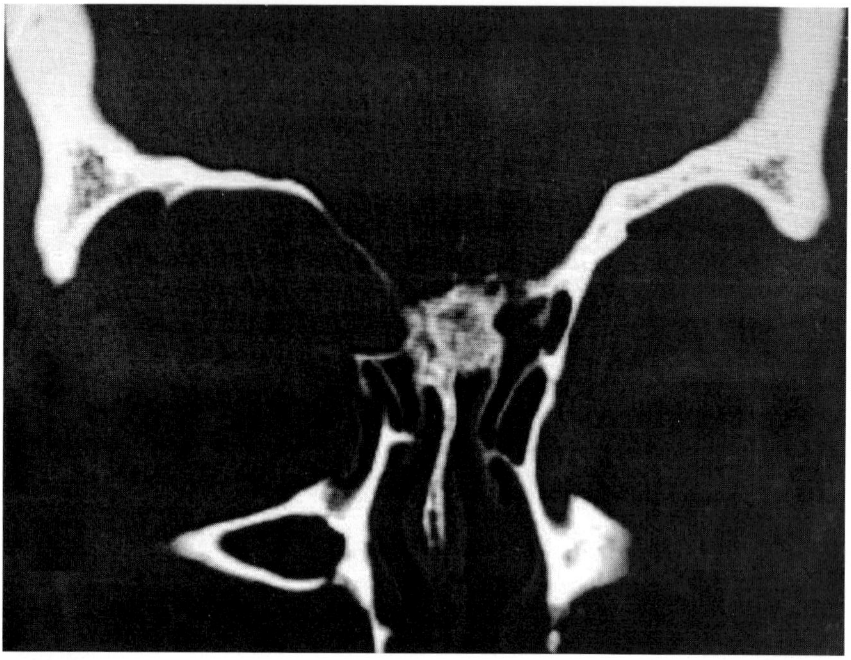

Figure 25 Right frontal mucocele eroding the medial orbital roof with inferolateral displacement of the globe.

Traditionally, mucoceles have been treated by frontal sinus obliteration or cranialization. This requires on osteoplastic flap of the anterior frontal sinus wall and removal of the entire mucocele and its lining. In cases of intracranial extension, the lining may be so adherent to dura that resection necessitates dural excision and repair (21). As experience grows with transnasal endoscopic surgery, these open procedures are being replaced by endoscopic mucocele decompression. These techniques are challenging and require experience in endoscopic nasal surgery. However, studies have shown that appropriately selected cases treated in this manner have mucocele recurrence rates approaching 0% (22–24). The most important selection criteria are the location of the mucocele and whether or not it can safely be accessed transnasally. This is a function of both location within the frontal sinus and surgical acumen. Cysts that occupy the lateral recesses of the sinus are poor candidates for transnasal decompression. These lesions are most appropriately dealt with by open procedures. Centrally located lesions, regardless of size, are suitable for endoscopic decompression (Fig. 26). The approach requires removal of the anterior frontoethmoid

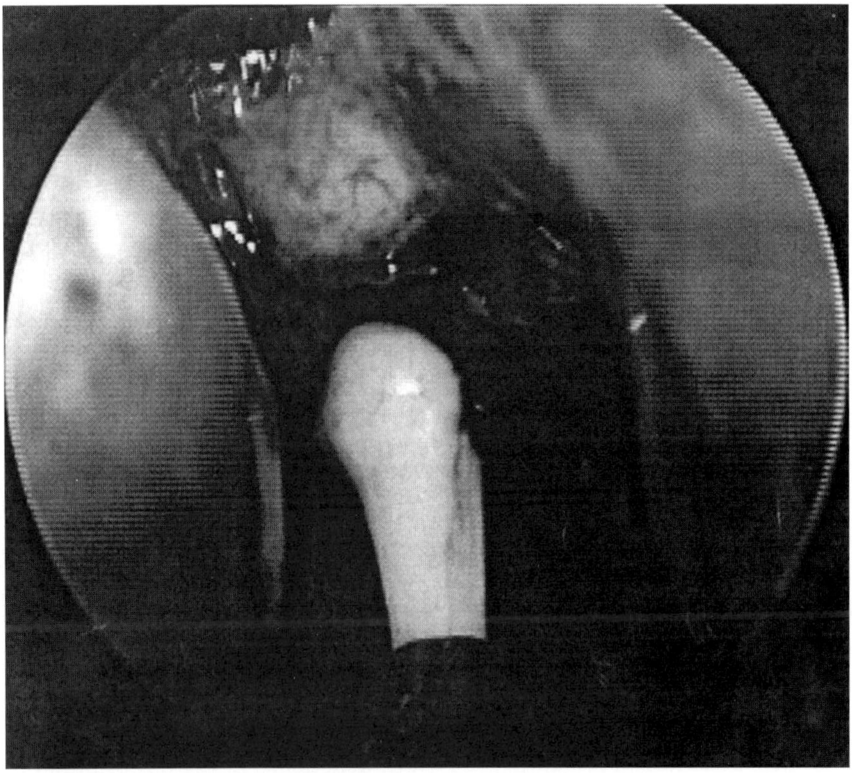

Figure 26 Transnasal endoscopic decompression of a frontal mucocele extending inferiorly into the anterior ethmoids.

air cells and exposure of the frontal sinus outflow tract. Details of the procedure are beyond the scope of this chapter and may be found elsewhere (21,25). Once the mucocele has been exposed it is widely marsupialized into the nasal cavity. Intracranial extension is not a contraindication to transnasal decompression. In fact, an endoscopic approach may be preferable in such cases because it may obviate the need for dural resection. To prevent inadvertent intracranial injury, instrumentation within the mucocele cavity should be avoided. The interior of the mucocele may be examined with the help of an angled endoscope. Stenting of the marsupialized mucocele's neck is controversial. It should be considered when the opening is not mucosally lined or less than 5 mm in diameter (26). Stents may be required for up to 12 weeks. Despite the recent success reported with transnasal endoscopic mucocele decompression, it must be remembered that open procedures are perfectly acceptable alternatives. In fact, when experience is lacking in endoriasal surgery, they should be considered the most appropriate.

2. Frontal Osteomyelitis

First described by Sir Percival Pott in 1755 (27) and commonly referred to as Pott's puffy tumor, osteomyelitis of the frontal bone is uncommon. It results from thrombophlebitis of the calvarium's diploic veins or, less commonly, from erosion of the anterior sinus wall by mucopyocele. The resultant subperiosteal abscess presents as localized forehead swelling and headache. Rarely are patients toxic. The abscess, if neglected, may result in concomitant orbital infection. Adequate treatment requires drainage of the abscess and debridement of all devitalized bone. Patients require prolonged culture-directed antibiotic therapy. Serial gallium scans are helpful to monitor effectiveness of therapy. Once the infection has been treated, the sinus should be obliterated.

B. Intracranial Complications

The frontal sinus is responsible for the majority of intracranial sinogenic infections. Brain absence (46%) and meningitis (29%) are the most frequent (28). Others include subdural absences, epidural abscess, and superior sagittal sinus thrombosis. As previously highlighted, the valveless transosseous venous channels of Breschet predispose infections of the frontal sinus to subdural extension. Trauma may result in dehiscence of the posterior sinus wall, mucocele formation, or chronic obstructive frontal sinusitis, all of which lead to these unfortunate sequelae.

The majority of patients will present with high fever and headache. The initial presentation often lacks localizing signs or symptoms and, therefore, the diagnosis requires a high index of suspicion. These complications should also be considered and ruled out in all patients suffering infectious extracranial complications. Contract and noncontrast CT scan of the brain is required to confirm the diagnosis. MRI is a useful adjunct in certain cases. In particular, magnetic resonance venography may prove valuable when septic superior sagittal sinus thrombophlebitis is suspected.

Early diagnosis is paramount. The incidence and severity of the late sequelae of intracranial infection, including seizure disorders, cognitive and motor deficits, and hydrocephalus, increase when treatment is delayed.

1. Brain Abscess

Brain abscess is thought to be the consequence of septic thrombophlebitis of the veins of Breschet and intraparenchymal implantation of septic emboli.

The abscess usually forms at the junction of the brain's gray and white matter. Initially, cerebritis develops around the septic intraparenchymal vein. Slowly, necrosis occurs and an abscess forms. This is usually a lengthy process, taking up to 14 days, thus explaining the relatively silent clinical presentation of frontal lobe abscess. If left untreated, these collections expand and cause increased intracranial pressure. Eventually they will lead to death as they rupture into the ventricular system. Frontal lobe abscess has been associated with a 19% mortality rate (29).

Patients usually present with lethargy, low-grade fever, mood changes, and headache. Localizing signs of intracranial infection are a late manifestation and indicative of increased intracranial pressure. Lumbar puncture (LP) is nondiagnostic. Owing to the increased intracranial pressures often present, LP is potentially harmful and should not be performed. The diagnosis is confirmed with CT scan (Fig. 27).

The management of brain abscess is controversial. Many will respond to medical therapy alone. Others will require either CT-guided or open drainage. Irrespective of the treatment plan, early neurosurgical consultation is imperative.

2. *Meningitis*

In the traumatized patient, meningitis is often the consequence of missed posterior wall fractures or posterior wall dehiscence in the incompletely obliterated sinus. As previously mentioned, when significant dehiscence of the posterior wall is encountered the sinus should either be cranialized or obliterated with vascularized tissue. Obliteration with fat often leads to fat resorption, re-epithelialization of the sinus, and mucocele formation.

Patients present with severe headache, high fever, meningismus, nausea, vomiting, and decreased mental status. Lumbar puncture (LP) confirms the diagnosis. However, a CT scan of the brain should be performed prior to the LP to rule out increased intracranial pressure. Although the primary management of meningitis is medical, the offending frontal sinus must be addressed. Timing of the intervention depends on the situation and condition of the patient. In the case of missed posterior-wall injury, the sinus must be obliterated. Otherwise, cranialization of the sinus should be considered once the meningitis resolves. Obviously, any abscess collection, whether intracranial or extracranial, should be drained as soon as the patient's condition permits.

C. Subdural Abscess

Subdural abscess is again the result of septic thrombophlebitis of the veins of Breschet that terminate in the subarachnoid space. These collections are

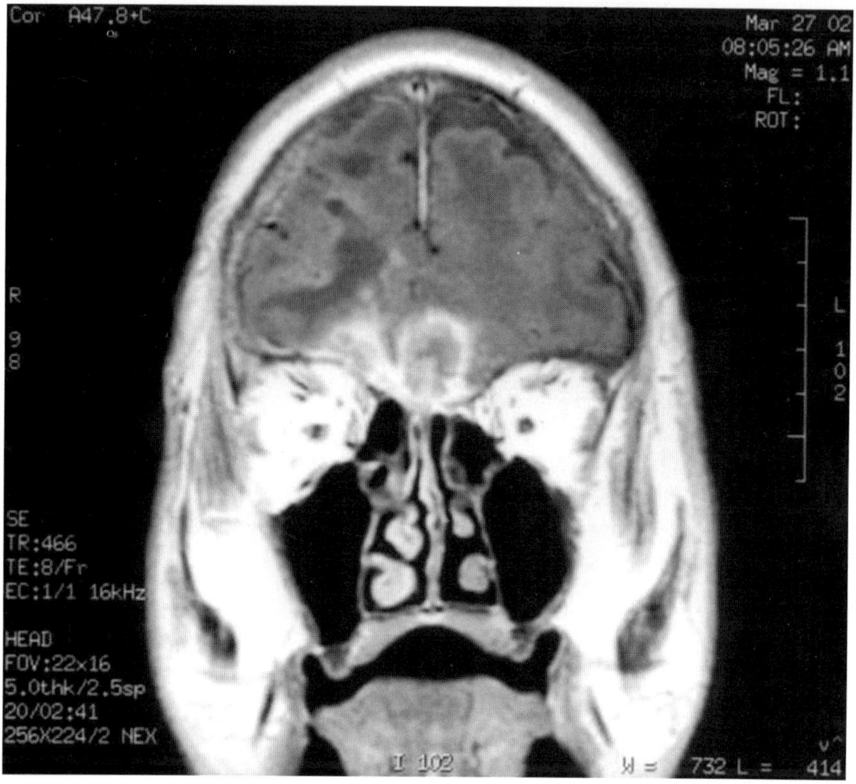

Figure 27 Frontal abscess secondary to frontal sinusitis. Note the bright ring enhancement at the periphery of the abscess.

often loculated and occur in the presence of an intact posterior frontal sinus wall. Patients are ill and present with high fever, meningismus, headache, and decreased mental status. The infection may result in septic dural vein thrombosis. This leads to increased cerebral edema that may cause venous infarction of the brain, transtentorial herniation, and death. Once again, CT confirms the diagnosis. Subdural abscess should be managed aggressively. The collection should be drained either through a burr hole or via craniotomy.

D. Epidural Abscess

Epidural abscess is an indolent infectious complication that may go undiagnosed for long periods. Neurological signs are most often absent and patients may only complain of mild headache and lowgrade fever. These collections may be associated with intact posterior frontal sinus walls but are most often the result of dehiscence. Treatment requires drainage. Aspiration is often possible through the sinus interior but on occasion may require craniotomy. Once the infection has been successfully managed, the frontal sinus often requires cranialization.

E. Superior Sagittal Sinus Thrombosis

Although a very rare occurrence, superior sagittal sinus thrombosis is an extremely serious complication. It is most frequently associated with fulminant bacterial meningitis. However, it may also result from acute and

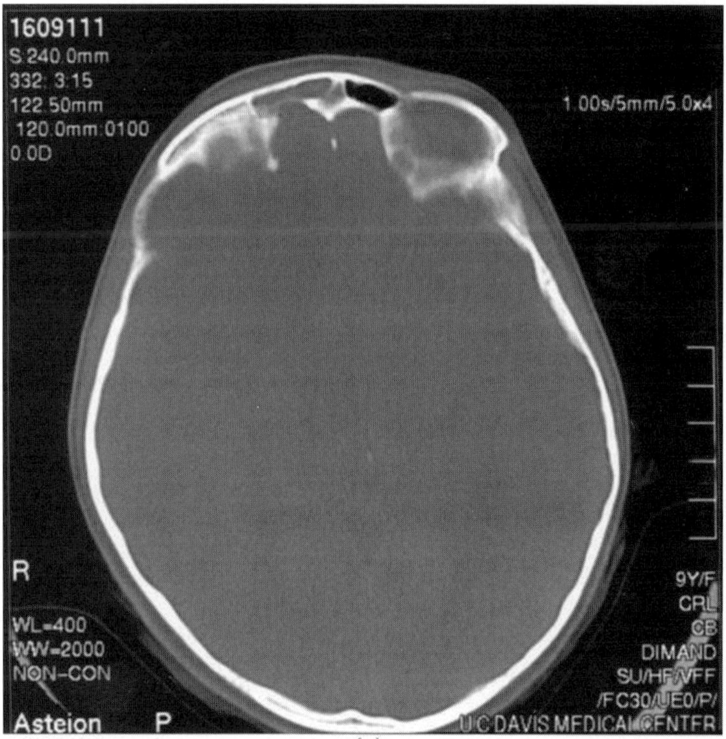

(a)

Figure 28 (a) Unilateral right frontal sinusitis. (b) Synchronous epidural and subdural empyemas. The epidural abscess is located immediately posterior to the frontal sinus and is characterized by a collection in the extradural space causing a broad-based concave depression in the frontal lobe. The laterally located subdural abscess is characterized by a collection over the cerebral convexity.

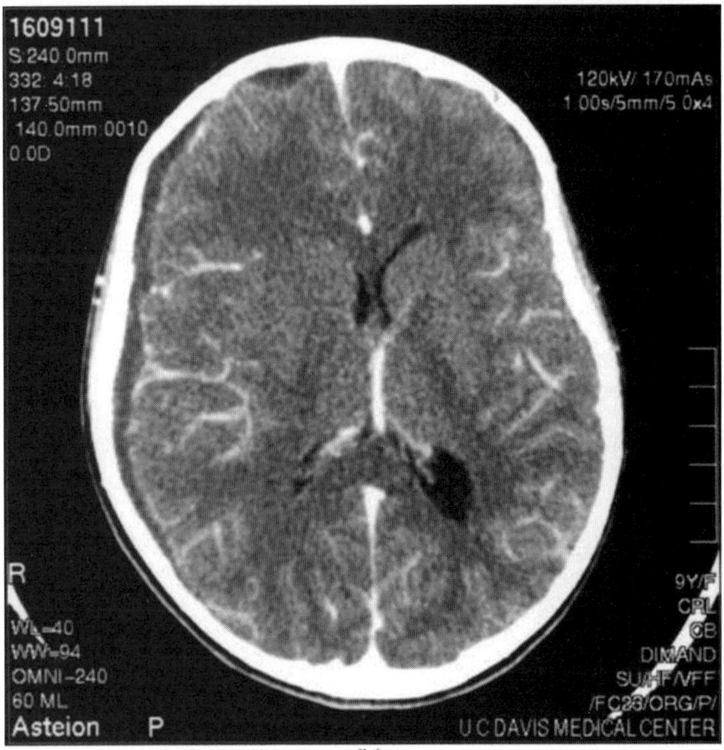

(b)

Figure 28 (*continued*)

chronic frontal sinusitis. The presentation is acute and includes high spiking fevers, decreased mental status, headache, seizures, and meningeal sings. As the septic thrombus propagates within the superior sagittal sinus, coma ensues. Death as a result of severe cerebral edema and venous infarction usually occurs once the thrombus extends beyond the proximal third of the sinus. Even when the thrombus is limited to the proximal third of the superior sagittal sinus, mortality rates as high as 80% have been reported (30).

The diagnosis is made with contrast CT scan. Findings include cortical vein thromboses, gyral-based hemorrhages, and the empty delta sign. This refers to a postcontrast filling defect within the sinus secondary to thrombus. CT and MR venography are valuable adjunctive imaging studies that help confirm the diagnosis. Treatment requires high-dose antibiotics. Administration of heparin and urokinase may help prevent propagation of the thrombus (31).

VIII. SUMMARY

A sound understanding of frontal sinus anatomy and pathophysiology is required for effective treatment of frontal sinus trauma. As illustrated herein, certain basic principles must be followed to appropriately manage these injuries. First and foremost, all injuries must be carefully evaluated and accurately classified. Inaccurate classification of the injury at hand often leads to unsuitable treatment and an increased incidence of complications. In addition, it is imperative to meticulously remove sinus mucosa whenever necessary and confirm nasofrontal duct patency. Failure to do so greatly increases the incidence of mucocele formation. The sinus should always be explored when posterior wall injury is suspected. Fractures of the posterior sinus wall should be managed with sinus obliteration or, in serve cases, cranialization. It must be emphasized that all intracranial dead space should be obliterated prior to cranialization of the frontal sinus. This often requires free fat grafts. If so, one should never hesitate to use a vascularized pericranial flap to augment the closure. The majority of complications from frontal sinus trauma manifest themselves months after initial care of injury. Despite appropriate treatment, vigilant follow-up and a high index of suspicion are needed. Unfortunately, owing to the demographics of this population, poor patient compliance and follow-up are commonplace. A systematic and thorough approach to the evaluation and treatment of these often seriously injured patients will help reduce the incidence of untoward sequelae. It behooves the surgeon to aggressively and appropriately manage every fracture with the assumption that continued follow-up of the patient will not occur.

REFERENCES

1. Van Alyea OE. Maxillary and frontal sinuses. In: English GM, Otolaryngology. Hagerstown, MD: Harper & Row, 1977.
2. Yuge A, Takio M, Masami T. Growth of frontal sinus with age—an x-ray tomographic study. In: Myers E, ed. New Dimensions in Otolaryngology—Head and Neck Surgery. Vol. 2. New York: Excerpta Medica, 1985:326–327.
3. Schaeffer JP. The Embryology, Development, and Anatomy of the Nose, Paranasal Sinuses, Naso-lacrimal Passageways, and Olfactory Organ in Man. Philadelphia: P. Blackston Son, 1920.
4. Lang J. Clinical Anatomy of the Nose, Nasal Cavity and Paranasal Sinuses. New York: G Thieme Verlag, 1989:62–69.
5. Novak R, Mehls G. Die aplasien der sinus maxillaries und frontales unter besenderer Berucksichtigung der pneumatisation bei spalttragern. Anat Anz 1977; 142:441–450.

6. Mosher HP, Judd DK. An analysis of seven cases of osteomyelitis of the fontal bone complicating frontal sinusitis. Laryngoscope 1933; 43:153.
7. Lotta JS, Schall RF. The histology of the epithelium of the paranasal sinuses under various conditions. Ann Otol Rhinol Laryngol 1934; 43:945–971.
8. Schenck NL. Frontal sinus disease. III. Experimental and clinical factors in failure of the frontal osteoplastic operation. Laryngoscope 1975; 85:76–92.
9. Donald PJ. The tenacity of the frontal sinus mucosa. Otolarnygol Head Neck Surg 1979; 87:557–566.
10. Nahum AM. The biomechanics of maxillofacial trauma. Clin Plast Surg 1975; 2:59.
11. Wallis A, Donald PJ. Frontal sinus fractures: a review of 72 cases. Laryngoscope 1988; 98(6):593–598.
12. Lakhani RS, Shubuya TY, Mathog RH, Marks SC, Burgio DL, Yoo GH. Titanium mesh repair of the severely comminuted frontal sinus fracture. Arch Otolaryngol Head Neck Surg 2001; 127(6):665–669.
13. Donald PJ, Ettin M. The safety of frontal sinus obliteration when sinus walls are missing. Laryngoscope 1986; 96(2):190–193.
14. Donald PJ. Frontal sinus ablation by cranialization: a report of 21 cases. Arch Otolaryngol 1982; 108:142.
15. Smith TL, Han JK, Loehrl TA, Rhee JS. Endoscopic management of the frontal recess in frontal sinus fractures: a shift in the paradigm? Laryngoscope 2002; 112:784–790.
16. Kuhn FA, Javer AR. Primary endoscopic management of the frontal sinus. Otolaryngol Clin North Am 2001; 34(1):59–76.
17. Donald PJ, Bernstein L. Compound frontal sinus injuries with intracranial penetration. Laryngoscope 1978; 88:225–232.
18. Nadell J, Kline DG. Primary reconstruction of depressed skull fractures including those involving the sinus, orbit, and cribriform plate. J Neurosurg 1974; 41:200–207.
19. Enepekides DJ, Donald PJ. Long-term outcomes of anterior skull base surgery. Curr Opini Otolaryngol Head Neck Surg 2000; 8:130–136.
20. Goldberg AN, Oroszlan G, Anderson TD. Complications of frontal sinusitis and their management. Otolaryngol Clin North Am 2001; 34(1):211–225.
21. Har-El G. Transnasal endoscopic management of frontal mucoceles. Otolaryngol Clin North Am 2001; 34(1):243–252.
22. Har-El G, Balwally AN, Lucente FE. Sinus mucoceles: Is marsupialization enough? Otolaryngol Head Neck Surg 1997; 117:633.
23. Josephson JS, Kennedy DW. Surgery of paranasal sinus mucoceles: operative techniques. Otolaryngol Head Neck Surg 1990; 1:133.
24. Lund VJ. Endoscopic management of paranasal sinus mucoceles. J Laryngol Otol 1998; 112:36.
25. Kuhn Fa. Surgery of the frontal sinus. In: Kennedy DW, Bolger WE, ZinReich SJ, eds. Disease of the Sinuses—Diagnosis and Management. Hamilton: BC Decker, 2001:281–301.
26. Rains BM. III Frontal sinus stenting. Otolaryngol Clin North Am 2001; 34(1):101–110.

27. Pott P. The Chirurgical Works of Percival Pott. London: Hayes W. Clarke & B. Collins, 1775.
28. Clayman GL, Adams GL, Paugh DR. Intracranial complications of paranasal sinusitis: a combined institutional review. Laryngoscope 1991; 101:234.
29. Singh B, Dellen Van J, Ramjettan S, Maharaj TJ. Sinogenic intracranial complications. J Laryngol Otol 1995; 109:945–950.
30. Southwick FS, Richardson EP, Swartz M. Septic thrombosis of the dural venous sinuses. Medicine 1986; 65(2):82–106.
31. Wasay M, Bakshi R, Kojan S, Bobustuc G, Dubey N, Unwin DH. Nonrandomized comparison of local urokinase thrombolysis versus systemic heparin anticoagulation for superior sagittal sinus thrombosis. Stroke 2001; 32(10): 2310–2317.
32. Donald PJ, Gluckman JL, Rice DH. The Sinuses. New York: Raven Press, 1995.

14

Maxillary Fractures

David A. O'Donovan
University of Miami and Jackson Memorial Hospital, Miami, Florida, U.S.A.

Oleh M. Antonyshyn
University of Toronto, Toronto, Ontario, Canada

I. HISTORICAL BACKGROUND

It is almost impossible to find a description of the management of fractures of the midface that does not commence with reference to the works of Rene Le Fort. At the turn of the last century, Le Fort was the first to document a tendency for specific fracture patterns of the midface to occur following direct facial trauma (1). His description of the effects of blunt facial impacts on 35 skulls, however, was made in an era when surviving the high-velocity impact of a modern motor vehicle accident could not have been imagined. The journey from his anatomical observations to the present-day management of complex facial trauma by advanced craniomaxillofacial techniques required a succession of often historically driven surgical advances.

The initial impetus for the clinical application of Le Fort's observations was the arrival of thousands of severe soft- and hard-tissue facial injuries produced by the new fragmentation missiles of World War I. Gillies (2,3) and Kazanjian (4) were instrumental at this time in recognizing the importance of the dental arch in stabilizing the midface through the use of a variety of extraskeletal fixation devices that are now for the most part obsolete. The advent of the antibiotic era during World War II, however, heralded the beginning of successful primary surgical intervention through the principles of anatomical reduction and internal bone stabilization.

As first described by Ipsen (5) in the early 1930s, Brown and McDowell (6,7) popularized internal K-wire fixation of facial fractures. Dingman and Natvig (8,9) subsequently introduced midface fracture immobilization by rubber band traction. In 1942, Milton Adams (10) was the first to propose the open reduction and internal fixation of facial fractures by using suspension wires to a stable cranial base.

Following World War II, Gillies extrapolated his experience from traumatic facial repair to the field of congenital facial anomalies and pioneered the elective Le Fort III osteotomy for Crouzon syndrome. This paved the way for Tessier's landmark description in 1967 of the cranial base approach to pediatric craniofacial skeletal deformities that heralded the birth of modern craniofacial surgery (11,12). High rates of long-term posterior midface collapse, however, shifted the focus away from craniofacial suspension in the 1980s to open reduction and internal fixation techniques that obviated the prolonged periods of intermaxillary fixation and ultimately reduced posttraumatic deformity rates. This approach, primarily popularized by Manson (13,14) and Gruss (15), is dependent upon accurate skeletal injury assessment by Computerized-Tomography (CT) scanning, wide exposure of all fracture sites, open mobilization and reduction of all bone segments, primary autogenous bone grafting, and stable internal fixation by plates and screws. These principles still comprise the basis of the almost universally subscribed to blueprint of modern craniofacial fracture management.

II. SURGICAL ANATOMY

The midface connects the cranial base to the occlusal plane. It provides the foundation for anterior facial projection while contributing to protection of the critical skull base and acting as an anchor for facial ligament and muscle attachment. The skeleton of the midface consists of a series of thickened vertical, sagittal, and horizontal bony structural supports (buttresses) that envelop a system of aerated cavities (sinuses).

The vertical structural supports of the midface consist of the nasomaxillary (medial), zygomaticomaxillary (lateral), and pterygomaxillary (posterior) buttresses (Fig. 1). The nasomaxillary buttress extends along the piriform aperture from the cuspid and anterior portion of the maxilla, through the frontal process of the maxilla, and up into the lacrimal crest and medial wall of the orbit to the frontal bone. The zygomaticomaxillary buttress extends from the maxillary alveolus above the first molar through the body of the zygoma up into the frontal process of the zygoma to the frontal bone. These medial and lateral buttresses provide the anterior

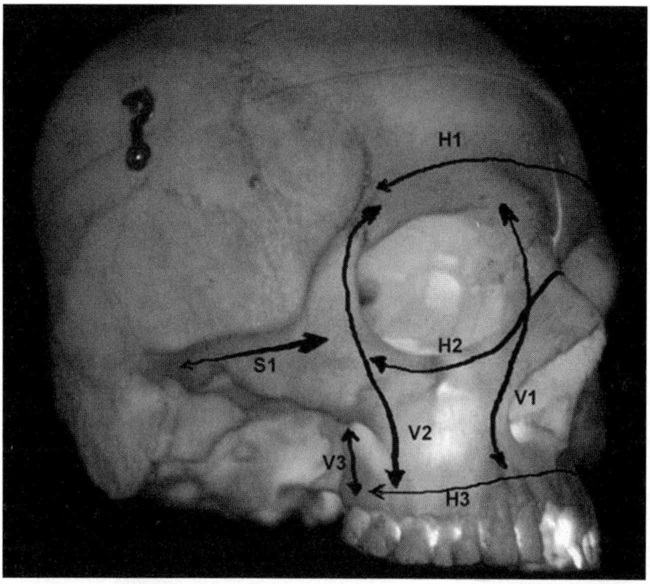

Figure 1 Transilluminated skull demonstrating air-filled sinuses within the midface, reinforced by dense skeletal buttresses. The vertical pillars, i.e., the medial or nasomaxillary buttress (V_1), lateral or zygomaticomaxillary buttress (V_2), and posterior or pterygomaxillary buttresses (V_3), dissipate forces directed toward the cranial base. The horizontal buttresses are oriented along the supraorbital rims (H_1), infraorbital rims (H_2), and dentoalveolar process and palate (H_3), providing further structural support to the functional spaces of the eyes, nose, and mouth. The zygomatic arches provide the only sagittal buttresses (S_1).

support. Posteriorly, the pterygoid buttress attaches the maxilla to the pterygoid plates of the sphenoid bone and provides posterior stabilization to the vertical height of the midface. The horizontal midface buttresses are comprised of the superior and inferior orbital rims and the hard palate. The zygomatic arches provide the only sagittal buttresses, rendering the midface susceptible to collapse and retrodisplacement particularly in the central segments (16).

Reconstruction of midfacial structural defects requires the reconstitution of these buttresses to restore normal pretraumatic load paths and thus the biomechanical parameters that are essential for maintaining skeletal structural integrity. These thickened bony columns provide the optimal sites for application of fixation plates to ensure maximal support and subsequent primary healing.

III. MIDFACE FRACTURE CLASSIFICATION

No description of the fracture patterns of the midface has succeeded that of Le Fort. Le Fort's classification though, is not a pure maxillary fracture classification as many other facial bones are involved. However, it should be noted that the majority of maxillary fractures are seldom isolated and are usually comminuted, involve numerous combinations of Le Fort–type fractures. Le Fort described three zones of transverse weakness in the midfacial skeleton that resulted in predictable fracture patterns (Fig. 2).

1. Le Fort I Fracture (30%):
   A horizontal fracture pattern that extends in a transmaxillary direction at the level of the piriform margin.
   Bilateral in nature and should result in a "floating palate" disconnecting the upper maxillary alveolus from the cranial base.

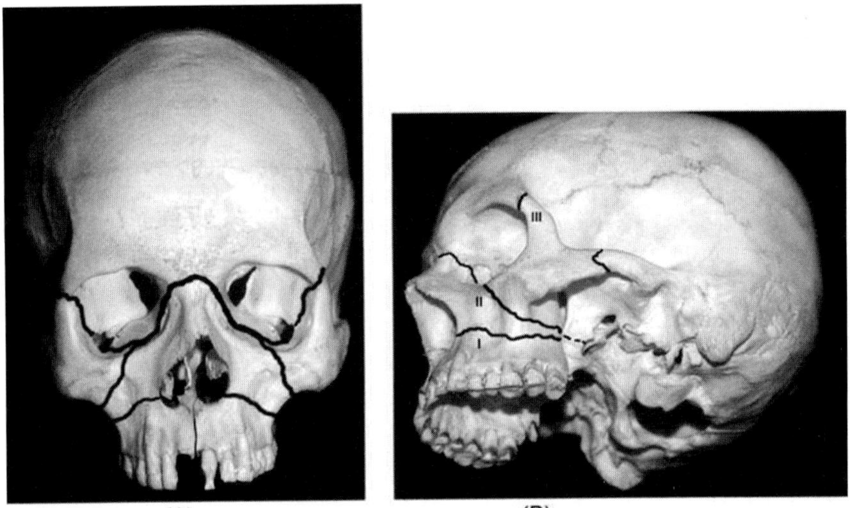

(A) (B)

Figure 2 Frontal (A) and lateral-oblique (B) views of the skull, illustrating Le Fort fracture patterns. The Le Fort I fracture (I) is a transverse disruption of the midface through the pyriform aperture. The Le Fort II fracture (II) separates the central midface (i.e., the nasal and maxillary bones) from the rest of the craniofacial skeleton. The Le Fort III fracture (III) dissociates the entire midfacial skeleton, including the central midface and orbitozygomatic complexes from the cranium. All maxillary fractures disrupt either the pterygoid plate (as shown by the dotted line in B) or pterygomaxillary junction.

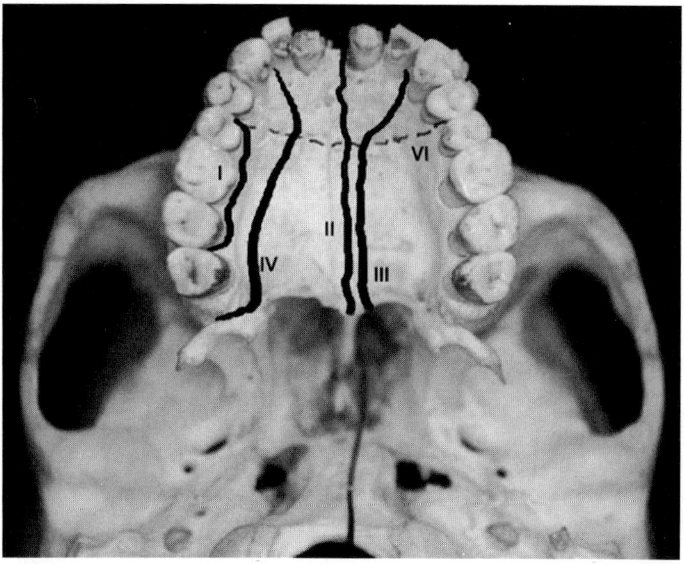

Figure 3 Palatal fracture pattern classification: (I) dentoalveolar; (II) sagittal; (III) parasagittal; (IV) para-alveolar; (V) complex (not shown), i.e., involving multiple fractures; (VI) transverse.

2. Le Fort II Fracture (42%)
   Pyramidal/subzygomatic fractures that produce dissociation of the central midface from the orbitozygomatic complex.
3. Le Fort III Fracture (28%)
   Also termed "craniofacial disjunction."
   Fracture produces a separation through the frontozygomatic suture and nasofrontal junction.

Vertical or palatal fractures of the maxilla have been comprehensively classified by Hendrickson et al. (17) (Fig. 3). These fractures are rare, occurring in only 8% of Le Fort fractures. However, they are important to recognize as the disruption of the maxillary arch significantly increases the potential for malunion and malocclusion.

IV. EPIDEMIOLOGY

Motor vehicle accidents are responsible for up to 60% of facial fractures, with assaults (24%), falls (9%), industrial accidents (4%), sports (2%), and gunshots (2%) making up the rest. Excluding nasal fractures, the midface is involved in approximately 40% of cases (18). Most authors agree that the distribution of frequency of Le Fort type fractures is in the order of type II > type I > type III (19–21). Sagittal fractures of the alveolar ridge or palate occur rarely in isolation and are present in less than 20% of maxillary fractures (22). Coincidental injuries are frequent, with associated head trauma (50%), cervical spine injuries (10%), concomitant chest or abdominal trauma (15%), and associated skeletal injuries (30%) being found in patients with midfacial fractures (23,24).

V. DIAGNOSIS OF MAXILLARY FRACTURES

A. Clinical Assessment

Midface fractures are usually diagnosed clinically and confirmed radiologically. Numerous factors can make the initial clinical assessment difficult, including the presence of facial edema, significant epistaxis, a severely impacted maxilla, or even an uncooperative or unconscious patient. In patients with a history of blunt facial trauma, suggestive clinical signs that should alert the physician to the possibility of a midfacial fracture include epistaxis, infraorbital ecchymosis or edema, increased vertical facial height ("equine facies"), or increased facial width with a loss of anterior projection ("dishpan facies"). The most precise assessment of the maxillary injury can usually be determined from the occlusal status. Malocclusion, maxillary mobility, and dental fractures are all indicators of possible underlying maxillary skeletal pathology. The occlusal pattern encountered will usually be dictated by the fracture orientation. Transverse Le Fort–style fractures allow the strong medial pterygoid muscles to produce a posteroinferior pull on the mobile segment resulting in a retrodisplaced maxilla (class III malocclusion), premature contacting molars, and a subsequent anterior open bite. Vertical fractures through the hard palate classically present with a crossbite from an increased maxillary arch width as a result of superolateral distraction of the mobile segments.

With a displaced maxillary fracture, a conscious patient will usually volunteer that his bite relationship is altered. In the unconscious patient, physical examination for apparent dental relationships and maxillary mobility is essential. With the patient's mouth open and head stabilized, the premaxilla is grasped between the thumb and index finger and mobility ascertained. If movement is present, palpation at the nasofrontal junction, lateral orbital rim, and infraorbital rim can often help determine the fracture level. Impacted maxillary fractures may not demonstrate mobility despite significant force being applied. If a maxillary fracture is suspected, a complete examination should include a full ophthalmological review, a record of an infraorbital neurosensory assessment, and inspection of the dental arch and palate for the presence of ecchymosis, mucosal tearing, and separation or avulsion of teeth. Premorbid orthodontic and ophthalmological histories are also useful if available.

B. Radiological Assessment

Plain-film x-rays are almost useless in providing an accurate assessment of the midfacial skeleton when compared to their power in evaluating mandibular injuries. A plain Water's view may show a discontinuity of the infraorbital rim or a clouding of the maxillary sinuses that can indicate skeletal pathology (25). A Panorex x-ray that shows the status of the mandibular condyles and a chest x-ray to detect inhaled dental fragments may also be useful. The best confirmation and delineation of a clinically suspected midfacial injury is by 3-mm to 5-mm axial CT images (26,27). If no cervical spine injury is a contraindication, coronal views should also be obtained, especially if associated orbital injury is suspected. If an unstable cervical spine precludes a formal coronal scan, slightly poorer-quality but workable reformatted coronal images can usually be obtained from the axial studies. The CT images provide the most accurate visual representation of fracture patterns, degree of comminution, and extent of bone loss. The CT scan is not solely for diagnostic purposes but also is of prime importance in planning the surgical reconstruction. Three-dimensional CT reconstructions can demonstrate the spatial relationships and the degree of displacement between the maxilla and the mandible and orbits. In addition, by displaying associated fractures regionally in the naso-orbito-ethmoid area, zygomatic arches, and orbital floors, the CT images can also dictate the surgical approach and planned plate fixation sites.

VI. INITIAL MANAGEMENT OF MIDFACIAL FRACTURES

Midfacial fractures very rarely cause airway obstruction but basic trauma management principles should be applied. Establishing an airway, controlling significant hemorrhage, and identifying and managing associated injuries (especially intracranial and cervical spine) are essential. Most patients do not require a surgical airway at time of presentation to the emergency room. Intraoperative airway management usually consists of a reinforced nasotracheal tube sutured to the nasal membranous septum to allow for fracture site exposure and intermaxillary fixation. If a nasal tube is contraindicated (e.g., severe nasal structural damage, significant skull base fracture), an oral endotracheal tube positioned behind the third molar and secured to a molar tooth with 26-gauge steel wire can be used. Rarely and usually in panfacial injuries is a tracheostomy required. Caution should always be used before passing any tube (nasogastric, etc.) through the nose of a patient with a midfacial fracture owing to the theoretical risk of an associated skull base fracture allowing the tube to be passed intracranially.

Owing to the very significant midfacial blood supply, maxillary fractures can result in life-threatening hemorrhage. In addition, the bleeding can be occult in nature with more blood passing from the nasopharynx into the oropharynx than is seen externally from the mouth or nose. Significant hypovolemia can develop before the extent of the bleeding is appreciated and often this is only following the violent emesis produced by large volumes of blood in the stomach. In the presence of severe bleeding, nasal packing can be lifesaving. Caution should be exhibited, however, in the presence of a displaced mobile maxilla as routine anterior nasal packing may further displace the segment and thus not offer any sustained pressure to control the bleeding. Posterior nasal packing using a Foley catheter inserted through both nares into the nasopharynx can be required (Fig. 4). The catheter's balloons should be air-inflated and are pulled anteriorly to close off the posterior choanae. The catheters are tied to one another externally, and in addition, the anterior nasal chambers are packed with a roll of gauze wadding to complete the tamponade (28). Should these measures fail to control hemorrhage, urgent selective angiography and embolization is indicated.

The presence of cerebrospinal fluid (CSF) rhinorrhea warrants a neurosurgical consultation and usually is an indication for prophylactic antibiotic coverage. The presence of a CSF leak can usually be determined clinically by examining the straw-colored nasal drainage for the presence of glucose or a positive halo sign. CT documentation of naso-ethmoid and cribriform plate fractures can also support the suspicion of a leak and can be proven by a prescan intrathecal injection of metrizamide (29).

Owing to the associated disruptions of the nasal and oral mucosa, maxillary fractures are generally deemed compound in nature and are routinely given broad-spectrum antibiotics to cover known oral contaminants. The timing of surgical intervention for midfacial fractures is usually determined by the patient's comorbid condition. In the situation where urgent neurosurgical intervention is required, immediate reconstruction of the midfacial skeleton at the same surgery can be considered and usually follows the completion of all dural and intracranial repairs

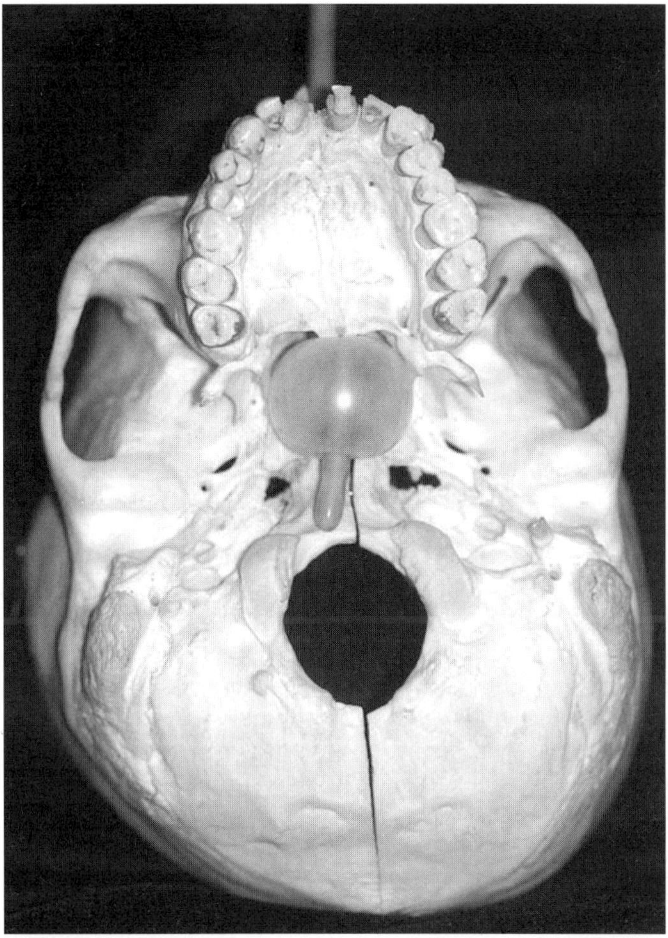

Figure 4 Hemorrhage associated with midfacial fractures is controlled by posterior nasal packing. Insertion of a Foley catheter into the nasal airway and inflation of the balloon with air (not water) effectively tamponades bleeding vessels as traction is applied to the catheter.

(30). Midfacial fracture repairs are routinely carried out on the earliest available surgical list. Extended delays in reconstruction may result in premature bony fusion that can make fracture reduction very difficult and may even necessitate the use of formal osteotomies to restore normal anatomy and ultimately can lead to adverse long-term results (31).

VII. SURGICAL MANAGEMENT OF MAXILLARY FRACTURES

A. Incisions

Fractures of the lower maxilla are best exposed through bilateral upper-gingivobuccal sulcus incisions. This approach allows subperiosteal access to the nasomaxillary and zygomaticomaxillary buttresses extending superiorly to the level of the infraorbital rims. Direct exposure of the inferior orbit is obtained through a transconjunctival or mid-lower eyelid. Both of these approaches are preferable to a subciliary incision owing to a lower risk of postoperative ectropion formation (32). Full exposure of the maxillary fracture sites requires a careful dissection of the mucosal lining from the lateral nasal wall and often a detachment of the caudal nasal septum from the maxillary crest. A complete release of the soft-tissue envelope is essential to allow maxillary fracture disimpaction. Dento-alveolar segmental fractures may require a vertical upper-buccal sulcus incision to help preserve the blood supply to the small tooth-bearing alveolar fragments.

Careful identification of all fragments is required when exposing comminuted buttress fractures. To ensure restoration of midfacial vertical height, retention of all significant-sized fragments should be emphasized to ensure an anatomical reduction. However, fragments too small for plate fixation should be discarded and replaced by primary autogenous bone grafts. Limiting the subperiosteal dissection in an attempt to preserve the vascularity of these small fragments should not be performed at the expense of adequate fracture exposure.

B. Maxillary Disimpaction and Occlusal Restoration

Restoration of the premorbid occlusal relationship is the first objective in maxillary fracture management (30,33). Realignment of a disrupted maxillary dental arch to an intact mandible enables anatomical reduction and fixation of the maxillary buttresses. Arch bars are attached to both the upper and lower dentition with 26-gauge interdental wire loops at the start of surgery. In patients with reasonably intact dentition, features including general arch shape, interincisal midlines, and wear facets are used as a guide to ensure appropriate restoration of occlusion. Premorbid dental history, photographs, and dental records can also add valuable information. In edentulous patients, maxillary fractures are less common as the teeth act as a conduit to communicate forces directly to the alveolar ridge and dentures act as a buffer to absorb some of the impact.

(A)

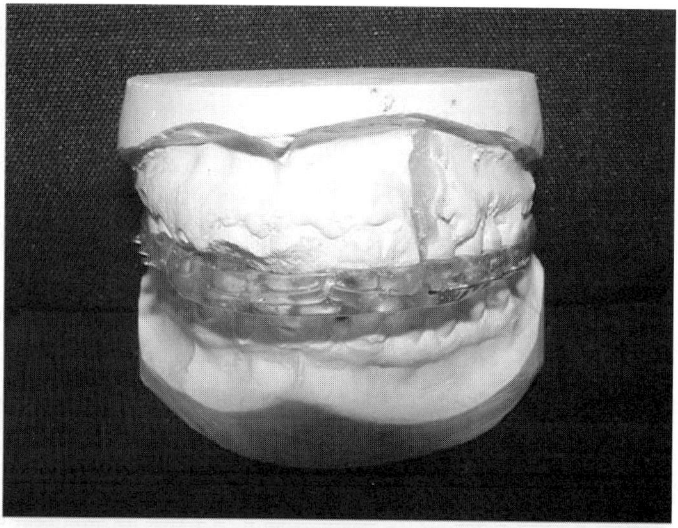

(B)

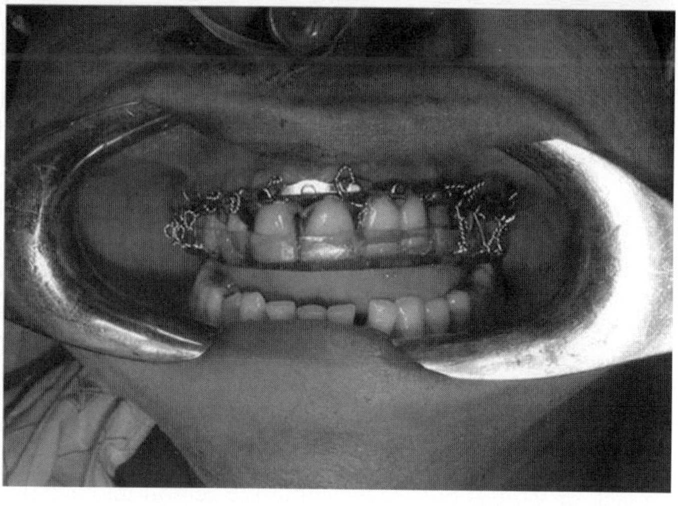

Figure 5 Preoperative splint fabrication is an extremely useful adjunct in selected cases. In this patient with a palatal splitting and mandibular fractures, preoperative impressions are taken to facilitate model surgery and restoration of preinjury occlusion. An acrylic splint (A) is then very effective in guiding and stabilizing the repositioning of dental segments intraoperatively (B).

Alternatively, owing to atrophy, the edentulous maxilla is thin and susceptible to fracture by smaller force loads. In the absence of teeth, either the upper denture, fixed by multiple lag screws to the hard palate or alveolar process, or a Gunning splint can be used as a guide to restore the premorbid arch relationship and set the correct facial vertical height. The lower denture is usually applied with a series of circumandibular 26-gauge steel wires. If, in the edentulous patient, dentures are not available, anatomical buttress alignment is performed followed by postoperative denture adjustment to manage minor occlusal discrepancies.

Complete disimpaction of the maxilla from its retrodisplaced position is essential to allow it to be passively opposed to the mandibular arch. A disimpaction (Rowe and Kelly) forceps or steel-wire loop passed through the anterior nasal spine can be used to provide the required anterior traction. If the maxilla has not been fully mobilized, postoperative posterior relapse will almost certainly occur as the static forces of the internal plate fixation will not withstand the dynamic posterior pull of the pterygoid muscles on the fracture segment. Owing to the unpredictability of maxillary fracture patterns, caution must be shown when disimpacting the severely impacted maxilla so as not to extend fractures into the cranial base or posterior orbit.

In certain circumstances the preoperative fabrication of an acrylic dental splint to guide the reduction, although time consuming, is extremely useful (Fig. 5). A preinjury anterior open bite, edentulous patient without dentures, and transverse disruption of the maxillary arch can all benefit from the use of a splint to prevent lingual or buccal inclination of dental alveolar segments or severe arch discrepancies postoperatively.

C. Sequential Approach to Maxillary Fracture Fixation (Table 1)

The anatomical arrangement of structural facial skeletal buttresses and, in particular, the lack of sagittal buttresses within the central midface predispose to a predictable fracture pattern. Loss of anterior projection in the central maxilla, with various degrees of rotation and vertical shortening, is a characteristic feature. Comminution is generally most severe in the central nasomaxillary region, with variable degrees of comminution also being found in the medial and lateral buttress regions.

The goal of midfacial fracture reconstruction is to restore the premorbid spatial position and orientation of the maxilla, and then to maintain this position by reconstructing a stable, three-dimensional, framework oriented along the structural buttresses. This is most effectively accomplished by an

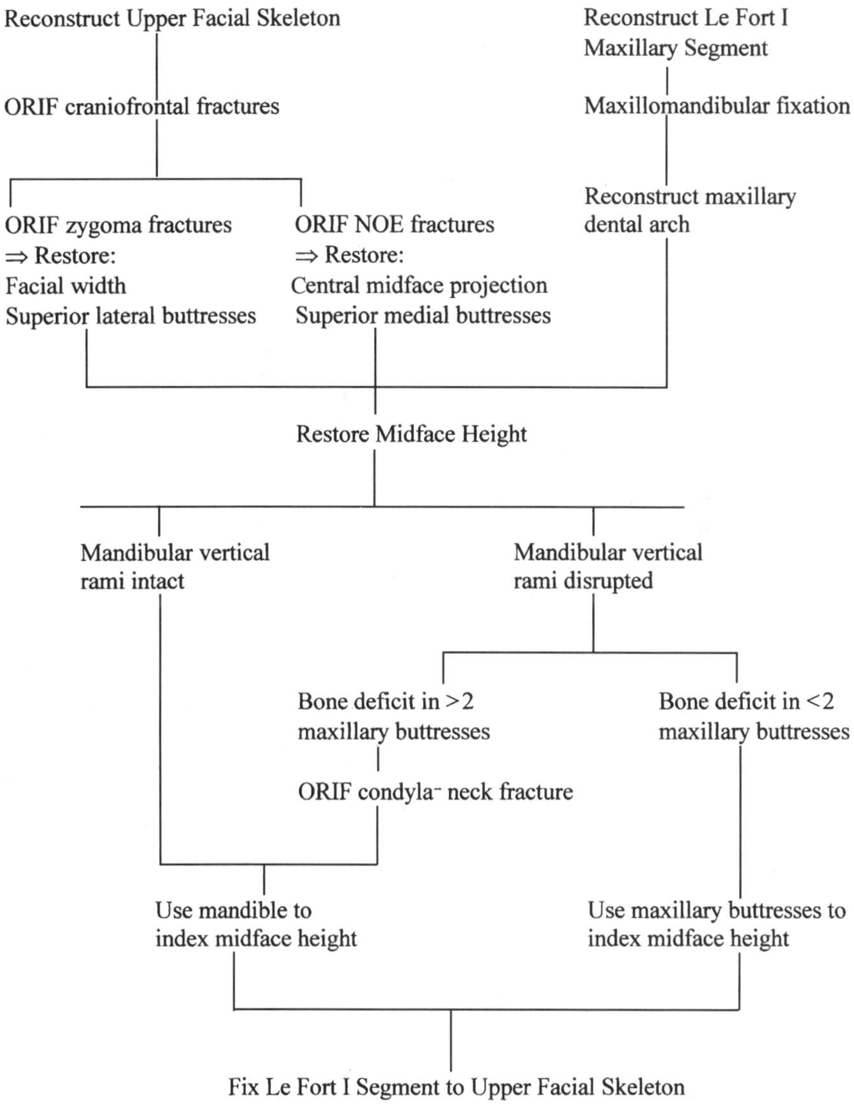

Table 1 Algorithm for Sequencing Midface Fracture Repair

orderly sequential approach, in which reliable peripheral skeletal landmarks are re-established first (Table 1). The presence of stable anatomically accurate references peripherally greatly facilitates the reconstruction of the central midface.

1. Restoration of the Upper Facial Skeleton

The upper facial skeleton is addressed first (Fig. 6). A coronal incision offers unparalleled exposure, while fracture segments tend to be large with minimal comminution or bone loss. Precise anatomical reduction and fixation are therefore easily accomplished. Further extension of the coronal dissection laterally and inferiorly exposes the zygomatic arch. Gruss et al. (35) first emphasized the importance of the zygomatic arch as the key to restoring midfacial width and projection. Using stable landmarks at the articulations with the arch, sphenoid, and frontal bones, the fractured zygoma can be precisely repositioned and fixed. This completes the reconstruction of the upper, outer facial frame, and re-establishes the projection and width of the midface.

The central portion of the upper face is more difficult to visualize. However, the presence of reliable stable landmarks superiorly at the craniofrontal base and laterally at the zygoma allows more accurate reduction of nasoethmoid fracture segments. Conceptually, completion of the upper facial reconstruction converts the complex panfacial disruption to a Le Fort I fracture, where the medial and lateral buttress landmarks are clearly and reliably established (36–38).

2. Restoration of the Dental Arches

Prior to the final reconstruction of the Le Fort I maxillary segment (usually the "occlusal segment"), the upper and lower dental arches must be re-established and fixated (39). The sequence for arch reconstruction is dictated by the relative comminution of the two structures (Fig. 7). The mandibular arch through larger segment sizes and easier access offers a more accurate three-dimensional reconstruction and is usually addressed first. Once stabilized, the mandible then acts as the foundation for the maxillary arch restoration. If a severely comminuted mandible exists or it has sustained significant bone loss, the maxillary arch is reconstructed initially and then used as a guide for the mandible. Failure to reconstruct the maxillary arch adequately prior to fixing the Le Fort I segment can lead to malocclusions with crossbite deformities.

If palatal or alveolar fractures exist and are not properly addressed, lateral rotation deformities in the outer dental segments can result. Impacted palatal fractures may or may not be accompanied by mucosal lacerations and can be easily missed, necessitating a thorough exploration of the palatal surface before definitive treatment. Open reduction at the piriform aperture and posterior palate with monocortical plate fixation should be ideally performed in conjunction with the initial application of an acrylic occlusal splint.

(A)

(B)

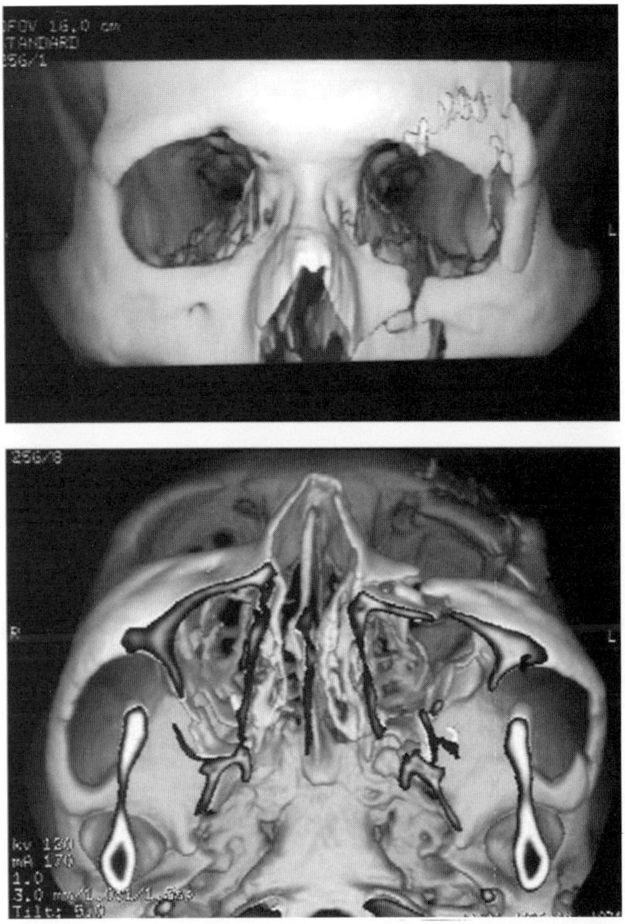

Figure 6 A 32-year-old man with a right Le Fort I fracture and left Le Fort I, II, and III fractures. Preoperative 3D-CT images demonstrate a left orbital blow-in fracture, with the supraorbital rim displaced into the orbital cavity (A). The left zygoma is comminuted and displaced inferolaterally (A), with exaggerated convex bowing of the zygomatic arch (B) resulting in increased facial width. Reconstruction proceeds from the top down. A combined intra- and extracranial approach through a coronal exposure (C) allows decompression of the left orbit and accurate reconstruction of the supraorbital rim and orbital roof fracture segments. Fractures of the zygoma and zygomatic arches are rigidly fixed under direct visualization (D) to ensure accurate restoration of midfacial width and projection. This approach allows predictable correction of the left hypoglobus, lateral canthal dystopia, and exaggerated facial width noted preoperatively (E), as demonstrated in the postoperative image (F).

(C)

(D)

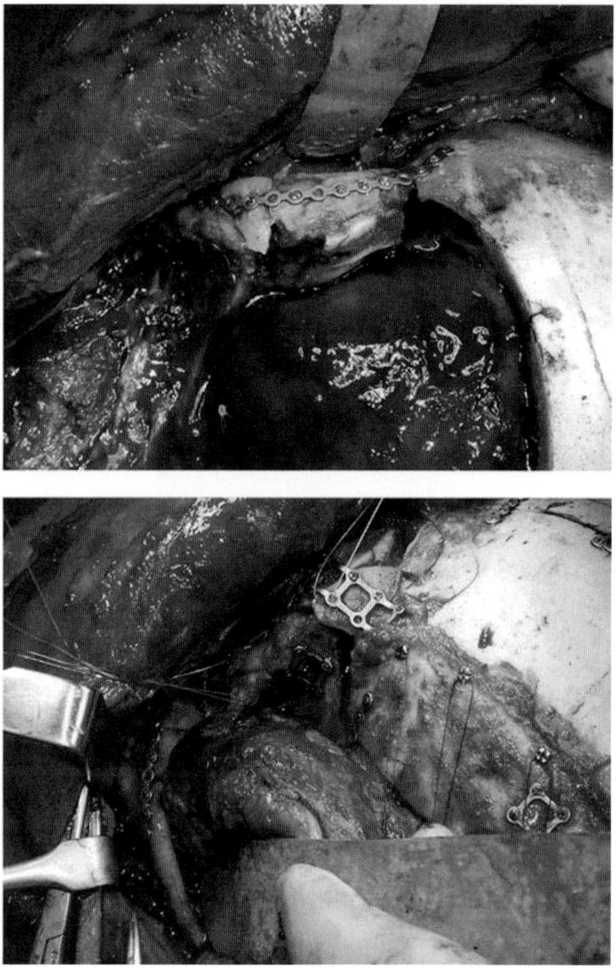

Figure 6 (*continued*)

3. Restoration of Midface Vertical Height

After the upper facial skeletal fractures are initially addressed and the dental arches are reconstituted, the residual maxillary injury is converted into a single-segment Le Fort I fracture. The final adjustment required prior to fixation of the Le Fort I segment is to ensure that the midfacial height has been properly restored. If the integrity of the mandibular ramus and condyles is intact, height restoration simply requires appropriate seating of the condyles

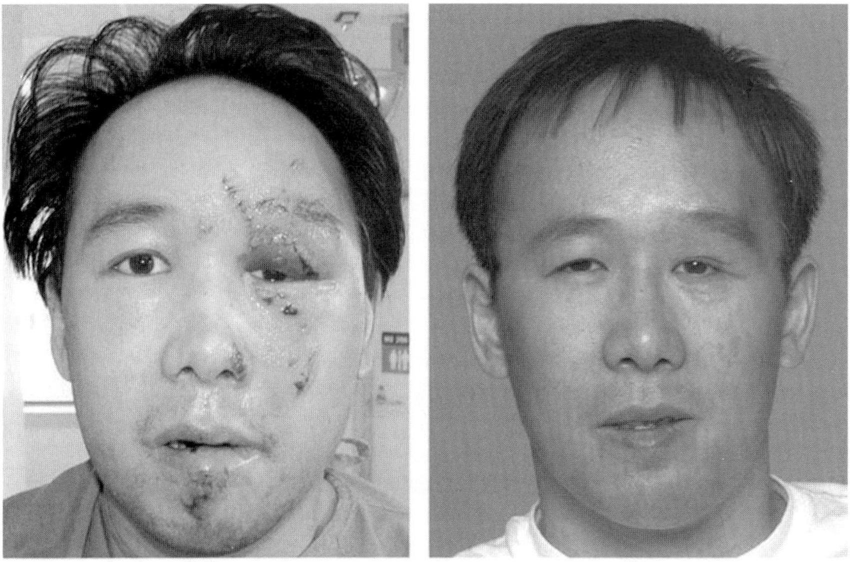

(E) (F)

Figure 6 (*continued*)

in the glenoid fossae followed by autorotation of the mandible to approximate the Le Fort I segment anatomically with the upper face (Fig. 8). If the mandibular vertical height is not available owing to concomitant ramus or condylar fractures, then precise anatomical reduction of the maxillary buttresses is used to guide vertical height restoration. If three or more buttresses are fractured and there is associated collapse of the mandibular vertical rami, open reduction and fixation of the mandibular component is required first to re-establish vertical proportions. As espoused by Manson, the mandible is the foundation for the lower midface upon which Le Fort fractures are reduced and stabilized (13). The importance of accurate mandibulomaxillary fixation prior to setting of the Le Fort I segment to avoid maxillary retrusion and an anterior open bite deformity postoperatively cannot be overemphasized. Premature posterior molar contact producing an anterior open bite can result if apparent reduction of the visible anterior buttresses is solely used as a marker for anatomical restoration. Failure to use the mandibular ramus to restore the height of the posterior buttress by mandibulomaxillary fixation results in this premature molar contact. It is also essential to ensure that the mandibular condyles are seated fully in the glenoid fossae prior to fixation (34). Inadvertent inferior or anterior

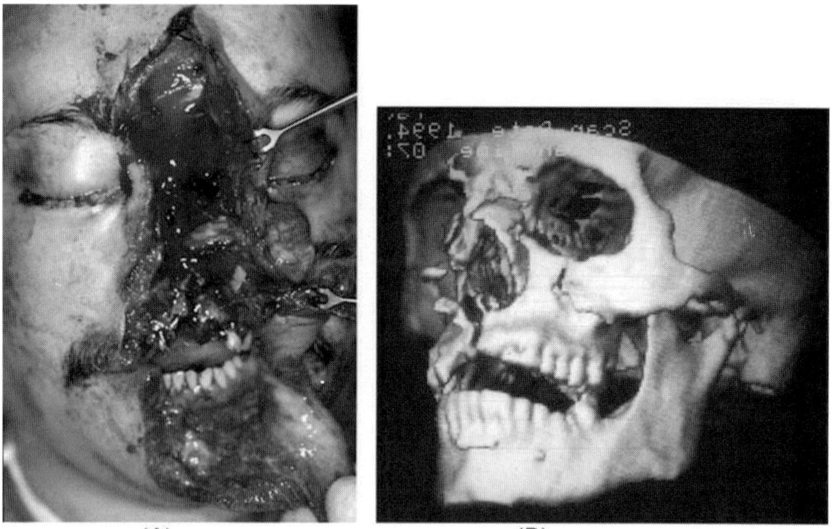

(A) (B)

Figure 7 A 27-year-old man with an avulsive facial injury (A) associated with right Le Fort I, II, and III fractures, left Le Fort II fractures (B), a palatal split, and a right mandibular body fracture. The palatal fracture is para-alveolar (Type IV) as demonstragted radiologically by the CT scan (C) and clinically by the mucosal tear and disrupted dental arch (D). Restoration of the dental arches (E) requires initial reduction and fixation of the mandibular fracture (F), followed by the maxillo-mandibular fixation and stabilization of the maxillary arch. The late postoperative result demonstrates restoration of normal midfacial width (G) and projection (H).

subluxation of the temporomandibular joint can produce either an increase in facial vertical height or posterior relapse of the maxilla when the mandibulomaxillary fixation is released.

4. Le Fort I Segment Reconstruction

Microplating of the maxillary buttresses in anatomical realignment is the final stage of maxillary fracture reconstruction. The medial and lateral buttresses require separate fixation plates that have to provide stabilization that will lead to bone healing of sufficient strength to overcome masticatory forces. The medial plate is placed along the thickened bone of the piriform fossae avoiding the thinner anterior maxillary wall bone. The lateral buttress plate is optimally placed along the thickened lateral maxillary edge up superiorly onto the zygomatic body. Care must be taken to avoid damaging the dental roots when drilling the inferior screw holes and similarly to

(C)

(D)

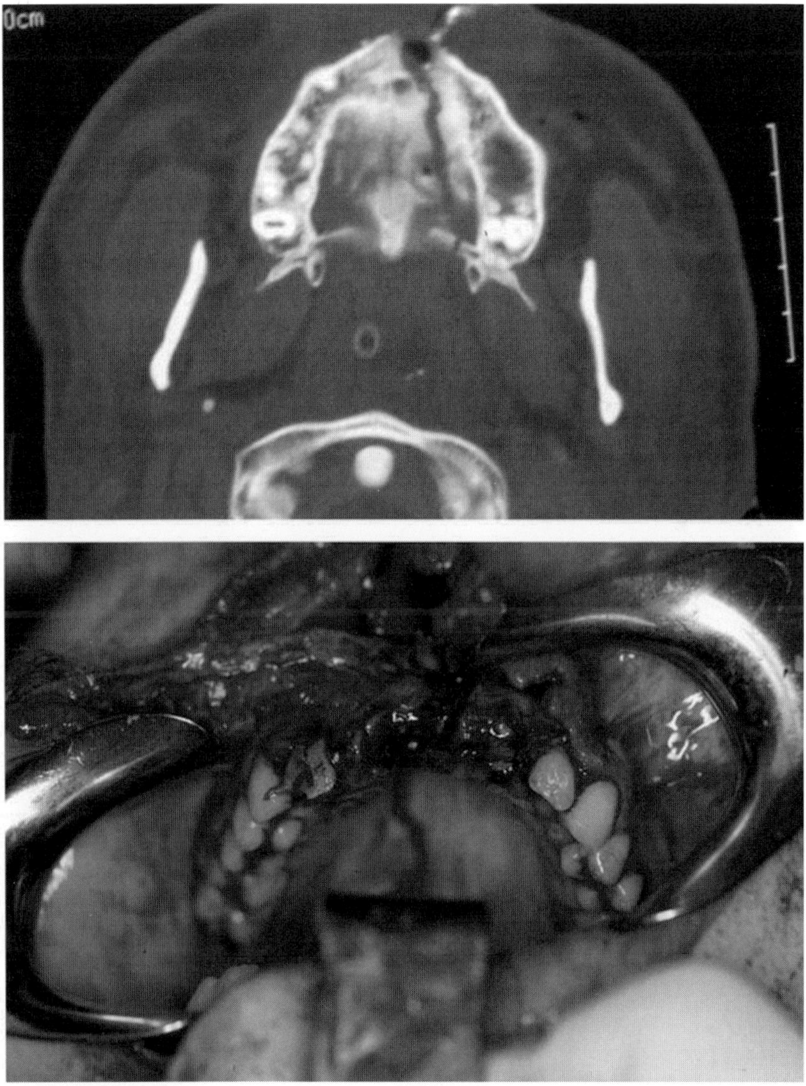

Figure 7 (*continued*)

protect a nasal endotracheal tube when placing drill holes for the medial plate. If the fracture is so inferior that the lateral plate cannot be placed without dental injury, a large plate should be place spanning from the zygomatic body to the thickened medial bone below the anterior nasal spine.

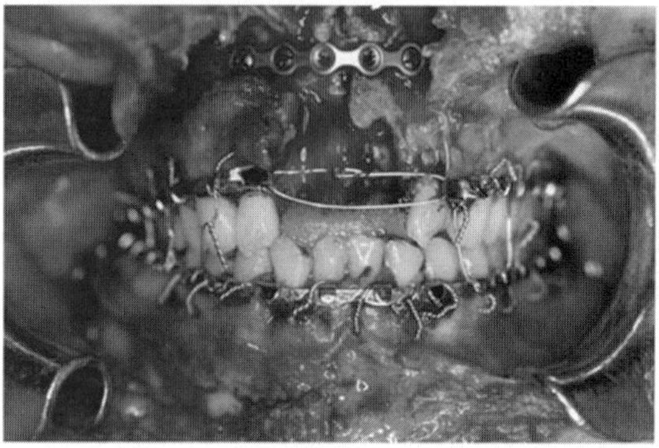

(E)

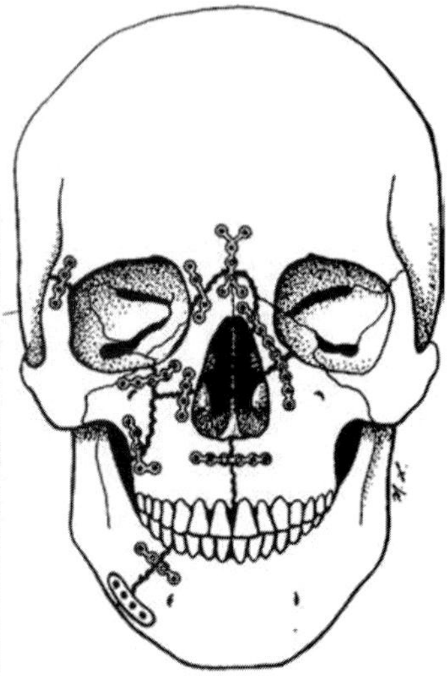

(F)

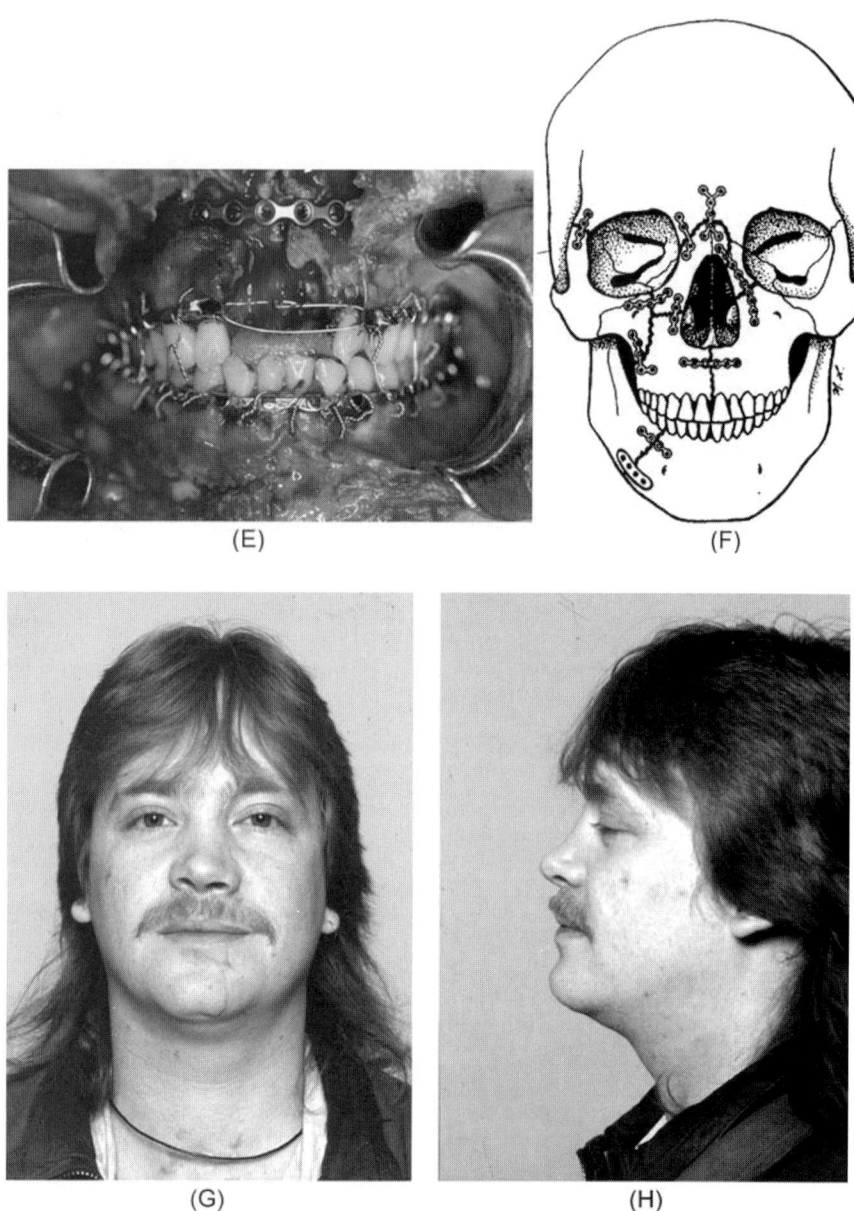

(G)

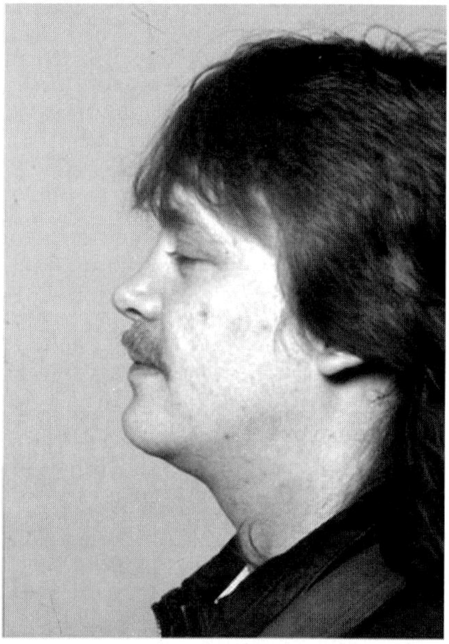

(H)

Figure 7 *(continued)*

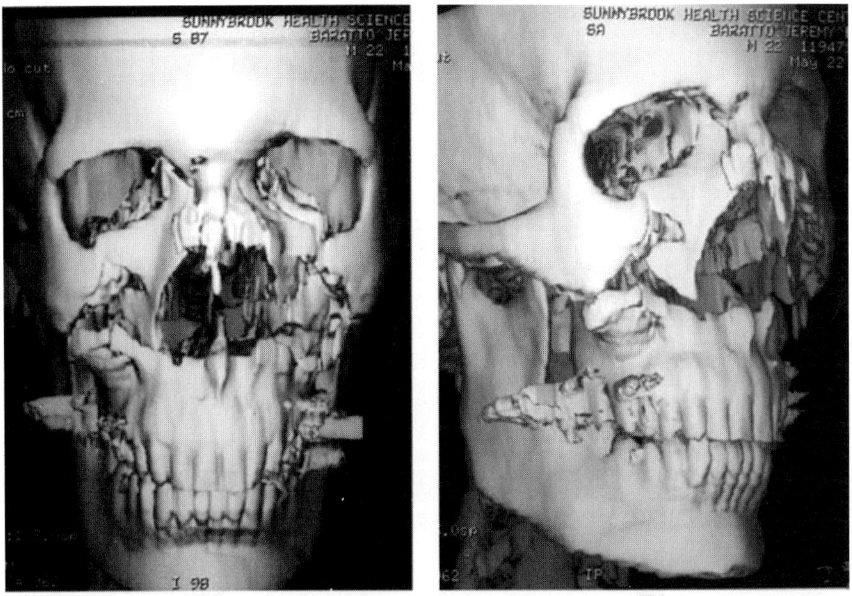

(A) (B)

Figure 8 A 25-year-old man with grossly displaced bilateral Le Fort I and II midfacial fractures associated with Type II NOE fractures (A,B). The NOE segments were reconstructed first to restore the upper facial skeleton. Maxillomandibular fixation approximated the Le Fort I segment to the mandible. An intact mandible and the right lateral (least comminuted) buttress were used as references to restore midfacial vertical height (C,D). Pre- and postoperative images illustrate the correction of midfacial height (E,F), projection (G,H), and restoration of occlusion (I).

Owing to the diminished bone stock in the edentulous patient, plates may have to be placed low on the alveolar ridge to get sufficient screw purchase. While dental injury is obviously not of concern in these circumstances, these plates may have to be removed after fracture healing to allow comfortable denture fixation.

VIII. PRIMARY BONE GRAFTING IN MAXILLARY FRACTURES

Tessier popularized the use of autogenous bone grafts for facial reconstruction in his pioneering descriptions of his craniofacial surgical techniques in the late 1960s (11,12). Bonanno and Converse first introduced the concept of

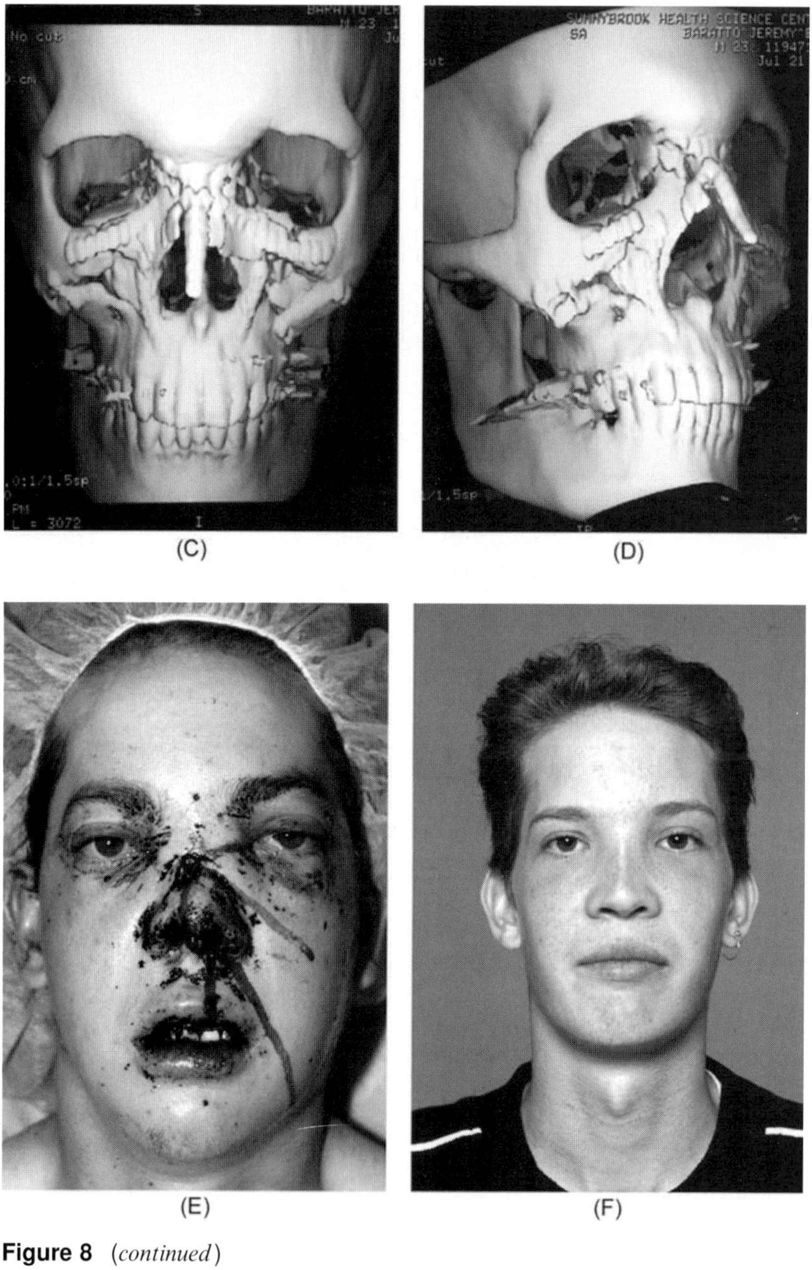

(C) (D)

(E) (F)

Figure 8 (*continued*)

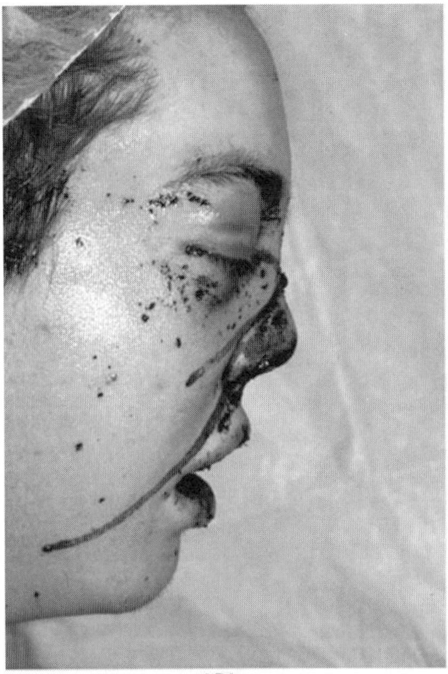

(G)

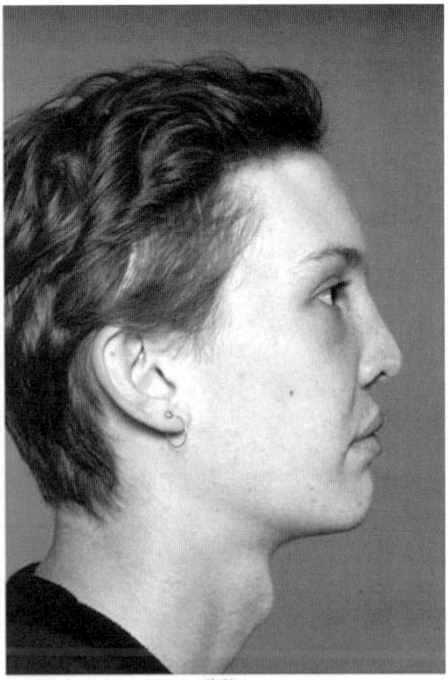

(H)

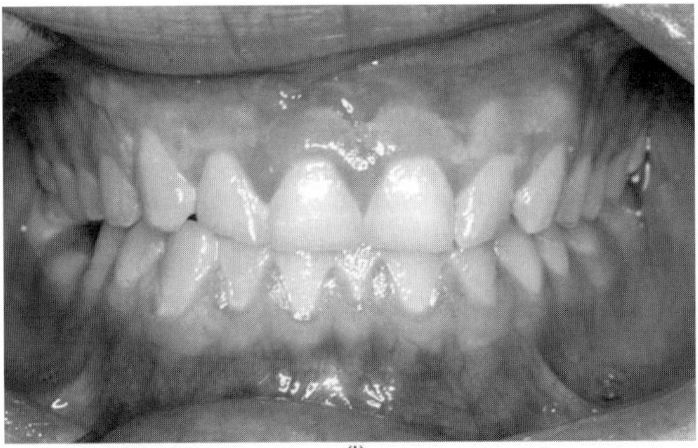

(I)

Figure 8 (*continued*)

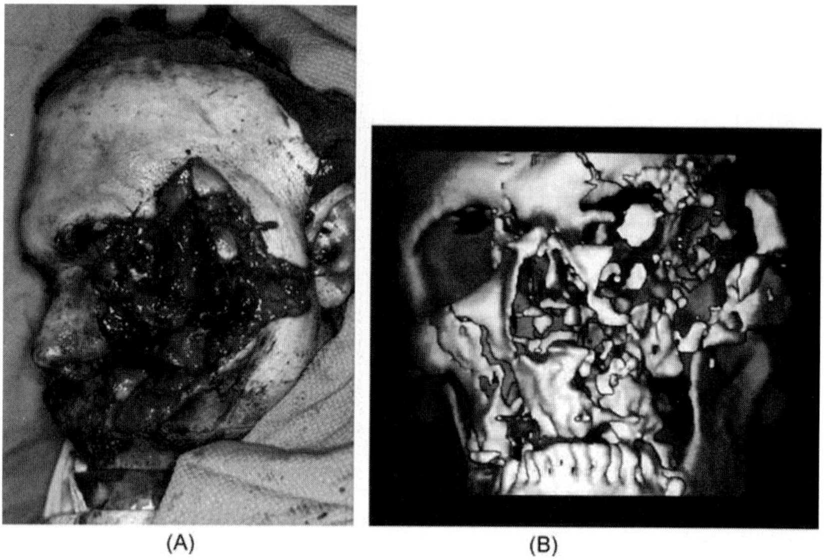

Figure 9 Gunshot wound to the face with right intraoral entry wound and left cranio-orbital exit wound. The left facial avulsion is associated with loss of eyelid, anterior cheek, and perioral tissues (A). A 3D-CT scan illustrates the degree of bone loss (B). All skeletal defects were reconstructed with primary bone grafting using split calvarial bone. Following dural repair with a large patch graft (C), a large bone graft (arrow) was used to reconstruct the anterior cranial fossa (D). The left temporalis muscle was fully mobilized as an island on its vascularized pedicles by osteotomizing the coronoid process (E). The posterior half (TP) of the muscle obliterated the orbital cavity while the anterior half (TA) obliterated the maxillary defect. Cranial bone grafts were employed in reconstructing the orbit (F) and use of existing skeletal landmarks at the zygomatic arch and frontal region permitted anatomically accurate (G) de novo construction of superior (s), lateral (l), and inferior (i) orbital rims. A cheek cervical flap (H) completes the cutaneous reconstruction. Postoperative result (I).

applying primary bone grafts to the maxillary tuberosity and pterygoid process in facial fracture management (40). Refinements of these techniques have since been described by Gruss (15,41–43) and Manson (14,44), who established primary bone grafting for reconstruction of the midfacial supporting pillars as a basic tenet of modern facial trauma management. The advantages of primary bone grafting include immediate correction of complex deformities allowing appropriate soft-tissue draping and subsequently minimizing secondary deformities (Fig. 9). It has also been shown that by stimulating new bone formation, bone grafts add to the mechanical stability

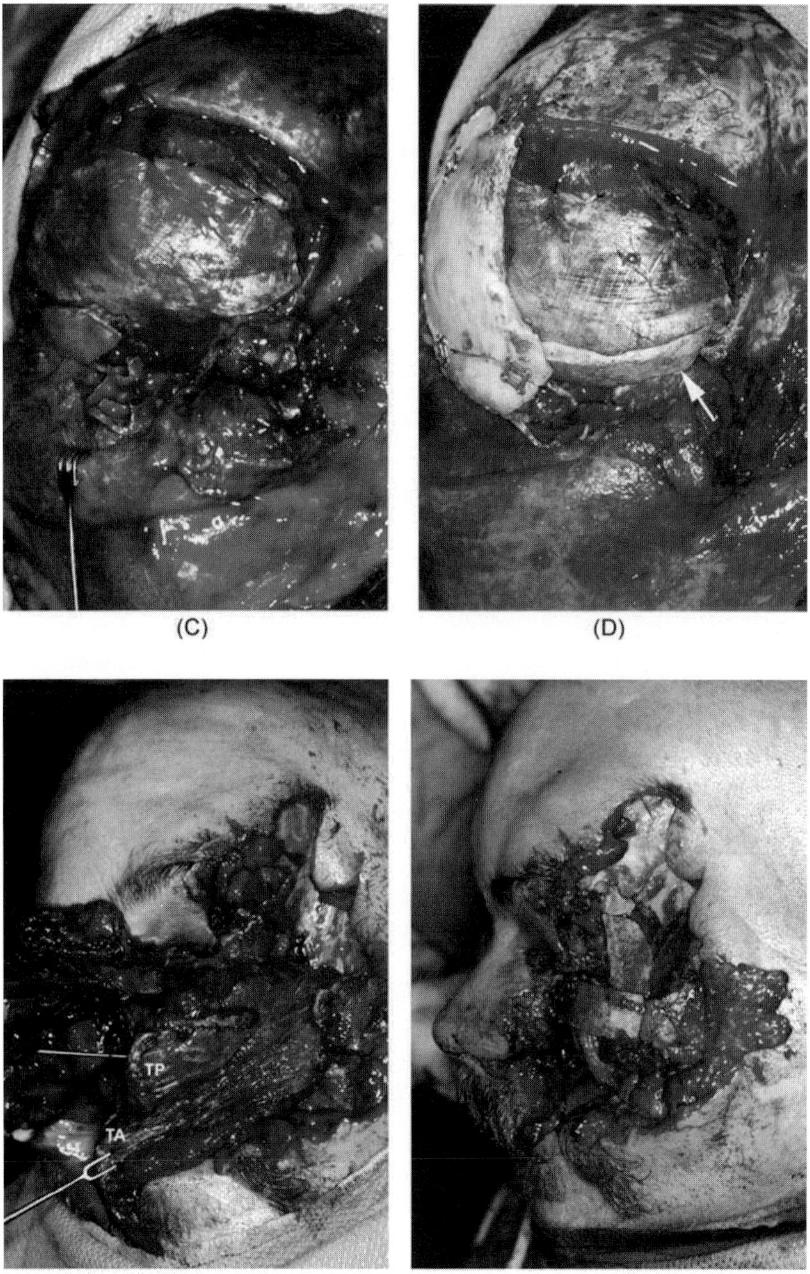

(C) (D)

(E) (F)

Figure 9 (*continued*)

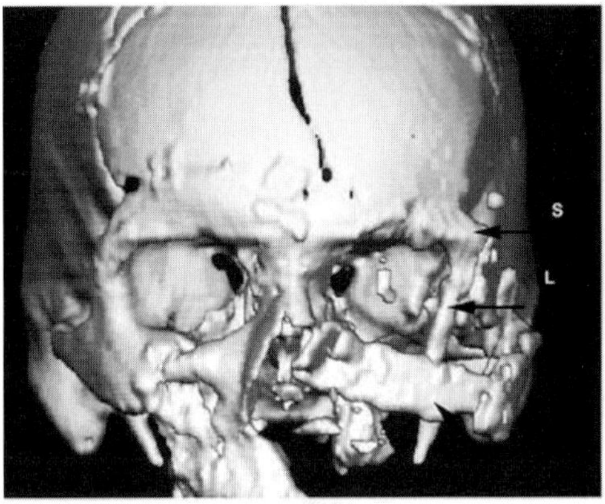

(G)

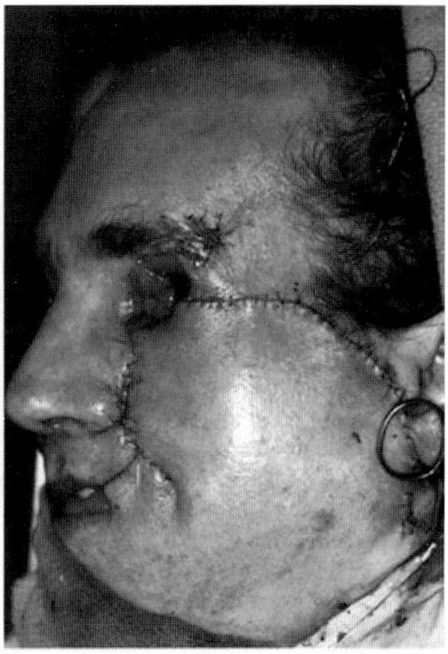

(H)

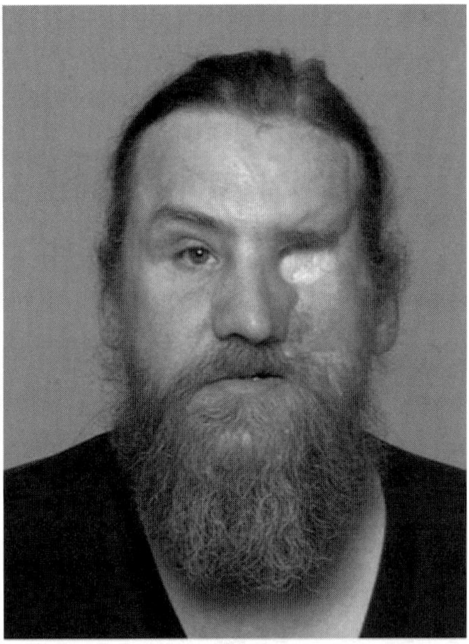

(I)

Figure 9 *(continued)*

of the fracture site and ultimately assist fracture union and consolidation. Gruss has stated that only bony defects up to 5 mm in size in the maxillary buttresses can be bridged by miniplates alone or else subsequent vertical collapse results (43).

The mandible is rarely treated by primary bone grafting owing to poor graft survival and high graft infection rates. The cranial vault, ribs, and iliac crest are the most common bone graft donor sites. Split calvarial bone grafts are the most popular and are thought to provide the strongest support for buttress reconstruction (45). Inlay grafts fixed by a miniplate to the remaining upper and lower bony segments are usually required for buttress defects whereas defects in the thin central anterior maxillary wall can be treated by onlay grafts secured to the surrounding bony margins (15). Though significant graft resorption may occur, the grafts supply sufficient stability during the healing phase to allow anatomical bony union while limiting secondary deformities from unwanted scar contracture. In a large series of over two hundred patients Manson found no increase in rates of infection, nonunion, or malunion between patients treated with primary bone grafts and those who were not (44).

IX. SOFT-TISSUE RECONSTRUCTION

Precise redraping of the facial soft-tissue envelope is essential to prevent postoperative facial asymmetries and to optimize the result of the bony reconstruction after midfacial repair. In particular, even minor surface deformities around the periorbital area can leave residual canthal dystopias and palpebral fissure irregularities that can be difficult to correct secondarily (46). Frequently medial or lateral canthoplasties and cheek subperiosteal soft-tissue resuspension are required (47). Early repair of the skeletal framework of the midface helps decrease facial edema, which makes accurate restoration of premorbid soft-tissue contours difficult and also prevents abnormal premature soft-tissue contractures from developing that can detract from the overall result.

X. POSTOPERATIVE PATIENT MANAGEMENT

The advent of rigid microplate facial fracture fixation reduced the requirement for postoperative intermaxillary fixation after midfacial fracture repair. With the tendency for occlusal drift due to muscular spasm, edema, and dental paraesthesia, all patients are treated with anterior interdental elastics to provide functional rehabilitation for at least 2 weeks postoperatively. Intermaxillary fixation is usually reserved for patients who have undergone extensive bone grafting of the maxillary buttresses. Patients with displaced sagittal palatal fractures are frequently treated with occlusal splints for up to 6 weeks. A soft diet and standard oral hygiene protocol with frequent antiseptic rinsing of suture lines are recommended until full healing has been achieved at about 4–6 weeks postoperatively. Arch bars are usually removed under neurolept anesthesia when no longer required.

REFERENCES

1. Le Fort R. Etude experimental sur les fractures de la machoire superieure, Parts I, II, III. Rev Chir Paris 1901; 23:201,360,479.
2. Gillies HD. Plastic Surgery of the Face. London: Frowde, Hodder & Stoughton 1920.
3. Gillies H, Millard DR Jr. The Principles and Art of Plastic Surgery. Boston: Little, Brown, 1957.
4. Converse JM, Kazanjian VH. Surgical Treatment of Facial Injuries. 2d ed. Baltimore: Williams & Wilkins 1982.
5. Ipsen J. Therapy of jaw fractures. Zentralbl Chir 1933; 60:2840.
6. Brown JB, McDowell F. Internal wire fixation for fractures of jaw: preliminary report. Surg Gynecol Obstet 1942; 74:227.
7. Brown JB, McDowell F. Internal wire fixation of jaw fractures: second report. Surg Gynecol Obstet 1942; 75:361.
8. Dingman RO, Natvig P. Surgery of Facial Fractures. Philadelphia: WB Saunders 1964.
9. Dingman RO. Use of rubber bands in the treatment of fractures of the bones of the face and jaws. J Am Dent Assoc 1939; 26:173.
10. Adams WM. Basic principles of internal wire fixation and internal suspension of facial fractures. Surgery 1942; 12:523.
11. Tessier P. Osteotomies totales de la face. Ann Chir Plast 1967; 12:273.
12. Tessier P. Definitive plastic surgical treatment of the severe facial deformities of craniofacial dysostoses: Crouzon's and Apert's diseases. Plast Reconstr Surg 1988; 82:872.
13. Manson PN, Hoopes JE, Su CT. Structural pillars of the facial skeleton: an approach to the management of Le Fort fractures. Plast Reconstr Surg 1980; 66:54–62.
14. Manson PN, Crawley WA, Yaremchuk M, et al. Midface fractures: advantages of immediate extended open reduction and bone grafting. Plast Reconstr Surg 1985; 76:1–12.
15. Gruss JS, MacKinnon SE. Complex maxillary fractures: role of buttress reconstruction and immediate bone grafting. Plast Reconstr Surg 1986; 78:9–24.
16. Manson PN, Clark N, Robertson B, et al. Subunit principle in midfacial fractures: the importance of sagittal buttresses, soft tissue reductions and sequencing treatment of segmental fractures. Plast Reconstr Sug 1999; 103: 1287–1307.

17. Hendrickson M, Clark N, Manson PN, et al. Palatal fractures: classification, patterns and treatment with internal rigid fixation. Plast Reconstr Surg 1998; 101(2):319–332.
18. Morgan BDG, Madan DK, Bergerot JPC. Fractures of the middle third of the face—a review of 300 cases. Br J Plast Surg 1972; 25:147.
19. McCoy FJ, et al. An analysis of facial fractures and their complications. Plast Reconstr Surg 1962; 29:381.
20. Kelly DE, Harrigan WF. A survey of facial fractures, Bellevue Hospital, 1948–1974. J Oral Surg 1975; 33:146.
21. Turvey TA. Midface fractures: a retrospective analysis of 593 cases. J Oral Surg 1977; 35:887.
22. Manson PN, et al. Sagittal fractures of the maxilla and palate. Plast Reconstr Surg 1983; 72:484.
23. Gwynn PP, et al. Facial fractures—associated injuries and complications. Plast Reconstr Surg 1971; 47:225.
24. Merritt R, Williams M. Cervical spine injury complicating facial trauma: incidence and management. Am J Otolaryngol 1997; 18:4.
25. Finkle DR, et al. Comparison of the diagnostic methods used in maxillofacial trauma. Plast Reconstr Surg 1985; 75:32.
26. Neuman PR, Zilkha A. Use of the CAT scan for diagnosis in the complicated facial fracture patient. Plast Reconstr Surg 1982; 70:683.
27. Robbins KT, et al. Radiographic evaluation of mid-third facial fractures. J Otolaryngol 1986; 15:366.
28. Ellis E, Scott K. Oral-facial emergencies: assessment of patients with facial fractures. Emergency Medicine Clinics of North America. WB Saunders, Philadelphia 2000; 18:3.
29. Schaefer SD, Diehl JT, Briggs WH. The diagnosis of cerebrospinal fluid rhinorrhea by metrizamide CT scanning. Laryngoscope 1980; 90:871.
30. Forrest CR, Antonyshyn OM. Acute management of complex midface fractures. Oper Tech Plast Reconstr Surg 1998; 5(3):188–200.
31. Gruss JS, Antonyshyn OM, Phillips JM. Early definitive bone and soft tissue reconstruction of major gunshot wounds of the face. Plast Reconstr Surg 1991; 87(3): 436–450.
32. Manson PN, et al. Single eyelid incision for exposure of the zygomatic bone and orbital reconstruction. Plast Reconstr Surg 1987; 79:120.
33. Kelly KT, Manson PN, Vander Kolk CA, et al. Sequencing Le Fort fracture treatment (organization of treatment for a panfacial fracture). J Craniofac Surg 1990; 1(4):168–178.
34. Gruss JS, Bubak PJ, Egbert MA. Craniofacial fractures: an algorithm to optimize results. Clin Plast Surg 1992; 19(1):195.
35. Gruss JS, Van Wyck L, Phillips JH, Antonyshyn OM. The importance of the zygomatic arch in complex midfacial fracture repair and correction of posttraumatic orbito-zygomatic deformities. Plast Reconstr Surg 1990; 85(6):878–890.
36. Markowitz BL, Manson PN, et al. Panfacial fractures: organization of treatment. Clin Plast Surg 1989; 16(1):105.

37. Manson PN. Some thoughts on the classification and treatment of Le Fort fractures. Ann Plast Surg 1986; 17(5):356–363.
38. Manson PN. The management of midfacial and frontal bone fractures. Georgiade GS, Riefkohl L, Levi LS eds. Plastic Maxillofacial and Reconstructive Surgery. 3d ed, Baltimore: Williams & Wilkins, 1997:351–376.
39. Pollock RA, Gruss JS. Craniofacial and panfacial fractures. Foster CA, Sherman JE, eds. Surgery of Facial Bone Fractures. New York: Churchill Livingstone 1987:235–253.
40. Bonanno PC, Converse JM. Primary bone grafting in the management of facial fractures. NY State J Med 1975; 75:710.
41. Gruss JS, MacKinnon SE, Kassel E, et al. The role of primary bone grafting in complex craniomaxillofacial trauma. Plast Reconstr Surg 75:17, 1985.
42. Gruss JS. Complex nasoethmoid-orbital and midfacial fractures: role of craniofacial surgical techniques and immediate bone grafting. Ann Plast Surg 1986; 17(5):377–390.
43. Gruss JS, Phillips JH. Complex facial trauma: the role of rigid fixation and immediate bone graft reconstruction. Clin Plast Surg 1989; 16(1):93.
44. Manson PN, et al. Midfacial fractures: advantages of immediate extended open reduction and bone grafting. Plast Reconstr Surg 1985; 76:1.
45. Schmitz R, et al. Indications, techniques and clinical results of compression osteosynthesis in mandibular fractures (5yr experience). Fortschr Kiefer Gesichtschir 1975; 19:74.
46. Dawar M, Antonyshyn O. Long term results following immediate reconstruction of orbital fractures: a critical morphometric analysis. Can J Plast Surg 1993; 1:24–29.
47. Phillips JH, Gruss JS, Wells MD, et al. Periosteal suspension of the lower eyelid and cheek following subcilliary exposure of facial fractures. Plast Reconstr Surg 1991; 88:145–148.

15

Zygoma Fractures

Jose I. Garri and W. Scott McDonald
University of Miami School of Medicine, Miami, Florida, U.S.A.

I. INTRODUCTION

Because of the zygoma's prominent position in the face, trauma often results in fractures to it and associated structures. Its unique, almost keystone position adjacent to the maxilla, frontal bone, zygomatic arch, and sphenoid as well as the orbit, globe, and mandible, therefore, makes it one of key elements in restoring normal facial contour. This chapter explores the anatomy of the zygoma and associated structures, the pathophysiology of zygomatic fractures, and the various approaches to treatment.

II. HISTORICAL PERSPECTIVE

Records of attempts to treat fractures of the zygoma date back to the Smyth Papyrus (1650 B.C.) where descriptions and treatment suggestions are made for several types of zygomatic fractures. The treatment of zygomatic fractures took a major leap in 1751, when Duverney wrote about his observations on the anatomy of the region, types of zygomatic fractures he had observed, and presented two case reports (1). He proposed the use of the mechanical forces of the temporalis and masseter muscle to buttress the reduction of the fracture.

The first known description of the transantral approach to the zygoma was recorded by Lothrop in 1906 (2). Known today as the Caldwell-Luc approach, the technique made use of an antrostomy to approach the fracture. Lothrop's work was quickly followed by that of Keen, who in 1909 described the intraoral approach to reduction of zygomatic arch fractures (3). The use of an incision in the temporal area to reach and reduce zygomatic arch fractures was documented in 1927 by Gillies et al. (4). They introduced an elevator through this incision in the plane deep to the deep temporal fascia to reach the zygomatic arch.

Dingman and Natvig, in their seminal study published in 1964, demonstrated that reduced zygomatic fractures, if not stabilized, could become displaced again owing to external forces (5). Their suggestion: treat displaced fractures of the zygoma by open reduction and wire fixation. This builds on a wiring technique developed in 1942 by Adams, who first saw the benefits of internal fixation of zygomatic fractures (6).

The search for improved techniques for internal fixation progressed from the use of simple wiring to Kirschner wires in 1951 (7) and finally the utilization of bone plates. The 1970s saw the dawn of a new era of reconstruction of facial fractures with the development of osteosynthesis, which allowed for miniplate fixation. Michelet et al. reported on the success of this technique (8). The use of plates in the fixation of facial fractures has since become commonplace today.

III. ANATOMICAL CONSIDERATIONS

As previously mentioned, the zygoma is a cornerstone of facial anatomy and its integrity is mandatory for normal facial width, adequate prominence of the cheek, and a normal orbit. On anterior-to-posterior projection the zygoma is seen to articulate with the maxilla, the frontal bone, and the greater wing of the sphenoid bone within the orbit. (See Fig. 1.) Viewed from the side the temporal process of the zygoma joins the zygomatic process of the temporal bone to form the zygomatic arch. (See Fig. 2.) Several muscles attach to the zygoma and produce significant deforming forces, an important factor in displacement after fracture. These include the zygomaticus minor and major and the orbicularis oculi. The masseter muscle attaches to the lateral aspect of the zygomatic arch, and can produce significant displacement force should a fracture occur.

Reduction and stable fixation can be approached through the concepts of structural pillars or buttresses. This concept, used by Sicher and Debrul in 1970, and since expanded by Manson et al., relates the facial bones to the cranial base and proposes that stabilization of these buttress is necessary to maintain width and height of the midface (9,10). One of these buttresses, the zygomaticomaxillary, connects the lateral alveolus to the

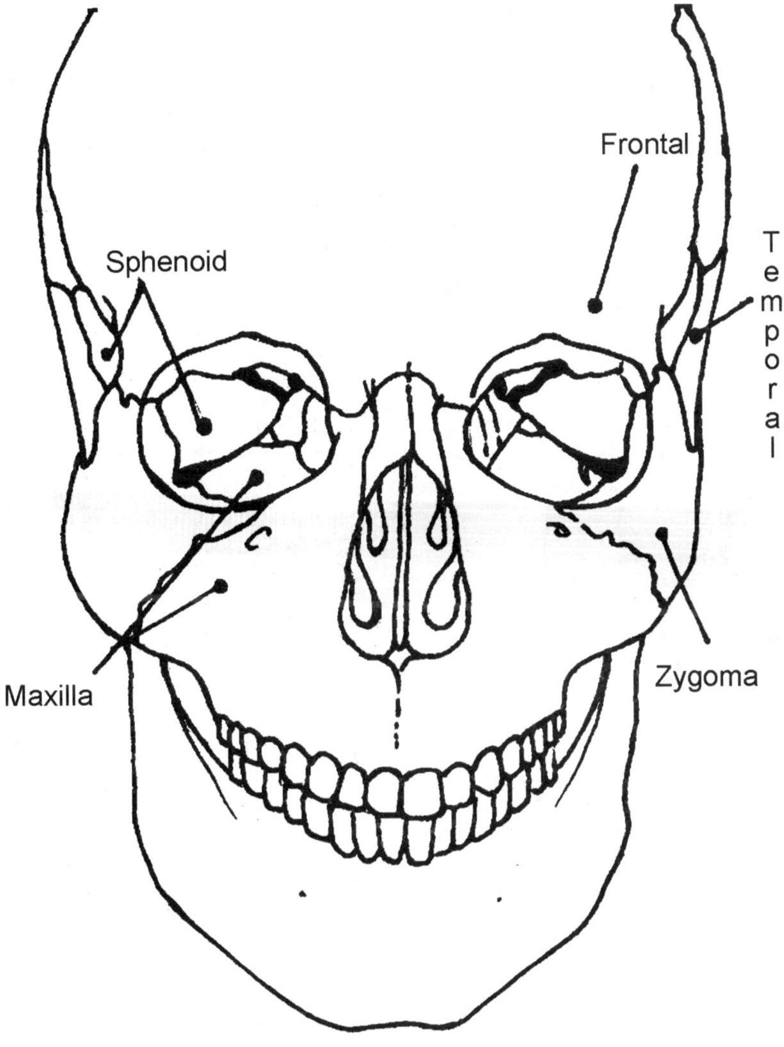

Figure 1 Frontal view of the zygoma.

zygomatic process of the temporal bone. Because of the zygoma's intrinsic strength fractures usually occur at the suture lines of the zygoma and rarely of the body.

Zygomatic fractures occur in two main varieties: those that involve the arch only and those that further involve the lateral and infraorbital wall. The latter category is often called zygomatico-orbital fractures,

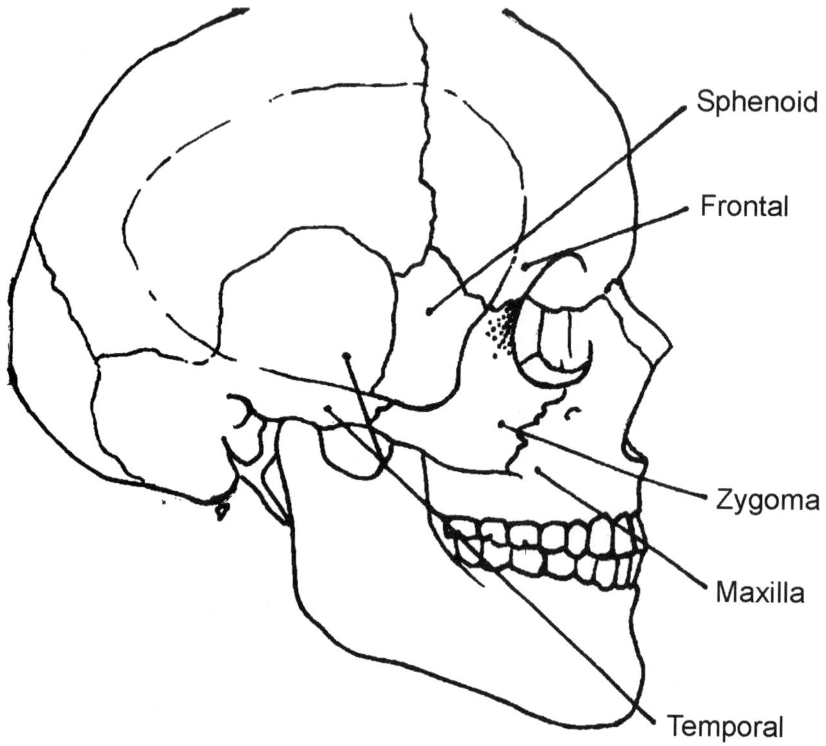

Figure 2 Lateral view of the zygoma.

malar fractures, or zygomaticomaxillary complex (ZMC) fractures. (See Fig. 3.) These fracture lines run through the infraorbital rim and posterolateral orbit, into the inferior orbital fissure, to the zygoma-sphenoid suture area, and on to the frontozygomatic suture line. It is crucial to achieve sufficient reduction of these fracture lines along with the important sphenozygomatic junction to obtain proper alignment of the zygoma (11,12).

Of note in this region is the presence of branches of the fifth and seventh cranial nerves. The temporal and zygomatic branches of the seventh nerve supply the facial muscles; the zygomaticotemporal and zygomaticofacial branches of the fifth nerve provide sensation to the malar region; the supraorbital and infraorbital branches of the fifth nerve supply sensation to the forehead, eyelid, nose, and upper lip. All must be elucidated carefully during surgery to avoid paresis and paresthesias.

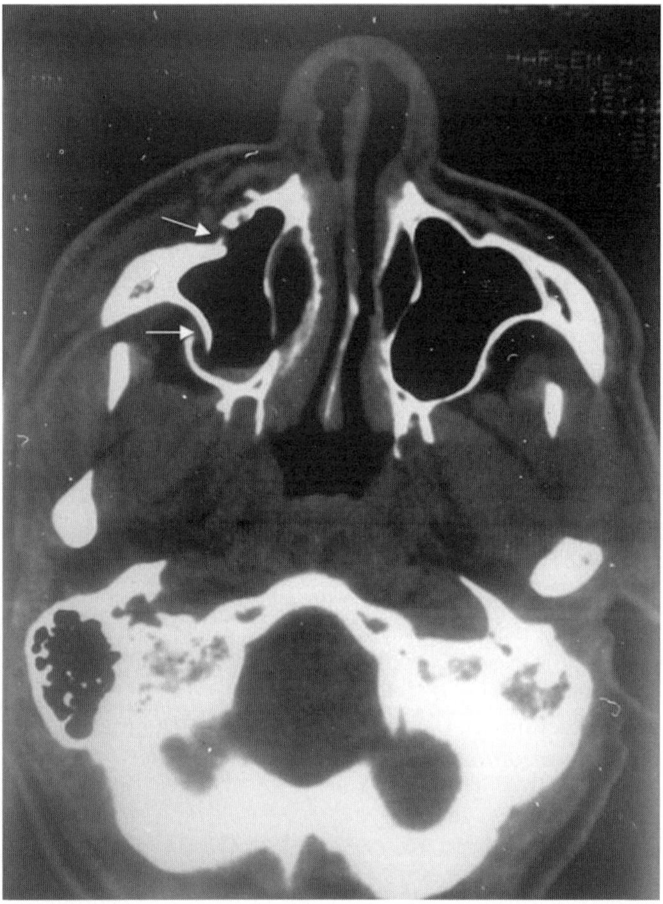

Figure 3 Axial CT scan view of zygomatic fracture.

IV. CLASSIFICATION

In 1961, Knight and North proposed an anatomically based classification system (13) that shed new light on the treatment and prognosis of zygomatic fractures.

No Changes Made Here
Group I: No significant displacement
Group II: Direct blows that buckle the malar eminence inward
Group III: Unrotated body fractures
Group IV: Medially rotated body fractures

Group V: Laterally rotated body fractures
Group VI: Complex fractures (presence of additional fracture lines across the main fragment)

Knight and North found that fractures in some areas were stable after a closed reduction without the need for fixation 100% of the time (groups II and V) while others (in groups IV, III, VI) remained unstable after reduction, so that some form of fixation became necessary.

Further research by Pozatek et al. noted that group V fractures were unstable about 60% of the time (14). In a study of patients who were submitted to closed methods of zygomatic elevation, Dingman and Natvig found that a significant number suffered from redisplacement of the zygoma if the reduction was not followed by fixation (5). They theorized that redisplacement took place as a result of the forces applied on the zygoma by the masseter muscle.

Manson and his colleagues have since developed a classification based on CT scan analysis (15). In this fractures are divided into low-, medium-, and high-energy injuries. In low-energy zygoma fractures, there is little or no displacement, and the incomplete fracture itself provides the stability. Middle-energy fractures demonstrate fractures at all buttresses, some displacement, and comminution. These frequently require eyelid and intraoral exposure to provide the necessary reduction and fixation. High-energy zygoma fractures are the most severe and often accompany Le Fort of panfacial fractures. These fractures can involve the glenoid fossa and produce significant posterior dislocation of the arch and malar eminence.

V. CLINICAL PRESENTATION

The symptoms of a patient with zygomatic fractures can vary depending on whether the damage is limited to the zygomatic arch, or whether it involves orbital structures. Generally, there are obvious signs of facial trauma, including swelling of the face and soft tissue injuries. The zygomatic depression associated with a fracture is sometimes hidden by edema, and does not become evident until the edema subsides, generally after several days. The depression in the area of the zygomatic arch caused by the fracture may be detected through palpation, which usually elicits tenderness. (See Fig. 4.)

Dysesthesia along the infraorbital nerve dermatome is often the result of a fracture line extending through the infraorbital foramen, or of damage to the orbital floor. The nerve travels just below the orbital floor, and it can be affected by displaced bony fragments in the area. Generally, the dysesthesia disappears on its own several days to weeks after fracture reduction and fixation, but it can also remain present for an indefinite period. A number of

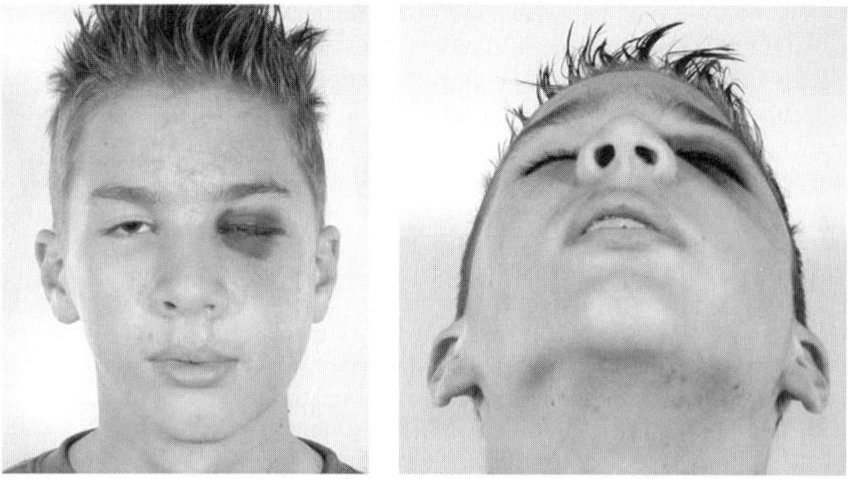

(A) (B)

Figure 4 (A) Zygomatic fracture. (Courtesy of S.A. Wolfe.) (B) Zygomatic fracture. (Courtesy of S.A. Wolfe.)

researchers have found a greater rate of success using open reduction and internal fixation in the restoration of sensory function than using closed reduction (16,17). These mere presence of infraorbital nerve dysfunction after a nondisplaced zygoma fracture should not be taken to mean that exploration and decompression are necessary, since most patients regain sensory function spontaneously.

After a fracture of the zygomatic arch trismus often occurs. This is generally as a result of impingement of the depressed arch on the coronoid process or the temporalis muscle. In such cases, elevation of the zygomatic arch and provision of adequate reduction are necessary. If left uncorrected, an old fracture may result in new bone formation under the zygomatic arch and ankylosis of the mandible. This can necessitate a coronoidectomy to free the mandible and restore movement.

When extensive zygoma fractures involve the bony orbit, eye-related pathosis may become apparent. Diplopia is an important finding to document if present prior to surgery. Causes include hematoma, extraocular muscle trauma, or entrapment in an orbital floor fracture and damage to the fine connective tissue system that surrounds the eye. In their series of 2067 zygomatico-orbital fractures, Ellis et al. found diplopia in approximately 12% of patients (18). When diplopia occurs after zygoma fractures that are not accompanied by entrapment and significant fractures in the orbital floor, it is usually due to hematomas and it will generally disappear.

Barclay reported an 8.4% incidence of diplopia, 60% of which were transitory (19). When symptoms of diplopia show no improvement after 1 or 2 weeks and there is a positive forced duction test and CT evidence of entrapped muscle or soft tissue, surgery is indicated. When diplopia is associated with enophthalmos, a substantial number of patients will note improved vision after correction of the enophthalmos.

Zygomatic complex fractures sometimes involve enophthalmos. To establish the presence of enophthalmos, compare the distance between the lateral orbital rim and anterior corneal surface of each globe using a Hertel exolphthalmometer. If the difference between the eyes is more than 3 mm, it is considered significant (20). When the lateral orbital rim cannot be used as a reference because of a displaced zygoma fracture, enophthalmos becomes more of a clinical finding. Zingg et al. demonstrated a 3–4% incidence of acute enophthalmos in a study conducted among 1000 patients (21). One of the major causes of enophthalmos is believed to be an expanded orbital volume that results from a displaced zygoma and loss of orbital floor. Other causes could be scarring and retraction of the globe and loss of the support generally offered by the intraorbital ligaments in the region.

An important consideration in the treatment of zygomatic fractures is the fact that anesthesia and surgery could aggravate some eye injuries. Before surgery, it is absolutely necessary to ascertain that there are no intraocular injuries. Some consider ophthalmological evaluation mandatory while others do so only in cases with obvious signs of eye trauma or in more complex zygomatic fractures. A thorough eye examination should include evaluation of visual acuity, funduscopy, and a test of extraocular muscle function including a forced duction test if there is a suspicion of entrapment. Eye injuries to consider and manage include globe rupture, laceration, and hyphema.

VI. RADIOGRAPHIC EVALUATION

When symptoms indicate the presence of zygomatic injury, the best way to confirm and evaluate the damage is through a radiographic survey, specifically CT scan. Plain radiographs have become a secondary alternative, although they can be of use in evaluating fractures. In addition, plain radiography is useful when used during surgery to determine whether or not the reduction of the fracture has been sufficient when the zygomatic arch is involved. The "facial series" taken in emergency rooms to determine whether or not there are facial fractures include the submentovertex view, the Waters veiw (Fig. 5) . The lateral view, and the posterolateral view (22).

The Waters view, which provides a very good look at the zygomatic buttresses and is considered the most helpful in the evaluation of zygomatic

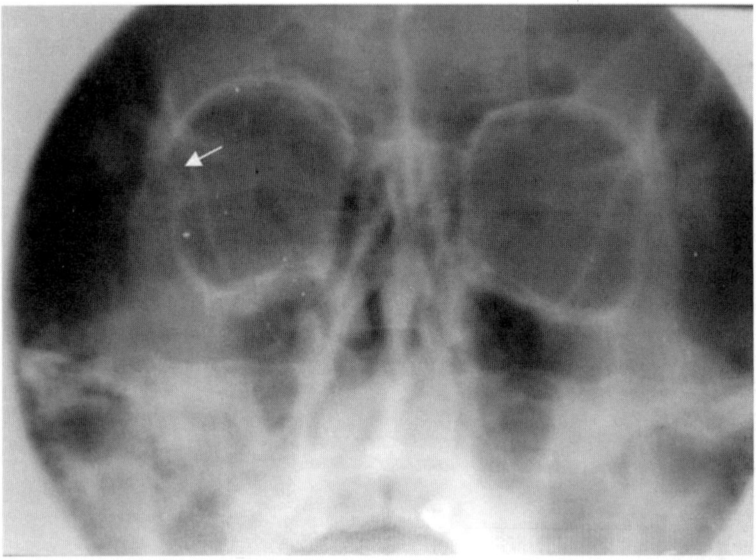

Figure 5 Waters view showing fracture of the zygoma. Note displacement at the frontozygomatic suture.

fractures, is taken at 30 degrees of occipitomental projection. It is not useful in the evaluation of the zygomatic arch, but reveals moderate displacement of fracture lines in the lateral orbital and infraorbital rim (23,24).

Of all the views in the facial series, the submentovertex is best for evaluating zygomatic arch fractures as it provides a view of the zygomatic arches away from the other bones of the skull. One advantage is that it can be done intraoperatively to evaluate the state of reduction of the zygomatic arch fracture. When this view is taken, the film is placed at the vertex of the head; the radiograph is shot pointing up from the chin area to the film cassette (25).

The CT scan has come to replace plain radiographs in the evaluation of trauma to the face. Patients with facial trauma often also have head injury, and since the CT scan is a quick and efficient way to evaluate those injuries, it can conveniently be extended to the bones of the face. In such cases, the CT scan images should be obtained at 3-mm intervals in both coronal and axial views and include the orbits. From the axial images, it is easy to study the zygomatic arch, orbital walls, and the maxillary sinus. The frontozygomatic suture and the infraorbital and lateral orbital rim are best studied in the coronal view. In cases where the patient cannot extend the neck, it is often not possible to obtain coronal views. An alternative, though not ideal, is to opt for reconstructed coronal views. Even though these

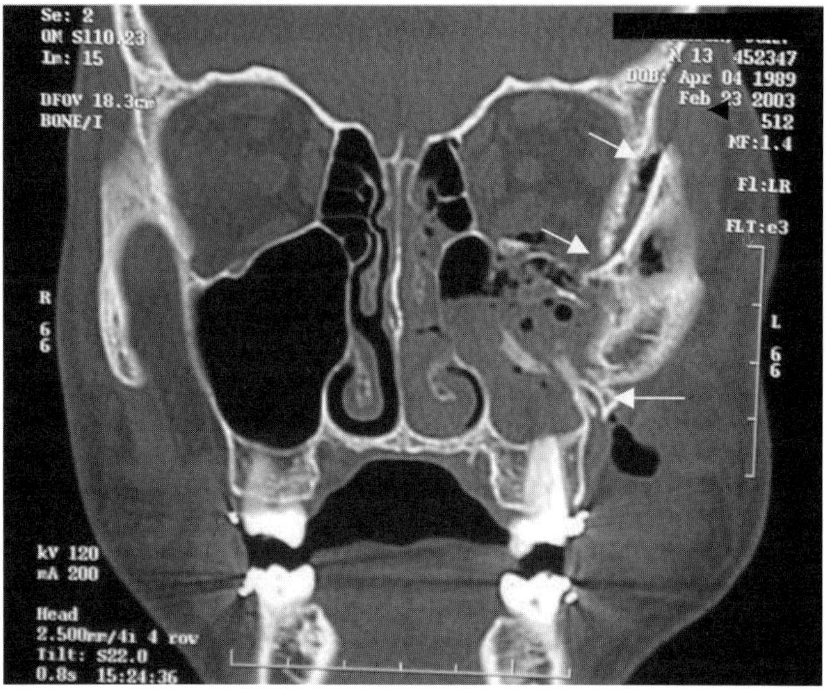

Figure 6 Coronal CT scan view of zygomatic fracture.

images tend not to be as sharp and rich in detail, they can at least indicate fracture location and alignment. (See Fig. 6.)

New computer technology has allowed radiologists to obtain three-dimensional images (26), which give added perspective in terms of how the fractures relate to the surrounding area. Another advantage is that the three-dimensional images can be manipulated on the computer screen for detailed study of fracture displacement.

Despite the current advantages of CT scans, there is still a potential for development. New technology is making intraoperative CT scan a possibility (27). With time, intraoperative CT scans should become more efficient and cost-effective, and are likely to lead to improved outcomes in the management and treatment of facial fractures.

VII. TREATMENT

The treatment plan for zygomatic fractures should be developed after a detailed physical examination and a radiographic evaluation are conducted,

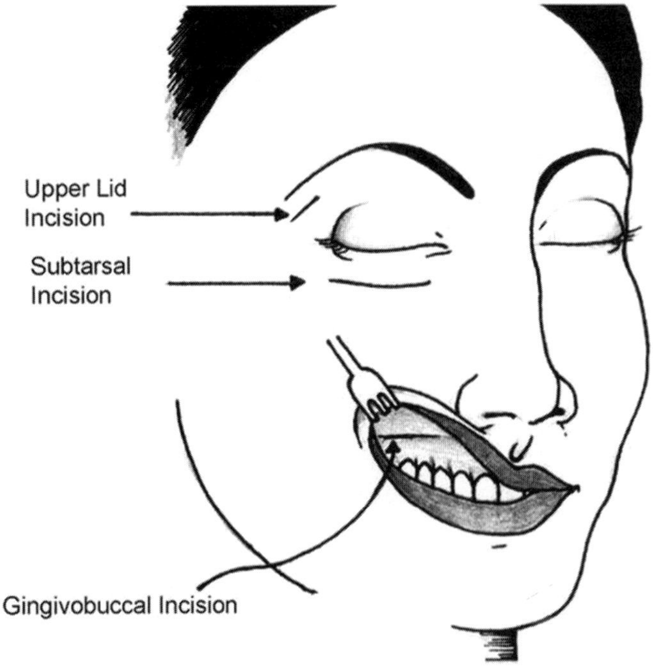

Figure 7 Different incisions for exposure to zygomaticomaxillary complex fracture.

and will depend on the patient's medical condition, the type of fracture sustained and any other injuries he/she might have incurred. The three main issues for the surgeon to consider are exposure, reduction and fixation. As in the treatment of all fractures, adequate exposure must be obtained in zygomatic fractures to achieve the best possible level of reduction and stabilization. (See Fig. 7.)

In cases of zygomatic arch or nondisplaced zygomatico-maxillary complex fractures, limited exposure is usually adequate, but grossly displaced or comminuted zygoma fractures generally require ample exposure through several incisions. To settle on a surgical plan, the surgeon must determine the location of the fracture and anticipate the amount of stabilization required.

A. Temporal and Supraorbital Approaches

If the fracture is limited to a depression of the zygoma arch, the temporal approach described by Gillies et al. is commonly employed (28). (See Fig. 8.)

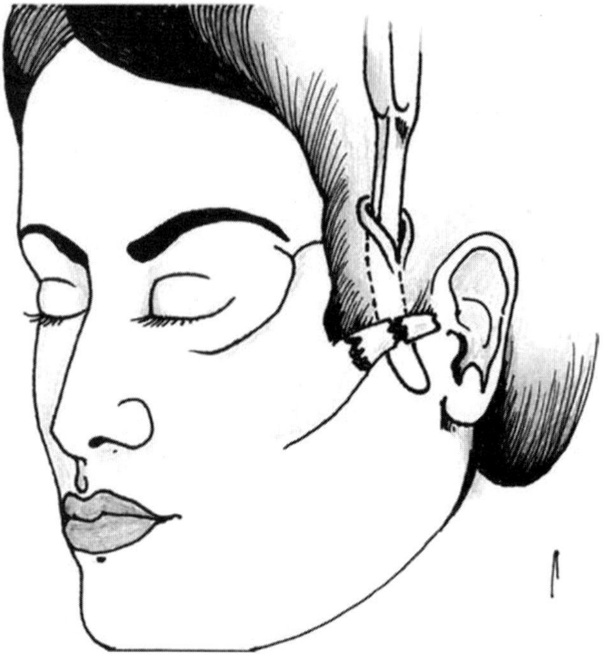

Figure 8 Gillies' approach to zygomatic arch reduction.

The procedure is effective for reducing a depressed zygoma arch and it leaves a very small scar on the hair-bearing area of the scalp. To begin the procedure, a small incision is made on the scalp behind the hairline and between the two branches of the temporal artery. From there, the dissection is carried to the deep temporal fascia, which is incised to introduce a urethral sound or an elevator deep to the fascia. The instrument is moved down until it lies deep to the fractured arch. The head must be made stable and traction applied to the instrument to reduce the fracture. Often, the surgeon will hear and feel the reduction of the fracture. This surgical approach is usually used on fresh, moderately displaced zygomatic arch fractures where stabilization is not anticipated.

In 1964, Dingman and Natvig described the supraorbital approach (29) to treat these fractures, a method that has been used efficiently since. It employs an incision at the side of the eyebrow or superior eyelid crease to give exposure to the region around the frontozygomatic suture. From this approach, it is also possible to insert an elevator deep to the zygomatic arch, to reduce a fracture. The Dingman and Natvig method is also useful in zygomatic complex fractures, as the exposure provides direct access to the frontozygomatic suture, which can be realigned and stabilized with wire or bone plate.

Neither of these two exposures, however, provides a very good, direct view of the arch. Kobienia et al. offered a solution to this problem, using intraoperative fluoroscopy to confirm adequate fracture reduction in patients with isolated zygomatic arch fractures (30). Intraoperative fluoroscopy or plain radiographs allow visualization of the arch and confirmation of fracture reduction, while decreasing the need for postoperative CT scans in patients with isolated zygomatic arch fractures.

B. Ginvigobuccal Sulcus Incision

It is also possible to reach the zygoma through a gingivobuccal sulcus incision, a procedure that allows ample exposure and leaves a completely hidden scar. This is a good way to approach acute comminuted fractures and malunited fracture-dislocation, where wide exposure of the anterior maxilla and zygoma is necessary. The surgeon must achieve the lateral extension of the periosteal elevation while carefully avoiding the infraorbital nerve and vessels. The incision offers a good way to reach the anterior maxillary wall for anything from fixation to bone grafting.

C. Lid Incisions

Surgeons can use one of three approaches to the infraorbital rim: the transconjuctival, the subciliary, or the subtarsal. Paul Tessier was the first to describe the transconjunctival approach for the management of fractures of the inferior orbital rim and orbital floor (31). However, this approach is of limited use when there is major fracture displacement and, therefore, need for extensive access. In these cases, surgeons may increase the amount of exposure through lateral canthotomy, but this will necessitate a careful repair.

Subciliary incisions, made on the skin just below the margin of the lid, date back to 1944 when they were first introduced by Converse (32). This incision is made less than 3 mm from the lid margin and either a cutaneous or myocutaneous flap can be dissected to reach the level of the orbital rim. This incision can also be combined with a lateral canthotomy for greater exposure to the orbital rim and zygoma. Among the drawbacks to subciliary incisions are findings of unacceptably high rates of skin necrosis, echymosis, and ectropion, particularly when a skin-only flap is used (33).

There is a lower complication rate—and similar exposure—with the subtarsal incision, made below the tarsal plate, preferably in a fold of the eyelid (34). The incision is hardly noticeable after healing and is our preferred approach when ample exposure of the lower rim and orbital floor is needed.

D. Coronal Incision

When zygoma fractures involve major posterior and lateral dislocation of the malar eminence and posterior and inferior depression of the zygomatic body, it is usually necessary to achieve coronal exposure to align the malar eminence and correct facial width especially with a comminuted unstable arch fracture. In these difficult fractures alignment of the sphenoid wing allows for good confirmation of anatomical reduction of the arch and malar eminence, as the sphenoid wing makes up the lateral wall of the orbit (35). Another advantage of the coronal incision is that it allows for ease of harvest of calvarial bone in the event that bone grafting is necessary to reconstruct sever comminuted fractures.

E. Endoscopic-Assisted Approach

Endoscopy is increasingly being used as an adjunct to or instead of open incisions. Lee et al. have determined that such procedures tend to reduce nerve injury, alopecia, scarring, and eyelid edema (36). Cadaveric studies have shown that this method is useful in treating comminuted fractures of the zygomatic arch, since it preserves the frontal branch of the facial nerve. The endoscopic approach uses the preauricular or temporal incision sites to gain access and view the damage, which is repaired with miniplate and screw systems. Chen and colleagues studied 15 consecutive cases and found that the use of miniplates in the reconstruction of the arch and zygoma had been adequate. Among the 15 patients, however, there were two cases of transient frontal nerve palsies (37).

To summarize, the goal of exposure is to allow for optimal reduction of the fracture and stable fixation. Through the physical examination and radiographic evaluation, the surgeon can gain an understanding of the displacement of a particular fracture and determine the necessary exposure. Although the reduction can at times be easily obtained, in grossly displaced and comminuted fractures, the application of force in multiple planes is necessary for fracture reduction. Thus, at times, the more displaced and comminuted the fractures, the more sites and extent of exposure is needed.

Once the surgeon achieves optimal reduction, the next step is ensuring stable fixation to protect the fracture against physiological forces and to promote healing. Fixation can be achieved through the use of wires or bone plates otherwise known as rigid fixation. Some have suggested that miniplates were much more efficient than interosseous wires in achieving malar and global symmetry (38). Another advantage of the miniplate was a lower complication rate such as sensory abnormalities of the infraorbital nerve. Lin et al. have shown that rigid fixation is preferable in that it allows for bone grafts to maintain their position and volume better (39). The principal cause of postoperative bone resorption is instability and motion between the ends of fragments. This is best avoided through rigid fixation with plates and screws, as this type of fixation best ensures three-dimensional stability. (See Fig. 9.)

As to the number of fixation points, three points are ideal but two points of fixation are adequate in most cases. Rinehart et al. used mechanical forces that simulated normal physiological loads on zygomatic arch fractures and found that at least two miniplates were needed for optimal fixation (40).

Surgeons can choose between a number of microplating systems. Titanium miniplates are strongest in distraction and compression across a central gap, as shown by a study that compared these plates with both biodegradable plates and screws and cyanoacrylate glue fixation systems (41). However, resorbable plates and screws are adequate in many situations, particularly when bone fragments are strong enough to fix in direct contact.

In our center, we approach zygomatic fractures through a superior lid incision, a buccal mucosa incision, and either a transconjunctival or mid-lower eyelid incision. This extensive exposure allows us to adequately reduce the fractures and provide fixation at the zygomate buttress, fronto-zygomatic suture, and infraorbital rim. If there is accompanying enopthalmus or a significant orbital floor fracture (greater than 2 cm in diameter), we will reconstruct the orbital floor preferably with calvanial bone.

Postoperative management is usually in the form of a soft diet and careful wound examination. Care should also be taken to protect the cornea from exposure and careful observation for increased intraocular pressure of hemorrhage is mandatory.

Complications of reconstruction of zygoma fractures include ectropion and canthal deformities. Ectropion deformities will frequently resolve with time and softening of the eyelid scars. Canthal deformities can occur after a poorly reconstructed canthal incision or misalignment of zygoma fracture. Enophthalmos and malunion of the zygoma are also possible and may require a secondary osteotomy for correction. Infection after zygoma fracture reconstruction is infrequent. One review noted a higher rate of infection after intraosseous wiring versus plating in facial bone fractures (42). In this series only 0.8% of these infections were in the midface. Sinusitis has been noted and such cases should be treated with satisfactory drainage and antibiotics.

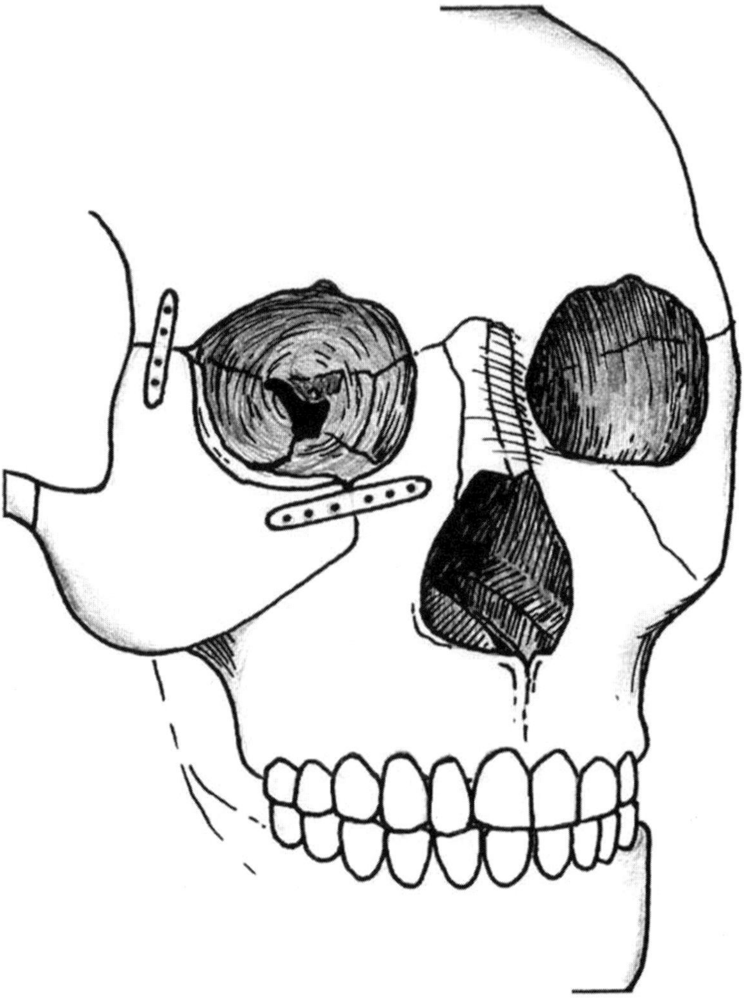

Figure 9 Bone plating of zygomatic fracture. At least two points of fixation are recommended.

One of the most common problems with plating facial fractures including the zygoma is the palpable plate. Orringer et al. found this to be the most common reason for removal of internal fixation devices (35%) (43). In zygoma fractures this is usually at the zygomatic frontal suture or the infraorbital rim.

VIII. CONCLUSION

In treating zygoma fractures, the following steps are necessary: First, a careful medical history should be developed, followed by thorough physical examination to ensure no other major injuries. Any findings during the examination should be confirmed through radiology; this will also give surgeons a more precise understanding of the injuries and help them determine the need for surgery. Once this is done, a decision should be made on the type of exposure needed and on the best way to achieve adequate fixation. During surgery, careful attention must be given to reduction and fixation and repair of any associated soft tissue injuries.

REFERENCES

1. Duverney JG. Traite des Maladies des Os. Paris: Dure L'aine, 1751.
2. Lothrop HA. Fractures of the superior maxillary bone caused by direct blows over the malar bone. Boston Med Surg 1906; 154:8.
3. Keen WW. Surgery: Its Principles and Practices. Philadelphia: WB Saunders, 1909.
4. Gillies HD, Kilner TP, Stone D. Fractures of the malar-zygomatic compound: with a description of a new x-ray position. Br J Surg 1927; 14:651–656.
5. Dingman RO, Natvig P. Surgery of Facial Fractures. Philadelphia: WB Saunders Co., 1964.
6. Adams WM. Internal wiring fixation of facial fractures. Surgery 1942; 12:523.
7. Brown JB, Fryer MP, McDowell F. Internal wire-pin stabilization for middle third facial fractures. Surg Gynecol Obstet 1951; 93:676.
8. Michelet FX, Deymes J, Dessus B. Osteosynthesis with miniaturized screwed plates in maxillo-facial surgery. J Maxillofacial Surg 1973; June; 1(2):79–84.
9. Sicher H, Debrul EL. Oral Anatomy. 5th ed. St Louis: Mosby, 1970:78.
10. Manson PN, Hoopes JE, Su. CT. Structural pillars of the facial skeleton: An approach to the management of Le Fort fractures. Plast Reconstr Surg 1980 Jul; 66(1):54–62.
11. Kelly KJ. Pediatric facial trauma. In: Achauer BM, Eriksson E, Guyuron B, et al, eds. Plastic Surgery: Indications, Operations, and Outcomes. St. Louis, MO: Mosby-Year Book, Inc., 2000; 2: 941–969.
12. Manson PN. Facial Injuries. In: McCarthy JG., ed. Plastic Surgery. Philadelphia, PA: WB Saunders Co., 1990; 2:867–1141.
13. Knight JS, North JF. The classification of malar fractures: an analysis of displacement as a guide to treatment. Br J Plast Surg 1961; 13:325.
14. Pozatek ZW, Kaban LB, Guralnick WC. Fractures of the zygomatic complex: an evaluation of surgical management with special emphasis on the eyebrow approach. J Oral Surg 1973 Feb; 31(2):141–148.
15. Manson PN, Markowitz B, Mirvis S, et al. Toward CT-based facial fracture treatment. Plast Reconstr Surg 1990 Feb; 85(2):202–212.

16. Taicher S, Ardekian L, Samet N, et al. Recovery of the infraorbital nerve after zygomatic complex fractures: a preliminary study of different treatment methods. Int J Oral Maxillofac Surg 1993 Dec; 22(6):339–341.
17. De Man K, Bax WA. The influence of the mode of treatment of zygomatic bone fractures on the healing process of the infraorbital nerve. Br J Oral Maxillofac Surg 1988 Oct; 26(5):419–425.
18. Ellis E, El-Attar A, Moos KF. An analysis of 2,067 cases of zygomatico-orbital fractures. J Oral Maxillofac Sur 1985 Jun; 43(6):417–428.
19. Barclay TL. Diplopia in association with fractures involving the zygomatic bone. Br J Plast Surg 1958; 11:47.
20. Manson P. Facial fractures. In: Smith JW, Aston S (eds), Grabb and Smith's Plastic Surgery. 4th ed Boston: Little, Brown, 1991:Ch 12:347–396.
21. Zingg M, Laedrach K, Chen J, et al. Classification and treatment of zygomatic fractures: a review of 1,025 cases. J Oral Maxillofac Sur 1992 Aug; 50(8):778–790.
22. Pogrel MA, Podlesh SW, Goldman KE. Efficacy of a single radiograph to screen for midfacial fractures. J Oral Maxillofac Surgery 2000; 58:24.
23. Ardekin L, Kaffe I, Taicher S. Comparative evaluation of different radiographic projections of zygomatic complex fractures. J Craniomaxillofac Surg 1993; 21:120.
24. Jacoby CG, Dolan KD. Fragment analysis in maxillofacial injuries: the tripod fracture. J Trauma 1980; 20:292.
25. Trapnell DH. Diagnostic radiography. In: Rowe NL, Williams J. LI. (eds), Maxillofacial Injuries. New York: Churchill Livingstone, 1985:138–139.
26. Fox LA, Vannier MW, West OC, et al. Diagnostic performance of CT, MPR, and 3DCT imaging in maxillofacial. trauma Comput Med Imaging Graph 1995; 19:385.
27. Stanley RB Jr. Use of intraoperative computed tomography during repair of orbitozygomatic fractures. Arch Facial Plast Surg. 1:19, 199.
28. Gillies HD, Kilner TP, Stone D. Fractures of the malar-zygomatic compound: with a description of a new X-Ray position. Br J Surg 1927; 14:651–656.
29. Dingman RO, Natvig P. Surgery of facial fractures. Philadelphia: WB Saunders Co., 1964.
30. Kobienia BJ, Sultz JR, Migliori MR, Schubert W. Portable fluoroscopy in the management of zygomatic arch fractures. Ann Plast Surg 1998 Mar; 40(3): 260–264.
31. Tessier P. The conjunctival approach to the orbital floor and maxilla in congenital malformation and trauma. J Maxillofac Surg 1973 Mar; 1(1):3–8.
32. Converse J. Two plastic operations for repair of orbit following sever trauma and extensive comminuted fracture. Arch Opththalmol 1944; 31:323.
33. Wray RC, Holtmann BN, Ribaudo JM, Keiter J, Weeks PM. A comparison of conjuctival and subcilliary incisions for orbital fractures. Br J Plast Surg 1977; 30:142.
34. Rorich RJ, Janis JE, Adams WP. Subciliary versus subtarsal approaches to orbitozygomatic fractures. Plast Reconstr Surg 2003 April; 111(5):1708–1713.

35. Zide BM, Jelks GW. Surgical Anatomy of the Orbit. New York: Raven Press, 1985.
36. Lee C, Jacobovicz J, Mueller RV. Endoscopic repair of a complex midfacial fractures. J Craniofac Surg 1997 May; 8(3):170–175.
37. Chen CT, Lai JP, Chen YR, Tung TC, Chen ZC, Rohrich RJ. Application of endoscope in zygomatic fracture repair. Br Jr Plast Surg 2000 March; 53(2):100–105.
38. Rohrich RJ, Watumull D. Comparison of rigid plate versus wire fixation in the management of zygoma fractures: a long-term follow-up clinical study. Plast Reconstr Surg 1995 Sept; 96(3):570–575.
39. Lin KY, Barlett SP, Yaremchuk MJ, et al. The effect of rigid fixation on the survival of onlay bone grafts: an experimental study. Plast Reconstr Surg. 1990 Sept; 86(3):449–456.
40. Rinehart GC, Marsh JL, Hemmer KM, Bresina S. Internal fixation of malar fractures: an experimental biophysical study. Plast Reconstr Surg 1989 Jul; 84(1):21–25.
41. Gosain AK, Song L, Corrao MA, Pintar FA. Biomechanical evaluation of titanium, biodegradable plate and screw, and cyanoacrylate glue fixation systems in carniofacial surgery. Plast Reconstr Surg 1998 Mar; 101(3):582–591..
42. Zachariades N, Papademetriou I, Rallis G. Complications associated with rigid internal fixation of facial bone fractures. J Oral Maxillofac Surg 1993 Mar; 51(3):275–278.
43. Orringer JS, Barcelona V, Buchman SR. Reasons for removal of rigid fixation devices in craniofacial surgery. J Craniofac Surg 1998 Jan; 9(1):40–44.

16

Mandibular Fractures

Anil P. Punjabi
Loma Linda University School of Medicine and Riverside County Regional Medical Center, Loma Linda, California, U.S.A.

Alan S. Herford
Loma Linda University Medical Center, Loma Linda, California, U.S.A.

I. INTRODUCTION

Fractures of the mandible are common. The goal of treatment of mandible fractures should be to return the patient to a preinjury state of function and aesthetics. The treatment of these injuries has evolved from closed treatment to open techniques with wire osteosynthesis to open techniques with rigid internal fixation with the goal of avoiding maxillomandibular fixation. Insight into the biomechanics and the biology of primary bone healing has contributed to the current trends of mandibular fracture treatment.

II. HISTORY

The treatment of closed reduction of mandibular fractures has a much longer history than open reduction. This is because before the advent of antibiotics and a sterile environment, the frequency of infections after open reduction was so high that closed reduction was the only real viable option for treatment.

The historical beginning of closed reduction is lost in time, with archeological evidence dating back thousands of years (1). The first written reference to monomaxillary wiring of teeth has been attributed to Hippocartes, but archeological proof exists that Phoenicians, Egyptians, and Etruscans wired teeth adjacent to the fracture sites (1). Intricate bandages were fabricated by Hippocrates, Galen, Soranus of Ephesus, Ambroise Paré, and others. The first mention of intermaxillary fixation was by Guglielmo Salicetti (1275), which was lost in the ages until it was revived by Gilmer in the United States in 1886. Gunning (1866) used custom-crafted vulcanite splints for the immobilization of fractured fragments (2). This splint was modified for the treatment of edentulous mandible. The development of arch bars by Winters, Jelenko, and Erich solved the problems associated with closed reduction and they remain currently popular for immobilization.

Though open reduction can be traced back 150 years it has become widely used only in the past several decades. The first method used was wires drilled through bone [Buck used a wire loop (1846), Kinlock used a silver wire (1859)] (1). Gilmer wired heavy rods on either side of fractures in 1881, but the first reference to the use of solid-steel bone plates held by four screws is attributed to Schede (1888). Other surgeons, including Mahe, Kazanjian, Ivy, and Cole, used variants of these. Infection, however, continued to be a major problem. Only after the introduction of penicillin did the use of metal pins, rods, plates, meshes, and bone clamps flourish and the golden age of open reduction had arrived. Though infection continued to be a hindrance it was not as much of a limiting factor.

Two schools of thought emerged. The first, espoused by the AO/ASIF (Arbeitsgemeinschaft fur Osteosynthesefragen/Association for the Study of Internal Fixation), required rigid stability with strong plates and screws and compression for primary healing (Luhr, Spiessl) (3). The other was the use of small, semirigid noncompression plates placed along the lines of ideal osteosynthesis on the mandible (Champy, Michelet) (4). Both systems have produced good clinical results, though the use of smaller plates is currently more popular.

In spite of the presence of these modern techniques, closed reduction has by no means fallen by the wayside and still remains a commonly used procedure.

III. INCIDENCE, ETIOLOGY, AND BIOMECHANICS

The anatomical architecture of the mandible as a curved beam predisposes the mandible to multiple fractures when struck. A blow delivered to the symphysis causes buckling at the condylar necks. The parasymphyseal region exposes the weakness at the contralateral angle or the condylar neck. It is, therefore, axiomatic that when a mandibular fracture is present, one should be suspicious of a second fracture unless proven otherwise.

Several points have emerged from studies on mandible fractures (5). Condylar fractures are most common. The angle is the second most common site of fracture, but if only one isolated mandibular fracture is present it is most commonly at the angle than at the condyle. Multiple mandibular fractures outnumber isolated fractures by a ratio of 2:1. Eighty percent of patients with fractures have teeth. Figure 1 shows the anatomical distribution of mandibular fractures (6).

A fracture is deemed favorable or unfavorable in the horizontal or vertical plane with reference to the direction of the fracture line and the action of the muscles on the fragments. Fractures, however, do not follow these simple patterns and basing treatment on this classification is impractical.

The causes of mandibular fractures include falls, interpersonal violence, motor vehicle accidents, pathology, and iatrogenic during tooth removal. Assaults are the most common cause of isolated mandible fractures (6).

Patients who have sustained a mandible fracture often have concomitant injuries. Mandibular fractures have been associated with cervical spine injuries, closed head injury, blunt carotid injury, and death (7–11). Mandible fractures sustained in motor vehicle accidents (MVA) have a high incidence of concomitant injuries. Fischer et al. (12) found that associated injuries occurred in the skull, face, neck, chest, abdomen, and upper and

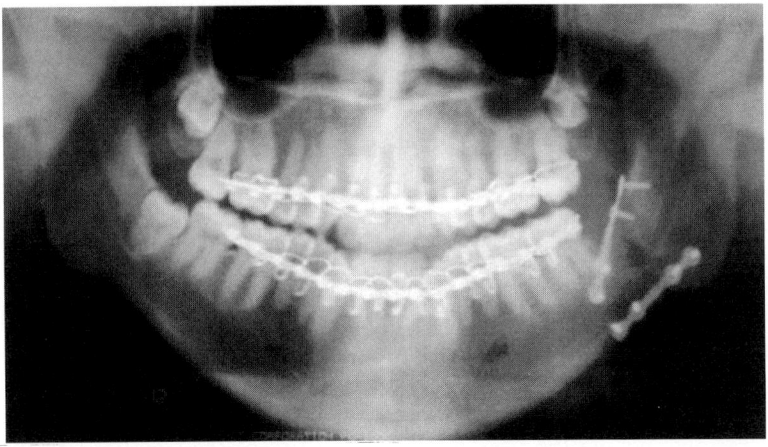

Figure 1 Left mandible fracture treated with superior and inferior border miniplates. The inferior border plate is usually not necessary.

lower extremity. Ninety-nine percent of their patients with mandible fractures sustained in an MVA had associated injuries.

IV. DIAGNOSIS

The gold standard for diagnosing a mandible fracture is a thorough history and physical examination. Careful inspection and palpation will reveal fractures in most cases. The clinical evaluation is supplemented by radiographic imaging for diagnosis and treatment planning.

Panoramic tomography is the standard imaging modality for evaluation of suspected mandibular fractures. The other methods include the mandible series, computed tomography, and zonography. Zonography is a tomographic technique used for imaging of the mandible with relatively good resolution; it is conducted with the patient in the supine position. This allows zonography to be applicable to the polytrauma patient, contrary to panoramic views, which are obtained with the patient in the upright position, thus limiting their use to ambulatory patients who can stand or sit upright.

Panoramic views are considered to be superior in detecting fractures to both plain radiography and nonhelical CT scans (13,14). Wilson et al. showed the sensitivity of helical CT to be 100%, compared to 86% for panoramic tomography, for diagnosing mandibular fractures (15). Coronal and oblique parasagittal reformatted views of the mandible provide details of fractures that are not clearly visualized in the axial plane alone.

Though getting a helical CT on every suspected mandibular fracture would be prohibitively expensive, this modality is specially useful on a case-by-case basis especially for imaging the posterior mandible, involving the ramus and condylar region.

V. CLOSED VERSUS OPEN TREATMENT OF MANDIBULAR FRACTURES

Mandibular fractures have been successfully treated by closed-reduction methods for hundreds of years. Maxillomandibular fixation (MMF) is used to immobilize the fractured segments and allow osseous healing.

When considering between open versus closed reduction of mandibular fractures the advantages should be weighed against the disadvantages. Considerations include the site and characteristics of the fracture and the morbidities of the treatment. Unwanted results including bony ankylosis or decreased mouth opening can be prevented by early mobilization of the mandible. Early mobilization helps to prevent possible ankylosis especially in patients with intracapsular fractures of the condyle. It is preferred to avoid maxillomandibular fixation when fractures involve the temperomandibular joint (TMJ) because postoperative physiotherapy can be started much earlier.

Advantages of closed reduction include simplicity, decreased operative time, and avoidance of damage to adjacent structures. Disadvantages of maxillomandibular fixation include inability to directly visualize the reduced fracture, need to keep the patient on a soft diet, and difficulties with speech and respiration. Open reduction of fractures via a transoral or transfacial approach can lead to morbidity by causing damage to the surrounding structures as a result of obtaining access for fracture reduction and treatment.

The traditional length of immobilization of fractures when treated by closed reduction has been 6 weeks. Juniper and Awty found that 80% of mandibular fractures treated with open or closed reduction and maxillomandibular fixation had clinical union in 4 weeks (16). They were able to show a correlation between the age of the patient and the predictability of early fracture union. Armaratunga found that 75% of mandible fractures had achieved clinical union by 4 weeks. Fractures in children healed in 2 weeks whereas a significant number of fractures in older patients took 8 weeks to achieve clinical union (17).

Although maxillomandibular fixation has long been considered a benign procedure it can be associated with significant problems. An excellent review of the deleterious effects of mandibular immobilization on the masticatory system is provided by Ellis (18). Closed reduction of mandibular fractures can adversely affect bone, muscles, synovial joints, and periarticular connective tissues.

The effects of immobilization on bone have been recognized in the orthopedic literature for many years as "disuse osteoporosis". Cortical and trabecular thinning, vascular distention, and increased osteoclastic activity have been described following joint immobilization (19). Changes involving the musculature include not only muscle atrophy but also changes in muscle length and function.

VI. RIGID FIXATION

In the early twentieth century surgical management of fractures was initially advocated by those in the orthopedic field with the goal of early functional mobilization (20). Open reduction became more common when orthopedic surgeons were able to see how poorly many fractures were reduced following closed techniques. Both this and the introduction of antibiotics led to an increase in open reductions of fractures to directly visualize the reduced osseous segments. In 1942 Adams' landmark article discussed the benefits of surgical exposure for purposes of reduction and fixation (21). In 1956 the Association for the Study of Internal Fixation (ASIF) was formed. A landmark publication in 1965 by Muller et al. described the technique of internal fixation of fractures for treatment of long-bone fractures with rigid fixation (22). Application and modification of these ASIF principles by Luhr (1970) and spiessl (1972) was the beginning of modern maxillofacial rigid fixation (23,24).

Rigid fixation in the mandible refers to a form of treatment that consists of applying fixation to adequately reduce the fracture and also permit active use of the mandible during the healing process. The four AO/ASIF principles are (1) anatomical reduction; (2) functionally stable fixation; (3) atraumatic surgical technique; and (4) immediate active function. Although many osteosynthesis systems are currently available to treat mandibular fractures, the principles of plate application are similar. An overview of the various types of plates follows.

A. Microminiplates

Microminiplates usually refer to small malleable plates with a screw diameter of 1.0–1.5 mm. Their use for mandibular surgery is limited because of their inability to provide rigid fixation and because they have a tendency for plate fracture during the healing process (25). These plates can work well in the midface where the muscular forces are much less than those acting on the mandible. A recent study found a 30.4% complication rate when 1.3-mm microminiplates were used to provide osteosynthesis for mandibular fractures (26).

B. Miniplates

Miniplates typically refer to small plates with a screw diameter of 2.0 mm. These plates have been shown to be effective in treating mandibular fractures. Typically a superior and inferior plate is required for adequate fixation. An exception to this is in the mandibular angle region where a superior border plate placed at the point of maximal tension is sufficient (Fig. 1). An advantage of these plates is that they are stable enough to obviate the need for maxillomandibular fixation and have a very low profile. They are less likely to be palpable, which reduces the need for subsequent plate removal. Typically screws are placed monocortically but may be placed bicortically when positioned along the inferior border of the mandible.

A minimum of two screws should be placed in each osseous segment. Smaller incisions and less soft-tissue reflections are required with these plates when compared to larger plates and they can be placed from an intraoral approach, thus eliminating an external scar. Because these plates are less rigid than reconstruction plates, their use in treating comminuted fractures should be avoided (27).

C. Compression Plates

Compression plates cause compression at the fracture site making primary bone healing more likely. These plates can be bent in only two dimensions because of their design and if they are not contoured properly they are unable to produce compression. It is important to avoid compressing oblique fractures. They also require bicortical screw engagement to produce even compression along the fracture line. This necessitates their placement at the inferior border to eliminate damage to the inferior alveolar neurovascular structures or the roots of the teeth. A higher incidence of complications has been noted in fractures treated with compression plates (28). Because of the relatively small cross section of bone surface in some fractures, interfragmentary compression is often not possible.

D. Reconstruction Plates

1. Conventional Reconstruction Plates

Reconstruction plates are recommended for comminuted fractures and also for bridging continuity gaps. These plates are rigid and have corresponding screws with a diameter of 2.3–3.0 mm. Reconstruction plates can be adapted to the underlying bone and contoured in three dimensions. A problem that may be associated with conventional reconstruction plates is loosening of the screws during the healing process leading to instability of the fracture.

2. Locking Reconstruction Plates

In 1987 Raveh et al. introduced the titanium hollow-screw osteointegrated reconstruction plate (THORP) (29). This system achieves stability between the screw and plate by insertion of an expansion screw into the head of the bone screw. This causes expansion of the screw flanges and locks them against the wall of the hole in the bone plate. Later Herford and Ellis described the use of locking reconstruction bone plate/screw system for mandibular surgery (30). This system simplified the locking mechanism between the plate and the screw (Locking Reconstruction Plate, Synthes Maxillofacial, Paoli, PA) by engaging the threads of the head of the screw with the threads in the reconstruction plate, thus eliminating the need for expansion screws (Fig. 2).

Locking plate/screw systems offer advantages over conventional reconstruction plates. These plates function as internal fixators by achieving

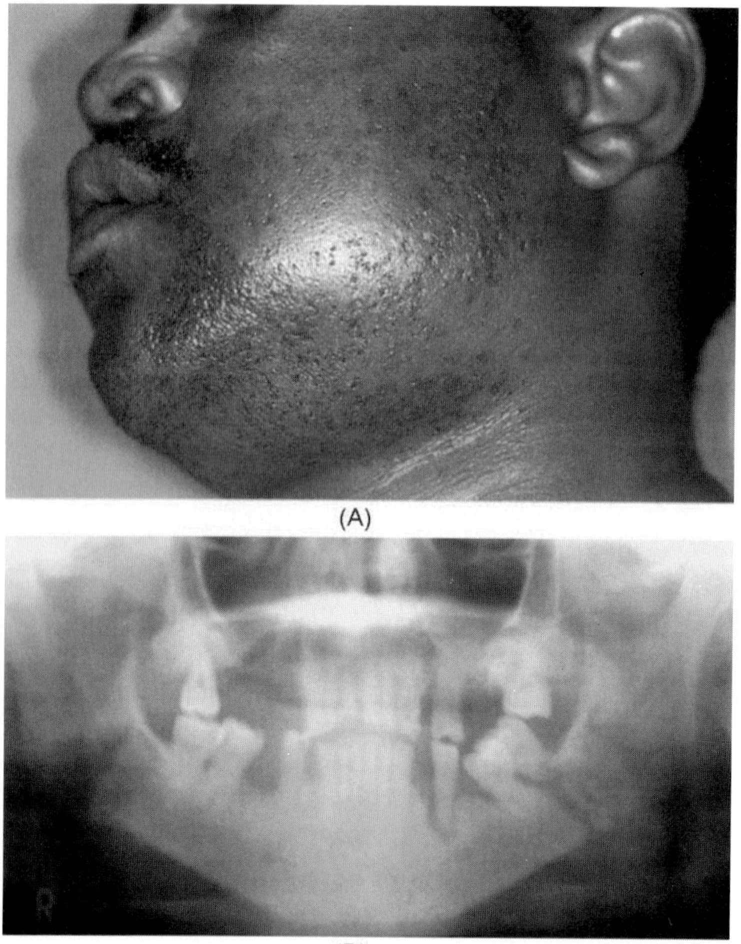

(A)

(B)

Figure 2 A, B. Infected left angle fracture. C. Extraoral open reduction showing bone gap after debridement. D. Reconstruction with a locking reconstruction plate.

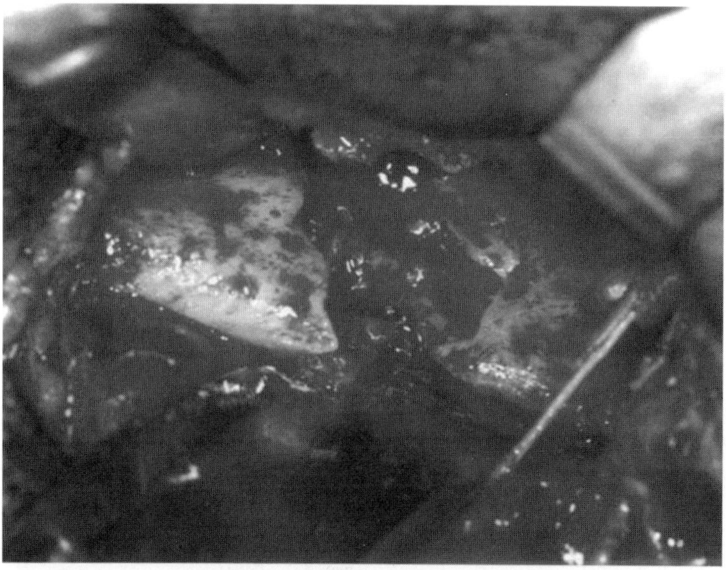

(C)

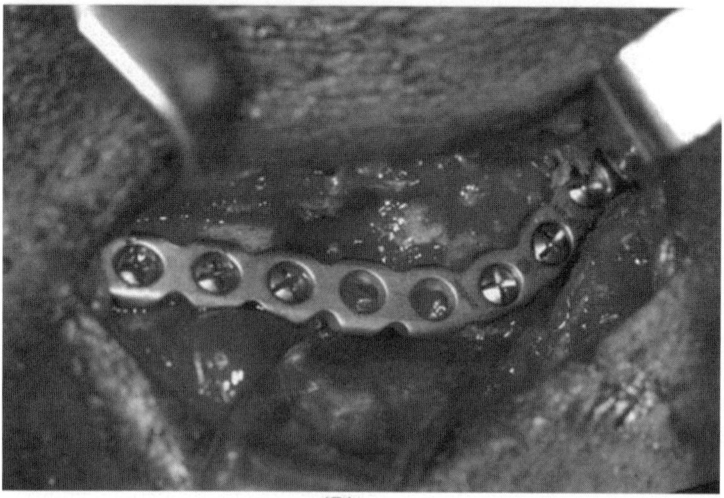

(D)

Figure 2 *(continued)*

stability by locking the screw to the plate and allow greater stability as compared to conventional plates (31). Fewer screws are required to maintain stability. The most significant advantage of this type of system is that it becomes unnecessary for the plate to intimately contact the underlying bone in all areas. As the screws are tightened they will not draw the plate and underlying bone toward each other.

E. Lag Screw Fixation

Lag screws can provide osteosynthesis of mandibular fractures (32,33). They work well in oblique fractures and require a minimum of two screws. The lag screw engages the opposite cortex while fitting passively in the cortex of the outer bone segment. This can be accomplished by using a true lag screw or by overdrilling the proximal cortex. This causes compression of the osseous segments and provides the greatest rigidity of all fixation techniques. The proximal cortex should be countersunk to distribute the compressive forces over a broader area and avoid microfractures.

The anatomy of the symphyseal region of the mandible lends itself to use of lag screws in a different technique. The lag screws can be placed through the opposing cortexes between the mental foramen and inferior to the teeth. Fractures should not be oblique with this technique because it may cause the fractures to override on each other (Fig. 3).

F. Bioresorbable Plates

Bioresorbable plates are manufactured from varying amounts of materials including polydioxanone (PDS), polyglycolic acid, and polylactic acid. These plates have not been found to predictably provide enough rigidity for treating mandibular fractures. It has been shown that the breakage of a poly-L-lactic acid (PLLA) plate occurred at 50% of the yield strength required to break a miniplate (34). Complications associated with these plates include inflammation and foreign-body-type reactions. We do not recommend use of the current bioresorbable plates for routine treatment of mandibular fractures. Consideration may be given for use in pediatric patients with the understanding of the possible complications (Fig. 4).

G. External Pin Fixation

Pin fixation was introduced in World War II for use with comminuted, compound, and infected fractures. Its use in the modern era of rigid internal fixation has waned, though it remains a valuable part of the armamentarium

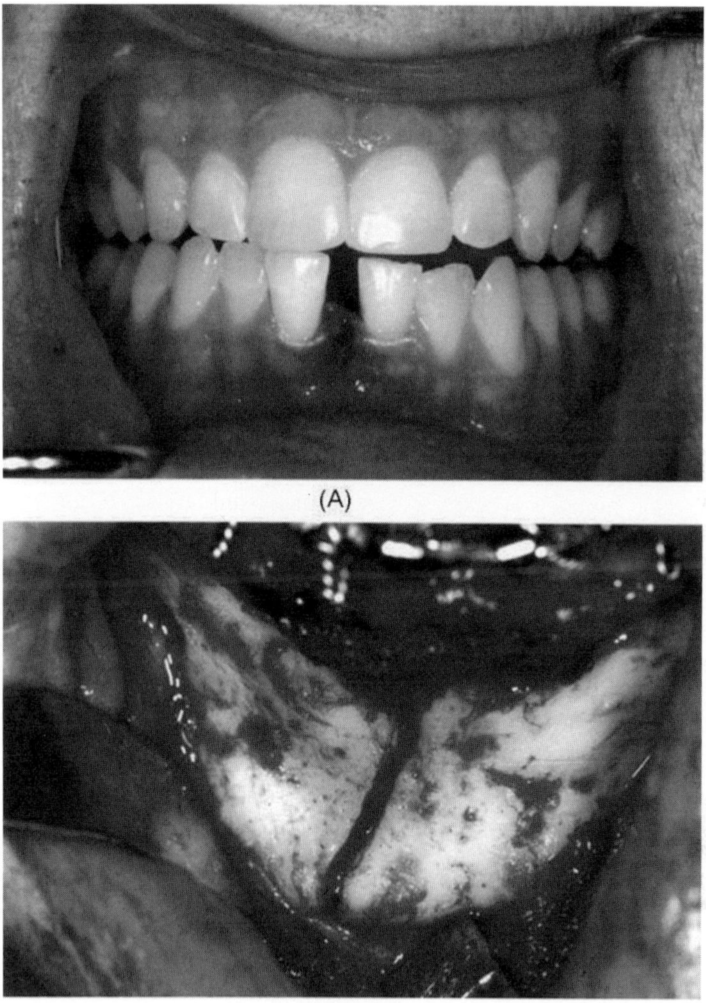

(A)

(B)

Figure 3 A. Symphysis fracture causing midline diastema. B, C. Intraoperative views showing fractured symphysis that is reduced and fixated with 2 lag screws. D, E. postoperative occlusion and radiograph.

in treatment of jaw fractures. It is useful in treatment of atrophic mandible fractures, pathological fractures, fractures associated with gunshot wounds, and mandibular fractures with concurrent cervical spine fractures that are in a halo.

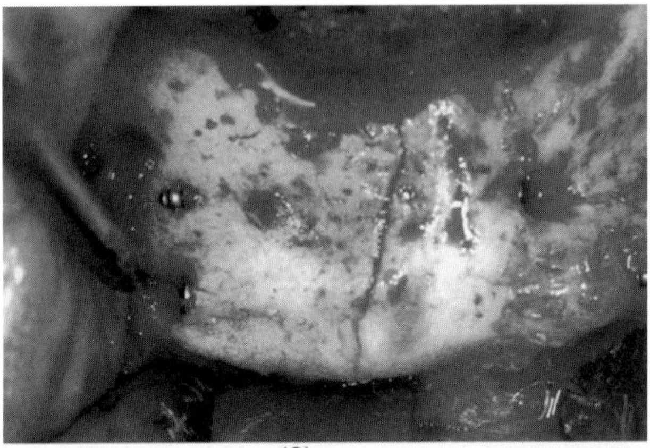

(C)

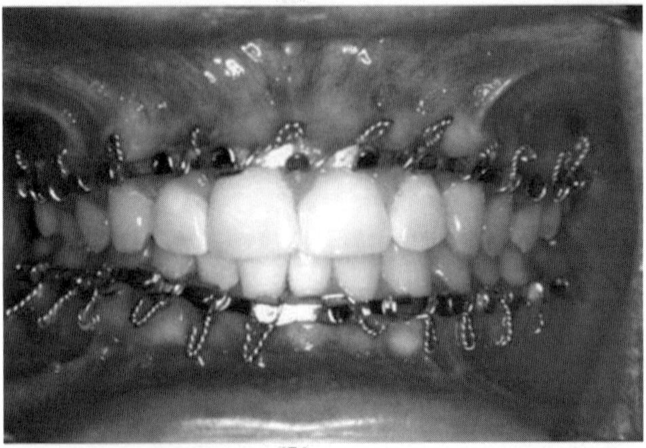

(D)

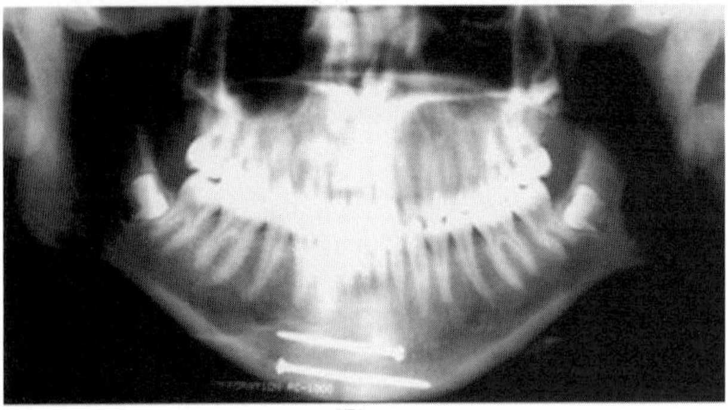

(E)

Figure 3 (*continued*)

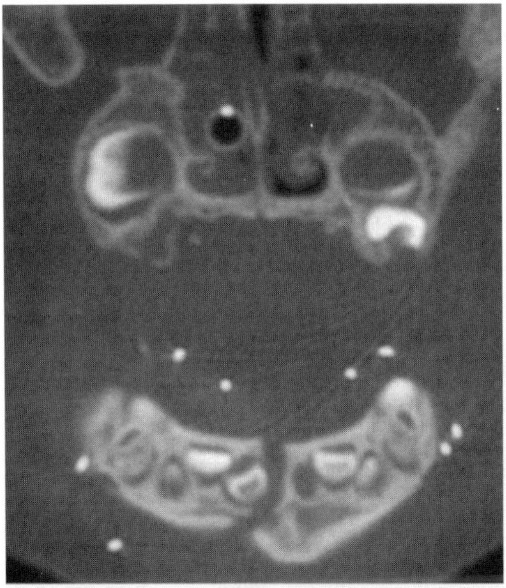

(A)

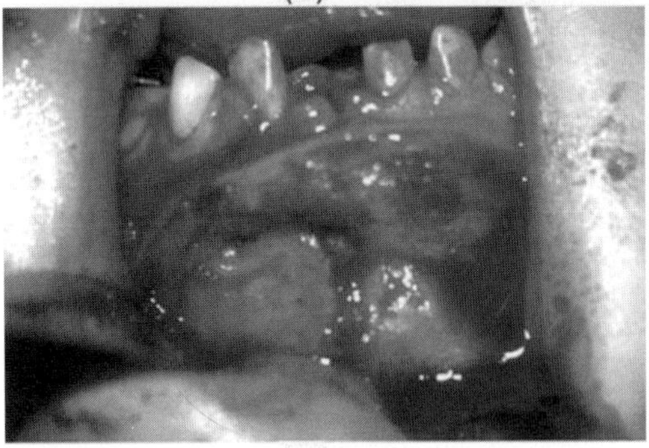

(B)

Figure 4 A, B. Radiographic and intraoperative view of a 3-year-old child with fracture of the symphysis. C. Fixation with resorbable plate.

The pins are inserted at least 1 cm from the fracture and at right angles to the bone. The pins are then connected in the biphasic system described by Morris and Hipp (35). Complications include pin loosening, infection, injury to the inferior alveolar nerve, and even injury to the facial nerve.

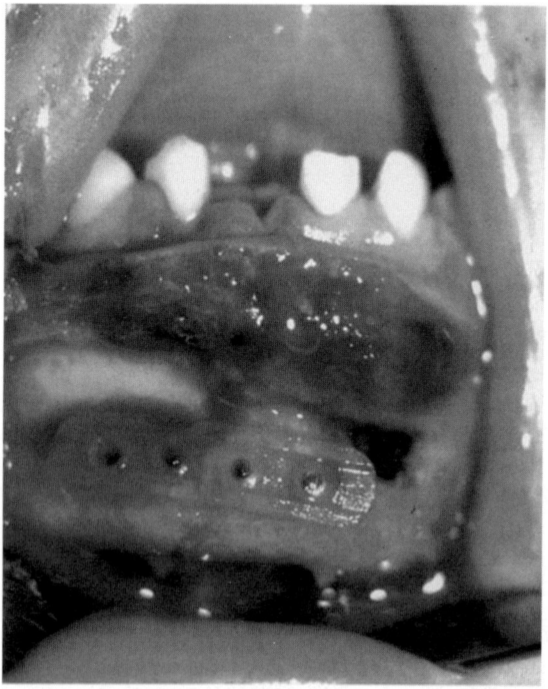

(C)

Figure 4 (*continued*)

VII. GENERAL PRINCIPLES

A. Surgical Technique

Intermaxillary fixation is placed prior to reducing a fracture. This allows for use of the occlusion to aid in anatomical reduction of the fracture. Use of full-arch bars combined with maxillomandibular fixation is the preferred method. The arch bars provide a way to maintain the occlusion postoperatively with elastic bands as needed during physiotherapy. The arch bars are removed after 6 weeks and after the patient has rehabilitated with an interincisor opening of 40 mm or more.

The surgical approach depends on the site of the fracture. Either a transoral, vestibular, or transfacial approach may be performed. A facial approach provides excellent access but also produces a facial scar and adds the risk of damage to the facial nerve. Most fractures, excluding those of the condyle, can easily be approached through a transoral incision.

A subperiosteal dissection with a periosteal elevator provides adequate access for reduction of the fracture and placement of fixation. Attention should be given to avoiding damage to the mental nerve, which exists the mental foramen near the apices of the premolar teeth. If additional exposure is needed, the nerve can be released by gently scoring the periosteum surrounding the nerve. Bone-reducing forceps are often helpful in reducing the fracture while adapting the bone plate. This also provides interfragmentary compression, making primary bone healing more likely.

The smallest bone plate that will provide adequate stability under functional loads during the healing period is chosen. A minimum of two screws on either side of the fracture is required. Larger, more rigid plates are required to treat comminuted fractures or continuity defects (30). The intermaxillary fixation that aided reduction of the fractures during plating is removed after the fixation is applied. A soft diet is recommended for at least 3 weeks after miniplate fixation. It is important during the postoperative period to regain preinjury function, including maximal mouth opening, with active physiotherapy.

B. Teeth in the Line of Fracture

Most teeth in the line of fracture can be saved if appropriate antibiotic therapy and fixation techniques are used. Indications for removal of teeth in the line of fracture include grossly mobile teeth, partly erupted third molars with pericoronitis, teeth that prevent reduction of the fractures, fractured tooth roots, entire exposed root surfaces, or an excessive delay from the time of fracture to treatment (36,37).

C. Antibiotics and Mandible Fractures

Zallen and Curry showed that mandibular fractures were associated with a 50% infection rate when patients did not receive antibiotic therapy. The infection rate was reduced to 6% for those patients who received antibiotics (38).

VIII. TREATMENT OF SPECIFIC FRACTURES

A. Symphysis Fractures

Simple symphysis fractures can be treated with two miniplates. Because of the torsional forces generated during function, a single miniplate is insufficient to predictably maintain rigid fixation during healing (39). One miniplate is placed at the inferior border and a second plate is placed superiorly. The superior plate is secured with a minimum of two monocortical screws in each segment whereas bicortical screws can be used on the inferior plate. More rigid fixation should be considered for comminuted fractures.

It is important to avoid "flaring" of the ramus in patients with a symphysis fracture and especially when combined with condyle fractures. This will be seen clinically as a dental crossbite of the posterior occlusion and also fullness of the mandibular angle region. This can be avoided by applying pressure at the angle region during fixation, overbending the plate(s), and directly visualizing the lingual aspect of the reduced fracture.

B. Body Fractures

Simple fractures involving the body of the mandible can be effectively treated with two miniplates. Care should be taken during the dissection to avoid damaging the mental nerve, which supplies sensation to the lower lip. If further reflection is necessary, the periosteum can be scored to release the nerve and allow improved visualization. Often a bone-reducing clamp can be applied prior to plate placement to aid in reduction of the fracture.

C. Angle Fractures

The angle region of the mandible is one of the most common sites of fracture. Often trauma to the lateral mandible will cause a fracture at the angle and also involve the contralateral mandible. Many reasons for the greater proportion of fractures to this site have been cited. These include the presence of impacted third molars, a thinner cross-sectional area in this region, and also the biomechanical lever arm in this area. A recent study looked at the incidence of fractures when teeth were involved. They found a significantly increased incidence of fractures involving the mandibular angle when there was an associated implacted third molar (40). The angle region is a weak point, because the bone anterior and posterior (body and ramus, respectively) are thicker than the bone in the angle region (41).

These fractures are associated with the highest rate of complications (16). Many techniques for treating mandibular angle fractures have been described. Because no teeth are present in the posterior (proximal) segment, arch bars cannot be used to stabilize the segments and there is no control over the proximal segment. Closed-reduction techniques are often associated with rotation of the ramus. With the introduction of plate-and-screw osteosynthesis many surgical methods have been described. Those who advocate large bone plates are attempting to eliminate interfragment mobility and thus allow for primary bone union (29,42). Others have questioned the need for absolute rigidity for treatment of angle fractures (43,44).

In 1973, Michelet et al, described the use of small, malleable bone plates for treatment of angle fractures (4). This led to a change from the previous belief that rigid fixation was necessary for bone healing. Later, Champy et al. validated the technique by performing several clinical investigations (39). They determined the most stable location where bone plates should be placed based on the "ideal lines of osteosynthesis". The "Champy technique" involves placing a small bone plate along the superior border and using monocortical screws to secure the plate and avoid damage to the adjacent teeth or inferior alveolar neurovasular bundle. Absolute immobilization is not provided with this form of treatment (semirigid fixation). Clinical studies have shown that the amount of stability of the fractures is significant enough to eliminate the need for maxillomandibular fixation (44). The superior border plate neutralizes distraction forces (tension) on the mandible while preserving the self-compressive forces that occur during function.

A recent prospective study looked at eight methods for treating mandibular angle fractures (44): (1) closed reduction; (2) extraoral ORIF with a large reconstruction plate; (3) intraoral ORIF using a single lag screw; (4) intraoral ORIF using two 2.0-mm minidynamic compression plates; (5) intraoral ORIF using two 2.4-mm mandibular compression plate; (6) intraoral ORIF using two noncompression miniplates; (7) intraoral ORIF using a single noncompression miniplate; and (8) intraoral ORIF using a single malleable noncompression miniplate. The results revealed that extraoral ORIF with a reconstruction plate and intraoral ORIF using a single miniplate are associated with the fewest complications (7.5% and 2.5%, respectively). This finding is interesting because the single miniplate is less rigid than the other forms of fixation, yet it is associated with the fewest complications. A possible explanation is that less extensive dissection is required and more of the blood supply is maintained.

D. Condyle Fractures

Fractures of the condyle can involve the head (intracapsular), neck, or subcondylar region. The head of the condyle may be dislocated outside of the fossa. The most common direction of displacement is in an anteromedial direction because of the pull from the lateral pterygoid muscle, which inserts on the anterior portion of the head of the condyle.

No other type of mandibular fracture is associated with as much controversy regarding treatment as those involving the condyle. Factors considered in deciding whether to treat a condyle fracture open or closed include the fracture level, amount of displacement, adequacy of the occlusion, and whether the patient can tolerate maxillomandibular fixation. Those who advocate open treatment cite advantages including early mobilization of the mandible, better occlusal results, better function, maintenance of posterior height, and avoidance of facial asymmetries (45). Others prefer closed reduction mainly because of the possible complications associated with open reduction including damage to branches of the facial nerve and a cutaneous scar. Recently endoscopic subcondylar fracture repair has been described with encouraging results (46).

Nonsurgical management (closed reduction) does not require wiring the jaws together. Training elastics are helpful in maintaining the occlusion while allowing jaw physiotherapy during healing. Measurable criteria should be obtained whether treating by closed or open methods. These should include pain-free movement, normal mouth-opening capacity, normal jaw movement in all excursions, preinjury occlusion, a stable TMJ, and good facial and jaw symmetry (47).

Zide and Kent described the absolute and relative indications for open reduction of condyle fractures (48). Absolute indications include (1) displacement of the condylar head into the middle cranial fossa; (2) impossibility of obtaining adequate occlusion by closed reduction; (3) lateral extracapsular displacement of the condyle; and (4) invasion by a foreign body (e.g. gunshot wound) Relative indications include (1) bilateral condyle fractures in an edentulous patient; (2) unilateral or bilateral condyle fractures when splinting is not recommended for medical reasons; (3) bilateral condyle fractures associated with comminuted midface fractures; and (4) bilateral condyle fractures and associated gnathological problems (e.g. lack of posterior occlusal support).

The degree of displacement of the condylar fracture has been used in deciding between open or closed treatment. Mikkonen et al. and Klotch and Lundy recommended open reduction if the condylar displacement was greater than 45 degrees in a sagittal or coronal plane and Widmark et al. recommended opening such fractures if the displacement was greater than 30 degrees (49–51). Care must be taken when using the degree of fracture displacement as a guide for nonsurgical or surgical treatment. Ellis et al. looked at the degree of displacement of the condylar head from immediately after arch bar placement to 6 weeks postsurgery (52). In fractures that were treated in a closed manner, 54% had greater than 10-degree displacement in the coronal plane and 30% in the sagittal plane. Those patients who were treated by an open technique had a 16% (coronal) and 23.5% (sagittal) displacement of fractures with a $>$10-degree displacement.

Intracapsular fractures involving the condylar head are difficult to treat and most recommend close treatment of these fractures to avoid damage to adjacent structures. Fractures involving the condylar neck and subcondylar region can be approached with less morbidity. Many surgical approaches have been described with the most common being the retromandibular, submandibular, and preauricular approaches (53). A nerve stimulator can be helpful in identifying branches of the facial nerve during the dissection.

A recent prospective study compared the effect on facial symmetry after either closed or open treatment of mandibular condylar process fractures (52). It was found that treatment by closed methods led to asymmetries characterized by shortening of the face on the side of the injury. The loss of posterior height on the side of fracture is an adaptation that helps reestablish a new temporomandibular articulation. Loss of facial height on the affected side can lead to compensatory canting of the occlusal plane.

Treatment of condylar process fractures should be individualized (Fig. 5). Many factors, including the patient's own preference, should be considered. Whether surgical or nonsurgical treatment is chosen, we recommend early mobilization during the healing process.

E. Pediatric Fractures

The management of pediatric fractures is complicated by the presence of deciduous teeth and the growing mandible. Children tend to be less tolerant of MMF. An acrylic splint can be helpful in managing mandibular fractures in children (Fig. 6). This can be used without MMF to allow early postoperative physiotherapy to avoid ankylosis and /or growth disturbances, which are more common in pediatric patients (54).

Condylar process fractures in children younger than age 12 should be treated by closed methods in most instances. Damage to the condylar growth center can result in delayed growth and in facial asymmetry. Dalhlstrom et al. showed good restitution of the TMJ and no growth disturbances in 14 children 5 years after nonsurgical treatment of their fractures (55). Early animal studies showed that there was little sacrifice of mandibular growth and symmetry with induced condyle fractures when treated with closed reduction. Boyne compared three methods of fracture treatment in rhesis monkeys and found no difference between those treated with internal fixation (wire), MMF, or no treatment (56).

F. Edentulous Fractures

Fractures of the edentulous mandible most commonly involve the body region (Fig. 7). Changes that occur with age include decreased osteogenesis, mandibular atrophy, and reduced blood supply. With age the inferior alveolar artery contributes less and less to perfusion of the mandible (57). The lack of teeth makes it difficult to adequately reduce the fracture because MMF cannot be used to help reduce the bony fragments.

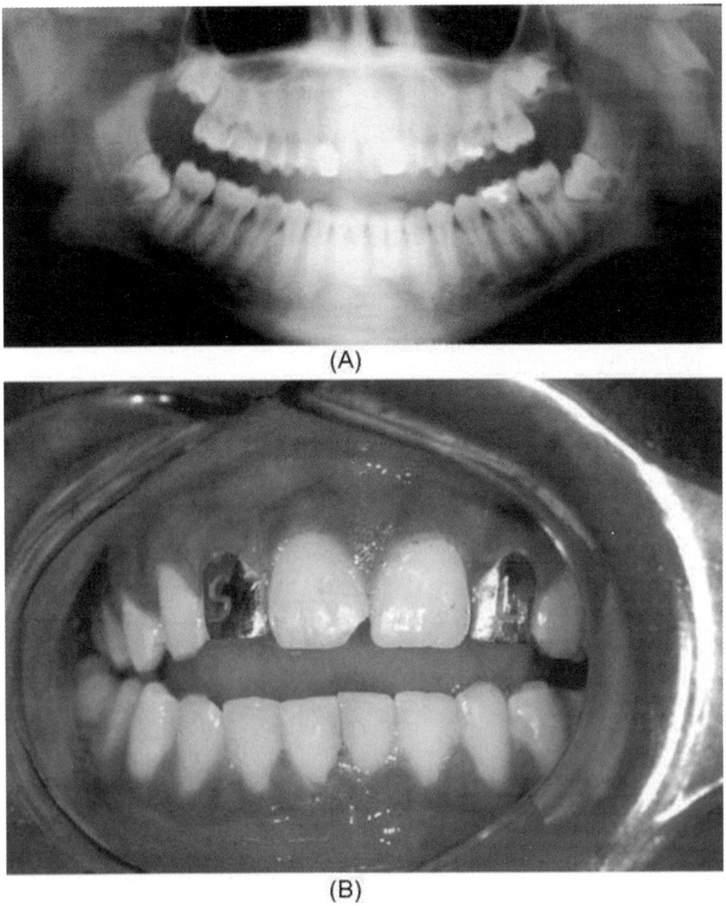

Figure 5 A. Displaced left condyle fracture. B. Anterior open bite. C, D. Postoperative occlusion and radiograph.

These fractures can be treated by either open or closed reduction methods. Closed techniques often entail wiring a mandibular prosthesis in place with circumandibular wires to stabilize the fracture. The second Chalmers J. Lyons Academy Study of fractures of the edentulous mandible reviewed 167 fractures in 104 edentulous mandibles. Fifteen percent of the patients developed a delayed fibrous union and 26% treated by closed-reduction techniques had problems with union. The fewest complications occurred with the patients who received transfacial open reduction and internal fixation (58).

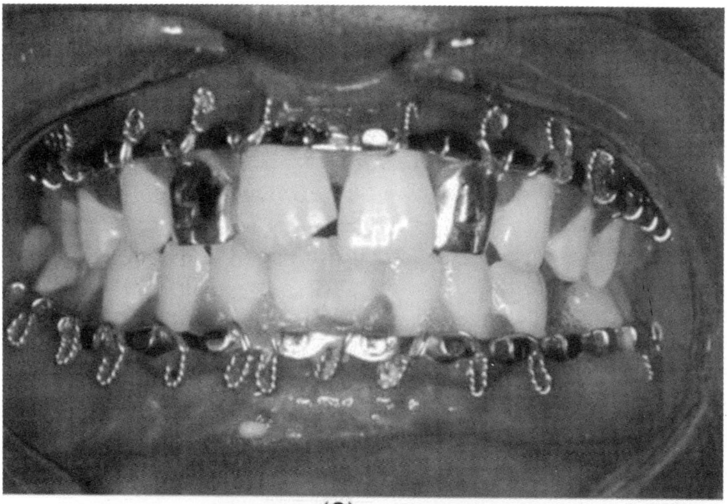

(C)

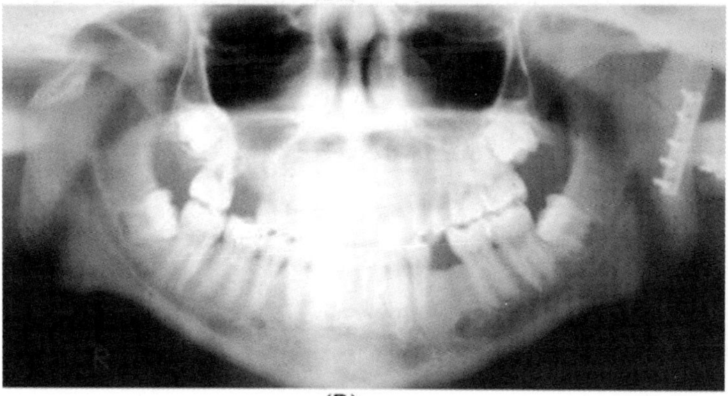

(D)

Figure 5 (*continued*)

Because of the mandibular atrophy and the decreased number of osteoprogenitor cells associated with these fractures, an iliac crest bone graft is often performed to aid in healing. The benefits of grafting should be weighed against the morbidity of graft harvest in elderly patients (58,59).

G. Infected Fractures

Infected mandibular fractures resulting from a delay in treatment can present certain challenges. Treatment by MMF, external fixation, and rigid

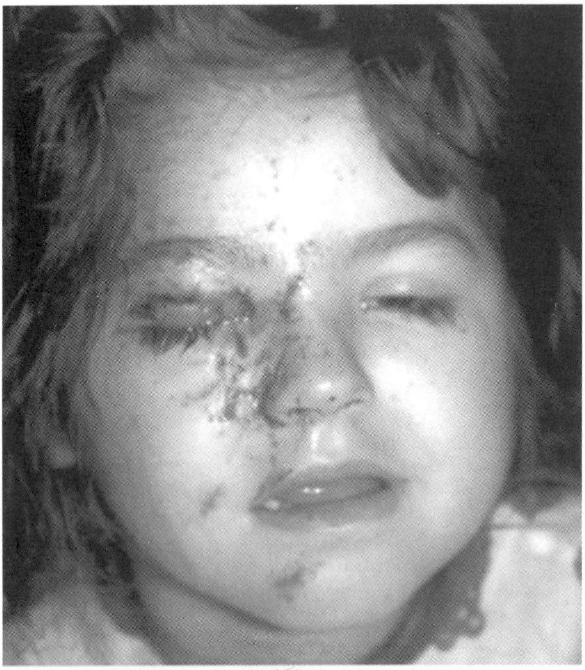

(A)

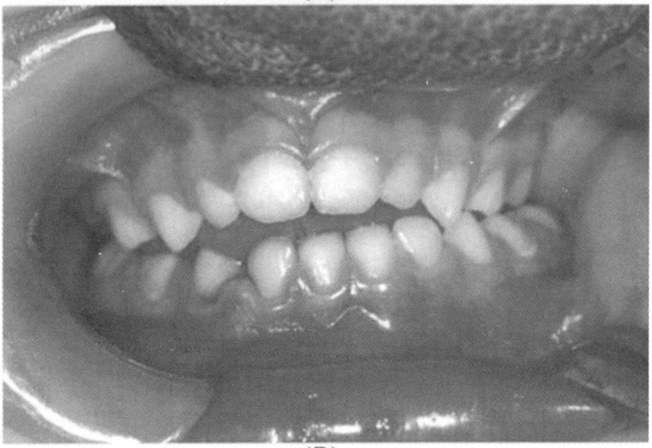

(B)

Figure 6 A. A 5-year-old child involved in motor vehicle accident. B–D. Anterior open bite resulting from a symphysis and condyle fracture. E. Dental models used for restoring preinjury occulsion. F–H Splint used for reduction and stabilization. I, J. Elastics used for restoring occlusion.

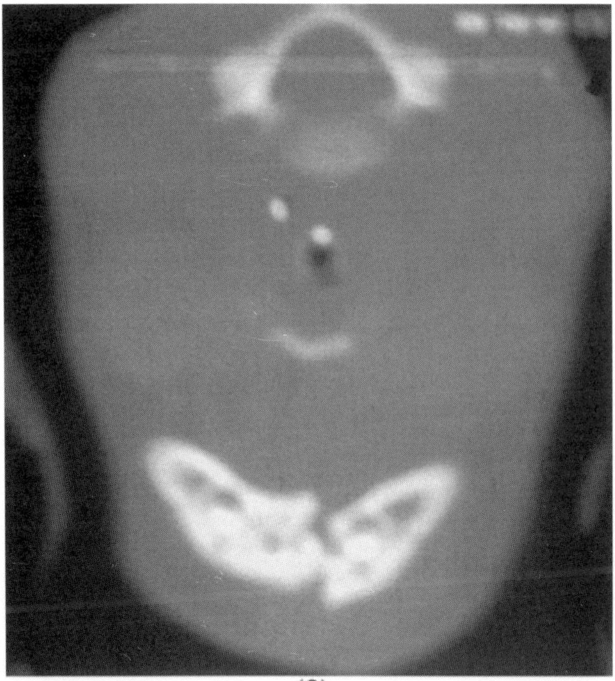

(C)

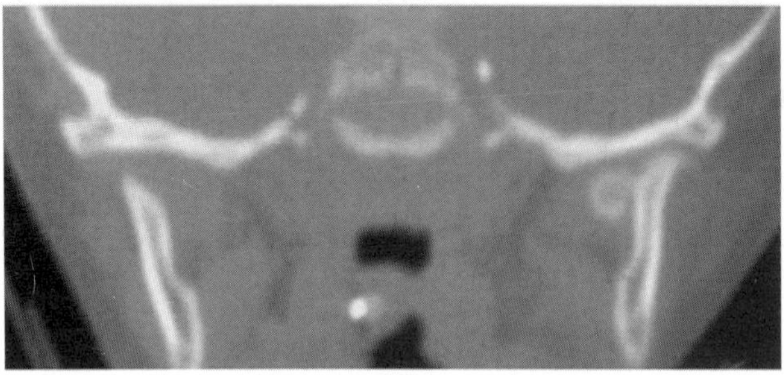

(D)

Figure 6 (*continued*)

internal fixation have been recommended. The goals of treating mandibular fractures that are complicated by an infection include resolution of the infection and achievement of bony union. Any airway compromise is managed initially and the fracture is treated subsequently.

Rigid internal fixation can predictably be used for treatment of infected mandibular fractures (60). Fracture union and resolution can be

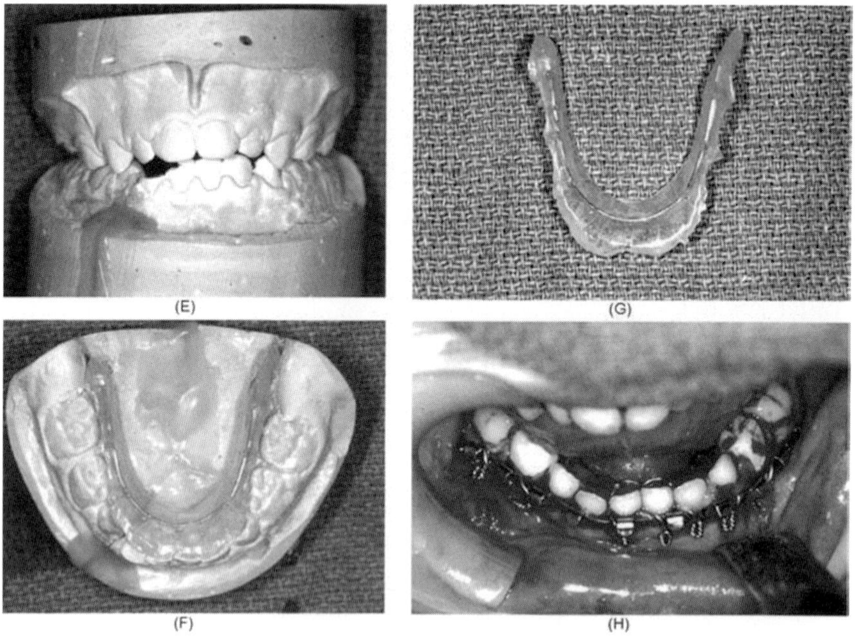

Figure 6 (*continued*)

attained with fixation. Even if the infection is prolonged, the fracture can heal as long as rigidity of the fracture is maintained. The plate can be removed after the bony union is achieved. Alternatively, if it is noted that plate or screw loosening has occurred and rigidity between the osseous segments is lacking, a nonunion is likely. The patient should be treated to regain rigidity and eliminate any loose hardware.

IX. TREATMENT PROTOCOL/ALGORITHM

The treatment of mandibular fractures has evolved with the experience gained and widespread acceptance of miniplates in mandibular fracture fixation. We retrospectively studied 32 male prisoners treated at our county facility who had a parasymphysis and contralateral mandible angle fracture. These patients were operated on by a single surgeon (AP) with an intraoral approach and fixated with 2.0 miniplates (Synthes Maxillofacial, Paoli, PA). Preoperatively, 11 patients had paresthesia on the side of the parasymphysis fracture, eight on the side of the angle fracture, six

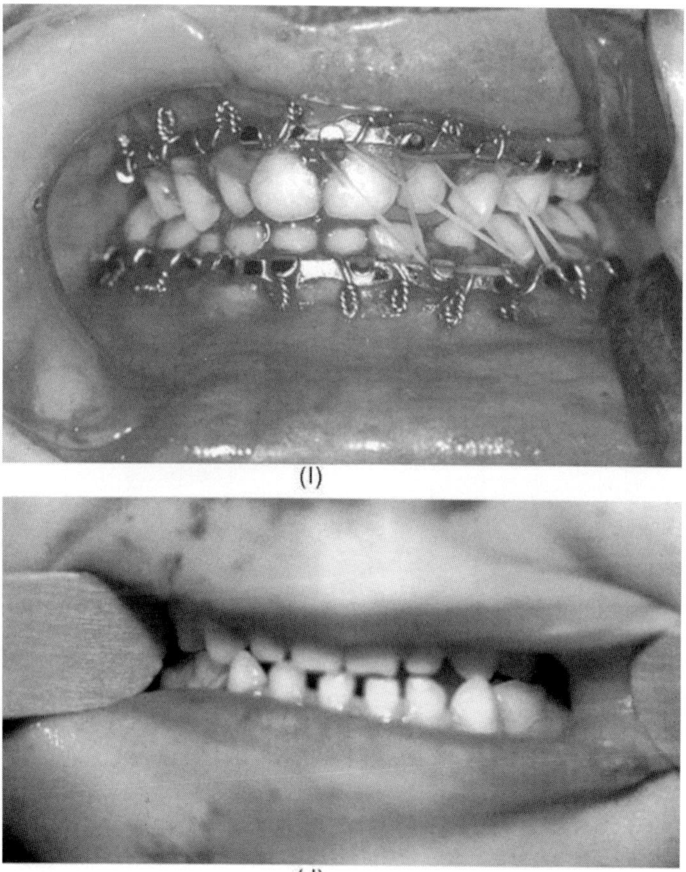

(I)

(J)

Figure 6 (*continued*)

bilaterally, and seven had no paresthesia. These patients were followed for 3 months postoperatively. If a third molar was present it was extracted prior to placement of the arch bars. The arch bars were then applied from first molar to first molar and the patient placed in maxillary mandibular fixation. The parasymphyseal fracture was exposed by a layered mucosal and muscular incision and access was obtained to the fracture, after careful dissection of the mental nerve which was identified in all cases. Two 2.0 miniplates, one at the inferior border of the mandible and the second above it, were placed. The inferior plate was fixated with bicortical screws and the superior plate stabilized with 4–6-mm monocortical screws. The superior plate was place above the mental foramen in 20 cases and there was

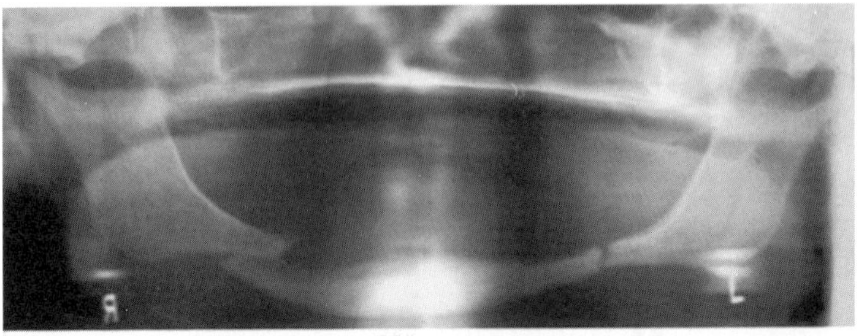

(A)

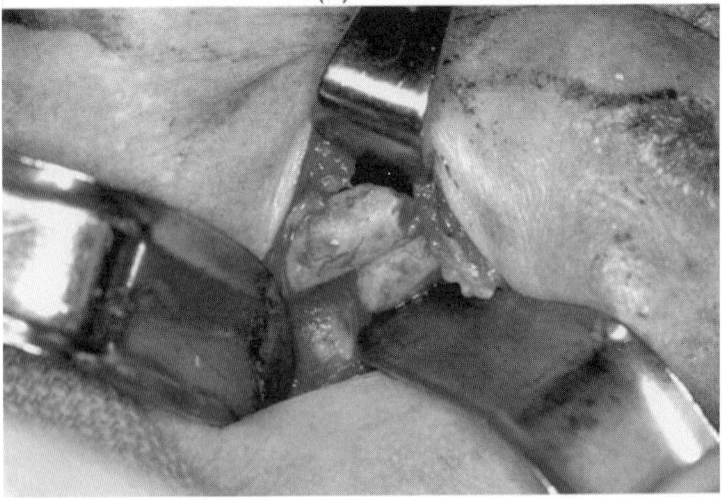

(B)

Figure 7 A. Bilateral fractures in an atrophic mandible. B, C. Extraoral open reduction with immediate bone grafting. D. Postoperative and preoperative radiographs.

adequate space inferior to the mental foramen in 12 cases. The wound was repaired with separate closure for the muscle and mucosa with resorbable suture (4-0 Vicryl). A chin compressive dressing was applied.

The angle was exposed by an incision along the external oblique ridge after which a single superior border four-hole 2.0 plate was adapted along the external oblique ridge and fixated to the proximal and distal fragments by means of two 6-mm screws on each side. The fracture was reduced under direct vision at the time of reduction and fixation of the parasymphyseal fracture. Closure is obtained with 4-0 resorbable suture (Vicryl). The MMF was removed prior to extubation though the arch bars were retained.

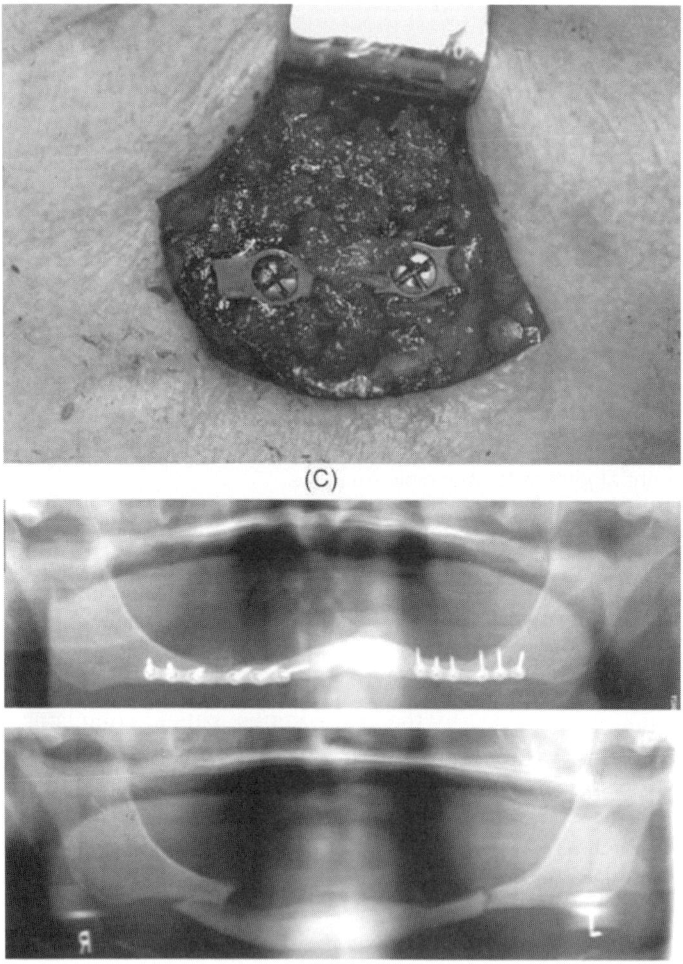

(C)

(D)

Figure 7 (*continued*)

All patients were discharged from the prison ward back to the prison on the first postoperative day. Eleven patients were placed in elastics at the 1-week appointment as they had premature occlusal contact. All 11 patients returned to satisfactory occlusion after 4 weeks of elastics, with eight requiring elastics for 2 weeks and the remaining three for 3–4 weeks. Two patients had plates exposed at 2 and 4 months. One of these was at the angle and the other at the parasymphysis. These were removed under local anesthesia in

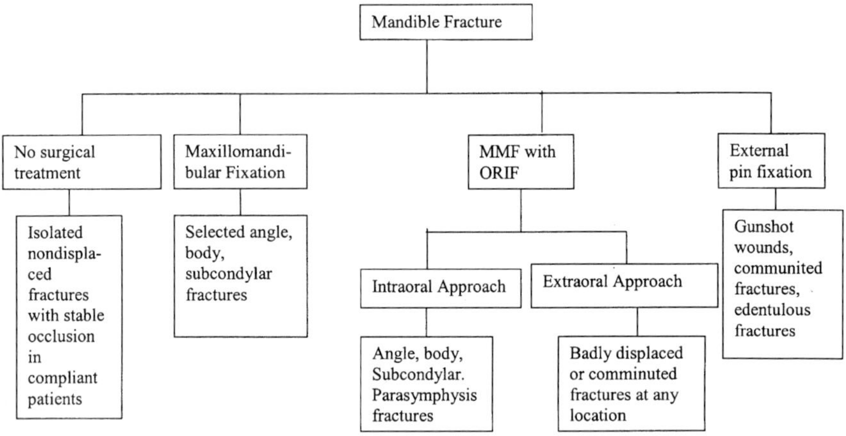

Figure 8 Treatment algorithm for mandible fractures.

the clinic. One patient developed infection at the parasymphysis and had to be returned to the operating room for debridement and an extraoral approach with placement of a locking reconstruction plate. Eight patients had residual paresthesia at 3 months. There were no malunions, nonunions, or malocclusion.

Treatment may be modified by the health status, patient compliance, patient tolerance for jaw wiring, other injuries, patient desires, and surgeon preference. Intraoral open reductions are performed in most cases except some comminuted fractures, infected fractures, or those complicated by concurrent pathology such as a tumor or cyst. Figure 8 is a flow chart for management of mandibular fracture.

X. COMPLICATIONS

A. Malocclusion and Malunion

Improper alignment of the fracture fragments results in facial asymmetry and malocclusion. Malunions occur in 0–4.2% of fractures (61). Malunions result from improper reduction, insufficient immobilization, poor patient compliance, and the improper use of rigid internal fixation (62). Nonrigid fixation techniques, such as maxillomandibular fixation or the use of miniplates, have resulted in a lower incidence of malunion because these are semiflexible systems that allow bony segments to be manipulated after fixation. Thaller found the least complications with immobilization and miniplates when compared with other treatment modalities (63).

Comprehensive management of malocclusion and malunion requires a full orthognathic workup. Standard osteotomies are performed at a different site from the malunion for restoration of preinjury occlusion. In general, treatment involves osteotomies at the healed fracture sites if they are within the dental arch, whereas fractures proximal to the dental arch are treated with ramus procedures. Bone grafting may be necessary (62).

B. Infection

Infection, the most common complication of mandibular fractures, is reported in 0.4–32% of all cases (61). Infections involving rigid fixation of mandibular fractures may not necessitate plate removal (minor) or may be major and require plate removal (loose hardware). There are many causes of postoperative infections, including mobility of the segments across the fracture site or loosening of screws securing the plate. Poor plate adaptation, inadequate cooling during drilling, or placing the screw in the fracture line itself can lead to increased chance of infection developing. Leaving a tooth in the line of fracture can also lead to an increased incidence of complications. Treatment of the infection requires antibiotics and determination of the stability of the fracture. The fracture site can heal and develop union in the face of infection as long as there is rigidity across the fracture site.

C. Delayed Union and Nonunion

Delayed union is failure of fracture union by 2 months. Infection, mobility, systemic disease, advanced age, and mandibular atrophy are contributing factors (61). Delayed union by definition means that the fracture will eventually heal without further surgery. Rigid internal fixation carries a lower incidence of delayed union compared to nonrigid fixation: 0–2.8% versus 1–4.4% (61).

Nonunion is the failure of a fracture to unite owing to arrested healing and requiring additional treatment to achieve fracture union. Mobility is the major cause of nonunion (62). More than 33% of nonunions involve infection (61). Large bony gaps, traumatized devitalized tissue, older age, intervening soft tissue, and systemic disease all can contribute to nonunion.

Mobility at the fracture site is manifested in nonunions. Debridement of the fracture fragments, bone grafting, usually from the iliac crest, and rigid fixation with internal or external fixation usually achieves fracture union (62).

D. Nerve Injury

Sensory nerve injury, particularly of the inferior alveolar and mental nerves, commonly occurs with mandibular fractures (63). In 11–59% of displaced mandibular fractures there is sensory nerve injury at diagnosis (64,65). Most injuries are neuropraxias secondary to stretching or compression and resolve spontaneously. Causes of inferior alveolar or mental nerve injury are displaced fractures, delay in treatment, and improper use of drill or screws. Closed reduction is associated with lower incidence of nerve dysfunction (62).

Facial nerve dysfunction infrequently results from mandibular trauma. Damage to the facial nerve in temporal bone fractures can lead to paralysis. Retrograde edema distal to the geniculate ganglion can cause temporary facial nerve loss after condylar fractures. Condylar dislocations can cause facial nerve injury distal to the stylomastoid foramen (62).

Injury to the facial nerve branches usually takes place iatrogenically during surgical treatment, though lateral displacement of the condyle can cause facial nerve injury (65). The marginal mandibular branch is the one usually injured. The surgical anatomy of this branch has been well described by Dingman and Grabb (67), and meticulous dissection under the platysma in the region of the facial artery with identification of the branches of the marginal mandibular can prevent injury to this nerve (66). The design of the preauricular incision in the approach to the condyle can be accomplished by observing the landmark work of Al-Kayat and Bramley (68).

REFERENCES

1. Sorel B. Open versus closed reduction of mandible fractures. Oral Maxillofac Clin 1998; 10:541.
2. Gunning TB. The treatment of fractures of the lower jaw by international splints. NY Med J 1866; 3:433.
3. Spiessl B. Internal fixation of the Mandible: A Manual of AO/ASIF Principles. Berlin: Springer-Verlag, 1989:3.
4. Michelet FX, Deymes J, Dessus B. Osteosynthesis with miniaturized screwed plates in maxillofacial surgery. J Maxillofac Surg 1973; 1:79–84.
5. Haskell R. Applied surgical anatomy. In: Williams JL, Rowe and Williams' Maxillofacial Injuries. New York: Churchill Livingstone, 1994:1–37.
6. Haug RH, Prather J, Indresano AT. An epidemiologic survey of facial fractures and concomitant injuries. J Oral Maxillofac Surg 1990; 48:926–932.
7. Haug RH, Wible RT, Likavec MJ, Coforti PJ. Cervical spine fractures and maxillofacial trauma. J Oral Maxillofac Surg 1991; 48:725–729.
8. Haug RH, Savage JD, Likavec MJ, Conforti PJ. A review of 100 closed head injuries associated with facial fractures. J Oral Maxillofac Surg 1992; 50: 218–222.
9. Punjabi AP, Plaisier BR, Haug RH, Malangoni MA. Diagnosis and management of blunt carotid artery injury in oral and maxillofacial surgery. J Oral Maxillofac Surg 1997; 55(12):1388–1395.

10. Plaisier BR, Punjabi AP, Super DM, Haug RH. The relationship between facial fractures and death from neurologic injury. J Oral Maxillofac Surg 2000; 58(7):708–712.
11. Ellis E, Moos KF, el-Attar A. Ten years of mandibular fractures: an analysis of 2,137 cases. Oral Surg 1985; 59:120–129.
12. Fischer K, Zhang F, Angel MF, Lineaweaver WC. Injuries associated with mandibular fractures sustained in motor vehicle collisions. Plast Reconstr Surg 2001; 108(2):328–331.
13. Chayara GA, Meador LR, Laskin DM. Comparison of panoramic and standard radiographs for the diagnosis of mandibular fractures. J Oral Maxillofac Surg 1986; 44:677–682.
14. Markowitz BL, Sinow JD, Kawamoto HK, et al. Prospective comparison of axial computed tomography and standard and panoramic radiographs in the diagnosis of mandibular fractures. Ann Plast Surg 1999; 42:163–168.
15. Wilson IF, Lokeh A, Benjamin CI, Hilger PA, Hamlar DD, et al. Prospective comparison of panoramic tomography (zonography) and helical computed tomography in the diagnosis and operative management of mandibular fractures. Plast Reconstr Surg 2001; 107:1369–1375.
16. Juniper RP, Awty MD. The immobilization period for fractures of the mandibular body. J Oral Surg 1973; 36:157.
17. Armaratunga NA de S. The relation of age to the immobilization period required for healing of mandibular fractures. J Oral Maxillofac Surg 1987; 45:111.
18. Ellis E. The effects of mandibular immobilization on the masticatory system: a review. Clin Plast Surg 1989; 16:133–146.
19. Geiser M, Trueta J. Muscle action, bone rarefaction and bone formation: an experimental study. J Bone Joint Surg 1958; 40B:282–311.
20. Labotte A. Le Traitment des Fractures. Paris: Masson, 1907.
21. Adams WM. Internal wiring of facial fractures. Surgery 1942; 12:523.
22. Muller M, Allgower M, Willenegger H. Technique of Internal Fixation of Fractures. Berlin: Springer-Verlag, 1965.
23. Luhr H. Operative behandlung suerfahren be: frakturen des zahnlosen unter kiefers unter besonderer berucksichtigung der kompressions osteosynthese. Chir Plast Recons 1970; 7:84.
24. Spiessl B. Rigid internal fixation of fractures of the lower jaw. In: Chapchal G, ed. Reconstructive Surgery and Traumatology. Basel: Karger, 1972.
25. Potter J, Ellis E. Treatment of mandibular angle fractures with a malleable non-compression miniplate. J Oral Maxillofac Surg 1999; 57:288–292.
26. Kim YK, Nam KW. Treatment of mandible fractures using low-profile titanium miniplates: preliminary study. Plast Reconstr Surg 2001; 108:38–43.
27. Edwards TJ, David DJ. A comparative study of miniplates used in the treatment of mandibullar fractures. Plast Reconstr Surg 1996; 97(6):1150–1157.
28. Iizuka T, Lindqvist C. Rigid internal fixation of fractures in the angular region of the mandible: an analysis of factors contributing to different complications. Plast Reconstr Surg 1993; 91:265–271.

29. Raveh J, Vuillemin T, Ladrach K, et al. Plate osteosynthesis of 367 mandibular fractures. J Craniomaxillofac Surg 1987; 15:244–253.
30. Herford AS, Ellis E. Use of a locking reconstruction plate/screw system for mandibular surgery. J Oral Maxillofac Surg 1998; 56(11):1261–1265.
31. Soderholm A-L, Lindqvist C, Skutnabb K, et al. Bridging of mandibular defects with two different reconstruction systems: an experimental study. J Oral Maxillofac Surg 1991; 49:1098.
32. Niederdellman H, Shetty V. Solitary lag screw osteosynthesis in the treatment of fractures of the angle of the mandible: a retrospective study. Plast Reconstr Surg 1987; 80(1):68–74.
33. Forrest CR. Application of minimal-access techniques in lag screw fixation of fractures of the anterior mandible. Plast Reconstr Surg 1999; 104:2127–2134.
34. Bos RRM, Boering G, Rozema FR, et al. Resorbable poly (L-lactide) plates and screws for the fixation of zygomatic fractures. J Oral Maxillofac Surg 1987; 45:751.
35. Morris JH, Hipp BR. Biphasic pin fixation. In: Williams JL, ed. Rowe and Williams' Maxillofacial Injuries. New York: Churchill Livingstone, 1994:329–340.
36. Neal DC, Wagner W, Alpert B. Morbidity associated with teeth in the line of mandibular fractures. J Oral Surg 1978; 36:859.
37. Shetty V, Freymiller E. Teeth in the line of fracture: a review. J Oral Maxillofac Surg 1989; 47:1303.
38. Zallen RD, Curry JT. A study of antibiotic usage in compound mandibular fractures. J Oral Surg 1975; 33:431.
39. Champy M, Lodde JP, Schmitt R, et al. Mandibular osteosynthesis by miniature screwed bone plates via a buccal approach. J Oral Maxillofac Surg 1978; 6:14.
40. Fuselier JC, Ellis E, Dodson TB. Do mandibular third molars alter the risk of angle fractures? J Oral Maxillofac Surg 2002; 60(5):514–518.
41. Shubert W, Kobienia BJ, Pollock RA. Cross-sectional area of the mandible. J Oral Maxillofac Surg 1997; 55:689–692.
42. Becker R. Stable compression plate fixation of mandibular fractures. Br J Oral Surg 1974; 12:13–23.
43. Ewers R, Harle F. Experimental and clinical results of new advances in the treatment of facial trauma. Plast Reconstr Surg 1985; 75:25–31.
44. Ellis E III. Treatment methods for fractures of the mandibular angle. Int J Oral Maxillofac Surg 1999; 28(4):243–252.
45. Ellis E, Throckmorton G. Facial symmetry after closed and open treatment of fractures of the mandibular condylar process. J Oral Maxillofac Surg 2000; 58(7):719–728.
46. Lee C, Mueller RV, Lee K, Mathes SJ. Endoscopic subcondylar fracture repair: functional, aesthetic, and radiographic outcomes. Plast Reconstr Surg 1998; 102(5):1434–1443.
47. Walker RV. Discussion: Open reduction of condylar fractures of the mandible in conjunction with repair of discal injury: a Preliminary report. J Oral Maxillofac Surg 1988; 46:262.
48. Zide MF, Kent JN. Indications for open reduction of mandibular condyle fractures. J Oral Maxillofac Surg 1983; 41:89.

49. Mikkonen P, Lindqvist C, Pihakari A, et al: Osteotomy–osteosynthesis in displaced condylar fractures. Int J Oral Maxillofac Surg 1989; 18:267.
50. Klotch DW, Lundy LB. Condylar neck fractures of the mandible. Otolaryngol Clin North Am 1991; 24:181.
51. Widmark G, Bagenholm T, Kahnberg KE, et al: Open reduction of subcondylar fractures. Int J Oral Maxillofac Surg 1996; 25:107.
52. Ellis E, Throckmorton G, Palmieri C. Open treatment of condylar process fractures: assessment of adequacy of repositioning and maintenance of stability. J Oral Maxillofac Surg 2000; 58:27–34.
53. Ellis E, Dean J. Rigid Fixation of mandibular condyle fractures. Oral Surg Oral Pathol 1993; 76:6.
54. Kaban LB, Mulliken MD, Murray JE. Facial fractures in children: an analysis of 122 fractures in 109 patients. Plast Reconstr Surg 1977; 59:15.
55. Dahlstrom L, Kahnberg KE, Lindahl. 15 years follow-up on condylar fractures. Int J Oral Maxillofac Surg 1989; 18(1):18–23.
56. Boyne PJ. Osseous repair and mandibular growth after subcondylar fractures. J Oral Surg 1967; 25(4):300–309.
57. Bradley JC. Age changes in the vascular supply of the mandible. Br Dent J 1972; 132(4):142–144.
58. Bruce RA, Ellis E III. The second Chalmers J Lyons Academy study of fractures of the edentulous mandible. J Oral Maxillofac Surg 1993; 51(8):904–911.
59. Boyne PJ, Upham C. The treatment of long standing bilateral fractures non- and mal-union in atrophic edentulous mandibles. Int J Oral Surg 1974; 3: 213–217.
60. Koury M, Ellis E. Rigid internal fixation for treatment of infected mandibular fractures. J Oral Maxillofac Surg 1992; 50:434–443.
61. Koury M. Complications of mandibular fractures. In: Kaban LB, Pogrell AH, Perrot D, eds. Complications in Oral and Maxillofacial Surgery. Philadelphia: WB. Saunders, 1997:121–146.
62. Punjabi AP, Thaller SR. Late complications of mandibular fractures. Oper Tech Plast Reconstr Surg 1998; 5:266–274.
63. Thaller SR. Management of mandibular fractures. Arch Otolaryngol Head Neck Surg 1994; 120:44.
64. Izuka T, Lindquist C. Sensory disturbances associated with rigid internal fixation of mandibular fractures. J Oral Maxillofac Surg 1991; 49:1264.
65. Marchena JM, Padwa BL, Kaban LB. Sensory abnormalities associated with mandibular fractures: incidence and natural history. J Oral Maxillofac Surg 1998; 56:822–825.
66. Brusati R, Paini P. Facial nerve injury secondary to lateral displacement of the mandibular ramus. Plast Reconstr Surg 1978; 62(5):728–733.
67. Dingman RO, Grabb WC. Surgical anatomy of the mandibular ramus of the facial nerve based on the dissection of 100 facial halves. Plast Reconstr Surg 1962; 29:266.
68. Al-Kayat A, Bramley PA. A modified pre-auricular approach to the temporomandibular joint and malar arch. Br J Oral Maxillofac Surg 1979.

17

Diagnosis and Management of Facial Fractures in Children

Corinna E. Zimmermann, Maria J. Troulis, and Leonard B. Kaban
Massachusetts General Hospital, Boston, Massachusetts, U.S.A.

I. GENERAL CONSIDERATIONS

A. Introduction

The incidence and etiology of craniomaxillofacial (CMF) trauma vary from one country to another and within regions of the same country. They are influenced by social, cultural, and environmental factors. The most common etiology worldwide in the nonpediatric population is motor vehicle accidents (MVA) followed by assaults, falls, and sports-related injuries. In children, the etiology varies with age-related activities and exposures.

In Western industrialized countries, considerable efforts have focused on the prevention of MVA-related injuries including legislation (speed limits, alcohol restriction, seat belt and helmet use), road construction measures, and vehicle safety modifications (safety glass, air bags). These measures have resulted in a significant decrease of incidence and mortality from MVA in some countries (1,2).

Interpersonal violence (3,4), in some countries the most common cause of adult maxillofacial (MF) trauma (5), is often associated with alcohol consumption, unemployment, and social problems. In addition, an increase in leisure time, sports facilities, and knowledge about exercise as an important health-promoting measure have contributed to an increase in sports-related trauma (6–12). Sports-related trauma is also a common cause of MF injuries in children and adolescents.

History and physical examination remain the most important diagnostic modalities for the majority of CMF injuries. The role of plain radiographs has changed, particularly in the pediatric population, because they fail to provide adequate detail and resolution and because overlap of adjacent structures obscures fractures (13–15). Today, computed-tomographic (CT) scanning has become the standard of care for imaging pediatric MF trauma patients (16,17). CT is quick and efficient, and the radiation dose continues to decrease as the technology improves. These studies provide fine, unobstructed anatomical detail required for diagnosis in children.

Until the mid-1970s, closed reduction and immobilization with maxillomandibular fixation (MMF) was the standard of care for all types of pediatric fractures (18–21). Today, observation or closed reduction is used only for greenstick and nondisplaced fractures or for fractures in the very young (17,22,23). Rigid internal fixation techniques are increasingly applied for the treatment of displaced fractures in pediatric patients because of the ability to accurately reduce the fractures and to eliminate the need for MMF (17).

B. Unique Features of the Pediatric Patient

The many differences between pediatric and adult patients have an important impact on the patterns of pediatric trauma in general and MF trauma in particular. Children have a higher surface-to-body volume ratio, higher metabolic rate, oxygen demand, and cardiac output, lower total blood volume, and smaller stroke volume than adults. Therefore, they are more at risk for hypothermia, hypotension, and hypoxia after blood loss and even mild airway swelling or mechanical obstruction. Airway maintenance, control of hemorrhage, and early resuscitation are therefore even more critical in children than in adults.

Compared to adults, children have a greater cranial-to-body mass ratio. The cranial-to-facial ratio is estimated to be 8:1 in infancy compared to 2.5:1 in adulthood (24). The relative "protection" of the face by the skull explains, at least in part, the lower incidence of midface and mandibular fractures in children, as well as the greater invidence of cranial injury in the younger age groups (22,25). It also explains why, with increasing age, the incidence of midface and mandibular fractures increases whereas the incidence of cranial injuries decreases (22).

In pediatric patients, bone is more elastic, suture lines are more flexible, and there is a thicker adipose layer covering the skeleton than in adults. These factors also contribute to the lower frequency of facial fractures and the greater number of greenstick and nondisplaced fractures in children. The lack of sinus pneumatization and presence of tooth buds within the jaw contribute to stability and lead to a lower incidence of midface fractures and minimally rather than severely displaced fractures (15,17,26).

The issue of postinjury growth disturbances, particularly after severe nasal-septal and condylar injuries, is an important consideration in the pediatric population. Adverse growth alterations over time after injury should be clearly understood when planning treatment. On the other hand, growth can also improve the result as with compensatory condylar growth and spontaneous occlusal adjustment after injury and treatment as deciduous teeth are shed and permanent teeth erupt.

The history is sometimes difficult to obtain from a child and the accompanying caretakers may not have witnessed the accident. Moreover, thorough clinical examination may be impossible in the uncooperative young trauma patient. In addition, because of the child's anatomy, plain radiographs are less helpful than in adults. This is particularly true for the midface region owing to poorly developed sinuses and the maxilla filled with multiple tooth buds. For these reasons, pediatric facial fractures are sometimes not suspected or are overlooked. The advent of CT scants has greatly increased diagnostic accuracy in pediatric MF trauma victims (27).

C. Etiology of Facial Fractures in Children

The etiology of facial fractures in children is age-dependent and the prevalence differs from adults. The major causes include falls, sporting accidents, and MVA (17,23,28–36). The actual percentages of the various etiologies reported depend on the age groups examined and on the types of fractures included (e.g., children below age 18 vs. children below 6, inclusion or exclusion of dentoalveolar and/ or nasal fractures). While low-velocity injuries (e.g., after falls) are common in the younger age groups, the number of high-velocity injuries (e.g., in MVA, sports-related trauma) increases with age. However, high-velocity MF injuries in children may be underreported because associated craniocerebral injuries result in death. Associated facial injuries are therefore not included in studies of pediatric MF trauma.

Falls are the most common cause of facial fractures in infants and preschool children (up to age 6) (23,29,32,37–41). The younger the child, the more likely the accident occurred in the home environment. With increasing age and outdoor exposure, falls tend to occur outside the protected area of the home and parental supervision (31). With increasing age and improving motor skills, sporting injuries become more common. The majority of facial fractures related to sports (rollerblading, skateboarding, soccer, skiing, snowboarding, bicycling, horseback riding, trampoline jumping, gymnastics) occur in children 10–14 years of age (40,42–47). Interpersonal violence is a rare cause of facial fractures in children and occurs mostly in adolescents (17,23,36,38,48).

Child abuse is an often underestimated cause of MF trauma. The head, neck, face, and mouth regions are affected in 50–75% of child abuse cases (49,50,51). Head injury from abuse is a significant cause (40–70%) of disability and death in children and facial fractures occur in 2.3% of cases of child abuse (52). Children of all ages are subject to abuse, but the groups most prone are newborns, infants, and preschool children (52–54), with a preponderance for boys. Parents or caretakers are the perpetrators in the vast majority of cases (90%), particularly in the younger age groups (52). Repeated injuries, multiple injury sites with inadequate history, or delayed presentation should raise suspicion for possible abuse. In most states, the law requires that emergency room personnel, surgeons, and other caregivers report the suspicion of child abuse to the authorities.

In the general population, motor vehicle accidents account for about 42,000 deaths in the United States annually (55) and for the vast majority of severe trauma cases with associated facial injuries (56). In children, MVA are the leading cause of death after the perinatal period (55). The incidence of facial fractures acquired in MVA is directly related to age (57). Apart from being a passenger in a motor vehicle, a child can be involved in an MVA as a pedestrian or bicyclist. In some studies, MVAs are the major cause of pediatric facial fractures in children 6 years and older (17,23,29,33,58–62).

D. Epidemiology of Pediatric Facial Fractures

1. Incidence

The incidence of facial fractures in children has decreased during the past three decades, particularly in victims below the age of 10 years (6). The incidence is much lower than in adults with only approximately 15% of all facial fractures occurring in the pediatric population. Most authors report that the incidence of facial fractures increases as children begin school (31,28,31) and again during puberty and adolescence owing to increased physical activity and sports participation (34,35,40,63–67). Facial fractures rarely occur below age 5 years (0.6–1.4%) (23,31–33,35,63,64,68–72). The peak incidence occurs during summer months (except for skiing injuries), when outdoor activity is greatest (9,17,23,40).

2. *Gender*

Worldwide and in all age groups, boys have a higher incidence of facial fractures than girls. The male preponderance, which has changed little during the past 40 years (6), ranges from 1.1:1 to 8.5:1 (9,17,22,23,27–34,38,40,41) (58,61–63,66–68,73) and has been attributed to a higher level of physical activity and more dangerous activities among boys (17,23,34,46,79). In the younger age groups, the etiology is similar in both sexes.

3. *Site and Pattern*

Fracture sites differ by age, because of the interrelationship between the etiology and force of the injury and the unique anatomical features of the child's stage of development. Whereas in infants (below age 2), the forehead is most prone to injury, the chin/lip region is more often involved in older children (39). Children below age 3 are more likely to sustain isolated fractures (17) that are greenstick or nondisplaced and are caused by low-impact/low-velocity forces.

When dentoalveolar and nasal fractures, both very common and often treated in the outpatient setting, are excluded, the mandible is the most commonly affected bone reported in hospitalized children (17,23,29,33), (35,38,48,56,61,65,66,68,80,81). The incidence of mandibular fractures increases with age (17,35,71,82).

The distribution of mandibular fracture sites varies with age and stage of dental development. In general, the condyle is the most frequently fractured mandibular site in children (23,29,31,34,35,38,71,73,82,83) and is more often affected than in adults (50% vs. 30%) (29). In about 20% of pediatric patients who sustain a condylar fracture, it occurs bilaterally (74,84,85). Apart from child-specific etiology (falls with impact forces to the chin being common), the child-specific anatomy of the condyle (short and highly vascularized with a high percentage of trabecular bone) is the underlying reason for the high incidence of these fractures. In adults, most condylar fractures are located in the subcondylar region followed by the neck and intracapsular region. In children below 6 years of age, condylar fractures are more often intra- rather than extracapsular in location. In children age 6 and above, most condylar fractures occur in the neck region (74).

Fractures in the condylar region are followed in number by symphysis, angle, and body fractures (23,31,35). The symphysis and parasymphysis regions of the mandible are more often affected than in adults, while body fractures are less common than in adults (81).

Midface fractures are usually the result of greater impact and/or high-velocity forces (e.g., MVA), often resulting in comminution and concomitant injuries or even death. Their incidence in children is low (20,22,29,31,35,36,70,72). Maxillary fractures at the Le Fort levels are the least common midface fractures and almost never seen before age 2. Children below age 6 sustain mostly alveolar fractures, acquired in low-impact falls and sports (40). The incidence of midface fractures increases after age 5 with increasing sinus development (17,35,40). The highest incidence of midface fractures within the pediatric population is seen in the older age group (i.e., age 13–15) (40).

Fractures of the orbital walls make up about 20% of pediatric facial fractures (17,22,29,73,75). They are probably due to transmission of forces from the bony orbital ring to the thin orbital walls (86). Orbital roof fractures occur in young children, in whom the frontal sinus is still underdeveloped, and are often associated with neurocranial injuries, whereas orbital floor fractures are more common in older children (17,87,88), in whom the maxillary sinus has expanded over the midpupillary line. The age at which the probability of an orbital floor fracture exceeds the probability of an orbital roof fracture is about 7 years (88).

Cranial vault fractures in children are rare. The frontal bone is most commonly involved (17), and fractures are generally more frequent in children below age 6, because of the relatively protruded position of the frontal bone (22). Frontal sinus involvement, however, is not seen below age 6 (89), as the sinus is very small (less than cherry-size) and has not even reached the orbital roof yet (90). The increasing incidence of frontal sinus fractures in puberty (89), mostly from MVA, parallels the extent of frontal sinus pneumatization. Multiple facial fractures and significant central nervous system injury are often associated with frontal skull and frontal sinus factures (89). Frontal skull fractures are sometimes grouped together with nasal factures as frontonasoethmoidal fractures (65), so their absolute incidence is not clear.

The nasal bones are the most fragile of the facial bones (91) and, as a protruding area, the nose is most likely to sustain injury in adults as well as in children (3,28–30,92). Yet, in many studies from large trauma centers, nasal fractures are not among the most common facial fractures in children (22,23,33,48), either because a great number of patients are seen and treated in an office setting, or because nasal fractures are grouped among midface fractures (17,30,36,38). When evaluated separately, nasal fractures are reported to comprise about 50% of all pediatirc facial fractures (28,29).

4. *Associated Injuries*

Facial fractures occur commonly in multiple-trauma patients and, conversely, patients who present with facial fractures often have other associated injuries (93). In children, concomitant injuries occur in 25–75% of facial fracture patients (17,22,25,27,40,41,60,69,73,75,77). Associated injuries include closed head trauma, neurocranial injuries, temporal bone fractures, extremity fractures, abdominal, thoracic, and spine injuries, as well as dental injuries, and soft-tissue lacerations.

The probability of associated injuries is proportional to the force of impact. Patients who are victims of MVA are at increased risk for associated injuries accompanying facial trauma (9,40). Patients with mandibular fractures have a higher incidence of associated injuries than those with nasal or orbital fractures, because the forces involved to create the fracture are higher (9,29,94). Children who sustain midface fractures are also likely to sustain associated injuries (17,27,40,60,73,75), particularly skull, brain, and cervical spine injuries (22,26,61,95). Finally, the more comminuted a facial fracture, the more the likelihood of an associated systemic injury (17).

E. Prevention

Preventive measures may reduce the number of accidents and/or minimize the severity of injuries. Legislation reducing speed limits, lowering the blood alcohol level for legal intoxication to 0.08 mg%, requiring shoulder and seat restraints and helmet use, as well as road construction measures and vehicle safety modifications (safety glass, padded dashboards, stronger frames, collapsible steering columns, air bags) have resulted in a decrease in the incidence of MVA-related injuries (1,2,96,97).

The use of seat belts can significantly reduce the number of deaths and the number and severity of CMF injuries in adults and children (96,98–102). The use of restraints has risen significantly owing to the passage of legislation during the past 20 years. However, compliance varies in different countries and is generally not high (27,57,68,103,104), particularly in the population most at risk, i.e., young males. Approximately 50–70% of all children sustaining injuries in MVA and up to 70% of children sustaining facial fractures are unrestrained (57,96,100–102).

It should be remembered that conventional seat belts may not offer proper protection for the pediatric passenger, because the anterior superior iliac spine is incompletely developed and the center of gravity is located higher than in adults. Children have greater body mass above the waist. Thus, conventional seat belts can cause abdominal and thoracic injury in a child (105). When age-appropriate restraints are used, protection is improved and specific restraint-related injury patterns do not occur (96).

Sports-related accidents are a common cause of facial fractures in children. Preventive measures in sports have not been emphasized nor have they been employed to the same degree as for MVA. For example, in several reported series, very few children who sustained bicycle-related head injuries, including facial fractures, wore protective helmets at the time of injury (31,46,79). Currently available helmets reduce the risk of head and midface injury but their design may not provide maximum protection for mandibular fractures (80,106).

The incidence and severity of sports-related injuries are inversely related to skill level and age (43,107). It is therefore necessary to emphasize preventive measures at an early age to develop appropriate habits (e.g., related to wearing a helmet) in the participants. It is also important to focus on the education of supervising adults, i.e., coaches, administrators, teachers, and parents.

F. Management of Facial Fractures in Children

Based on the anatomical and developmental considerations noted above, some basic principles in the management of pediatric facial fractures can be formulated. Care has to be taken to maintain an adequate airway, fluid and electrolyte balance, and nutritional intake throughout the treatment period. From a psychological standpoint, children must be treated appropriate to their developmental age. They will then be as cooperative as adult patients (108).

The overall treatment goal is to re-establish the preinjury skeletal and dentoalveolar anatomy and function through accurate occlusion-based reduction and fixation (109,110). In children, anatomical reduction must be accomplished earlier than in adults (87,111) because of the rapid rate at which bony union occurs (15,36). Immobilization by MMF, when required, is for a short period of time (2 weeks vs. 4–6 weeks) when compared to adults (31,63,75). Earlier mobilization is possible and recommended in children to make use of the remodeling capabilities and to avoid functional impairment after prolonged immobilization (31,63).

Immobilization, usually achieved via elastic dental "guidance," may be more difficult than in adults, because fewer teeth may be available, roots of deciduous teeth may be resorbed, enamel of deciduous teeth exhibits no retentive surfaces for etching techniques, and the crowns of deciduous teeth and partly erupted permanent teeth may be unfavorably shaped for the fixation of interdental wires and arch bars (112).

Observation, combined with a liquid to soft diet and analgesics as needed may be sufficient for greenstick and nondisplaced fractures. Independent of age (17), displaced fractures often require closed or open reduction and fixation. The likelihood of surgical intervention increases with the child's age (22). Intraosseous tooth buds and (erupting) teeth in the line of fracture should not be additionally traumatized during treatment. Fixation can be achieved with intermaxillary immobilization or internal fixation or a combination of these, depending on the type of fracture and the patient's stage of development. The mandible can often be reduced and immobilized with a Gunning splint secured with circumandibular wires or sutures.

G. Rigid Internal Fixation in Children

The introduction of rigid internal fixation into CMF surgery has revolutionized the treatment of facial fractures by allowing more accurate reduction and fixation of bone fragments and by minimizing the need for long-term MMF. Today, open reduction and rigid internal fixation (ORIF) has become the standard of care in the treatment of most CMF trauma cases even in children. With the use of plates and screws, stable three-dimensional reconstruction of the anatomy can be achieved. This promotes primary bone healing, shortens treatment time, allows for early release of intermaxillary fixation, favorable in the case of condylar fractures, and improves postoperative respiratory care, nutritional intake, and oral hygiene measures (17). Compared to intraosseous wire fixation, complication rates with respect to delayed union, pseudarthrosis, and malocclusion may be lower with rigid internal fixation (113).

The use of ORIF in children has been controversial, because of a number of possible disadvantages or potential complications. Disadvantages include the formation of artifacts on standard radiographs, CT scans, or magnetic resonance images. In addition, treatment by ORIF is more costly than closed reduction. Complications include the more general risks of palpability or visibility of plates through the child's thin skin, pain, and early or late infection. Child-specific risks include trauma to tooth buds or erupting teeth, the migration of plates or screws with risk of dural tear, cerebrospinal fluid leak, meningitis or even brain injury after translocation through the inner cortex of the skull, and, finally, growth disturbances (114–116).

Animal experiments on craniofacial development after rigid fixation and clinical studies in humans have yielded equivocal results. While adverse effects on growth were demonstrated in dogs (117) and rabbits (118–120), these may be overcome by compensatory regional bone growth (118,120,121). Moreover, it has been difficult to determine whether the initial trauma, the surgical procedures for reduction and fixation, or hardware removal have had the greatest adverse effect on growth (122,123). In humans, the effects of plates on facial growth are unknown and adverse effects have not been reported (111,124). However, some surgeons recommend the removal of plates and screws as early as 2–3 months after placement (71,115). Reasorbable plates and screws might offer an alternative for the growing skeleton in the future.

Cutaneous wound healing in children can be complicated by keloid formation. Therefore, large skin incisions should be avoided, unless facial lacerations already favor a particular trancutaneous approach.

II. SPECIFIC FRACTURE MANAGEMENT

A. Mandibular Fractures

A typical history in a young child is a fall, with a blow to the chin, causing a hematoma or skin laceration, dental injuries, and a symphysis/parasymphy-parasymphysis and unilateral or bilateral condylar fractures. Clinical signs are the same as in adults and may include displacement of the fragments, mobility, crepitus and hematoma, swelling, mucosal tears, limited mouth opening, malocclusion, pain, and sensory deficits in the distribution of the inferior alveolar nerve.

Panoramic, supplemented by posterior-anterior (PA) and lateral oblique, radiographic views usually confirm the diagnosis. CT scans are rarely needed for diagnosis of mandibular fractures but may help to determine three-dimensional displacement of the condyles.

The management of mandibular fractures in children has changed little over the years and differs from management in adults in that the stage of development of the skeleton and pediatric dentition must be considered (15,108). Isolated alveolar fractures of the mandible are treated by open or closed reduction and immobilization by splints and arch bars for 2–3 weeks. Although rarely necessary, long-term monomaxillary immobilization for up to 2 months to prevent malocclusion has been reported (66).

Greenstick and nondisplaced mandibular fractures without malocclusion are managed by close follow-up once or twice a week, a liquid to soft diet, avoidance of physical activities (e.g., sports), and analgesics.

Closed reduction and immobilization with either a mandibular splint alone or a splint with MMF is adequate for some displaced fractures, particularly in infants, when tooth buds within the mandible do not allow internal fixation with plates and screws (94). ORIF through an intraoral incision is possible in symphysis fractures as early as age 6, when the permanent incisors have erupted, and in parasymphysis fractures after age 9, when the buds of the canines have moved up from their position at the inferior border. Similarly, in body fractures, the inferior mandibular border can be plated, when the permanent premolar and molar tooth buds have migrated superiorly toward the alveolus (108).

In the case of condylar fractures, the great majority are treated with closed reduction and MMF for no more than 7–10 days. The immobilization period must be short to prevent ankylosis. Early mobilization also promotes remodeling of the condylar stump. There is some evidence that open reduction improves functional outcome (125). However, most authors advocate closed reduction. MMF is usually followed by a period of physical therapy consisting of mandibular opening exercises and guiding elastics. Recently reported endoscopic visualization, reduction, and fixation of condylar fractures may lead to more frequent use of open reduction. This is particularly advantageous in teenagers because it avoids MMF (126). Postoperative follow-up should be frequent to detect and treat early complications such as infection, malocclusion, malunion, or nonunion, which are fortunately rare in children. Follow-up should continue to monitor late complications such as damage to permanent teeth, which may occur in 50% of mandibular fractures (78), temporomandibular joint (TMJ) dysfunction (recurrent subluxation, noise and pain, limited condylar translation, deviation on opening, ankylosis), and growth disturbances (e.g., secondary midface deformity or mandibular hypoplasia or asymmetry). In contrast to condylar fractures, those of the mandibular body carry very little or no risk for growth abnormalities (78).

B. Midface Fractures

As in adults, history and physical examination are the primary diagnostic modalities in pediatric midfacial fractures, which tend to result from high-impact/high-velocity forces (e.g., abrupt deceleration in a MVA). Physical findings may include periorbital swelling and monocular or binocular hematoma, telecanthus, sensory abnormalities in the distribution of the infraorbital nerve (V_2), diplopia (due to edema or entrapment of intraorbital soft tissues with or without extraocular muscles, neuromuscular injury, hematoma formation, or globe displacement), painful limitation of mouth opening and pain upon forced occlusion, malocclusion (alveolar fractures or Le Fort midface injuries), facial asymmetry, and elongation of the middle third of the face. Mobility of the maxilla (Le Fort I level), at the infraorbital rim and nasofrontal suture (Le Fort II level) or at the frontozygomatic and nasofrontal sutures (Le Fort III level) may be palpable.

Plain radiographs are not useful in diagnosing pediatric midface injuries, because the region is obscured by lack of pneumatization of the sinuses and the presence of tooth buds in the maxilla. In addition, diagnosis of zygomatic arch fractures on a typical submental vertex view is impeded by the superimposition of the skull (13). Since fractures are easily overlooked on plain radiographs, CT imaging has become the standard of care in the diagnosis of midface fractures in children (27).

C. Zygomatic Complex Fractures

Zygomatic complex fractures are the most common midface fractures in children after nasal and alveolar maxillary fractures (36,40,124). The patient may report decreased jaw opening, blurred and/or double vision, and pain on eye movement (e.g., upward gaze) and maximal mouth opening or forced occlusion. Common physical findings are: cheek asymmetry, particularly when seen from below or behind, periorbital swelling and ecchymosis, hyposphagma, chemosis, enophthalmos, decreased ocular mobility, positive forced duction test, diplopia, paresthesia in the distribution of the infraorbital nerve (V_2), and limitations on mouth opening due to impingement on the coronoid process. Ophthalmological consultation should be obtained on initial presentation.

CT scans demonstrate separation at the frontozygomatic, zygomaticotemporal, and zygomaticosphenoidal sutures, the zygomatic buttress, infraorbital rim, orbital floor/roof of the maxillary sinus, lateral orbital wall, and fluid in the maxillary sinus.

Minimally and nondisplaced zygomatic fractures without functional deficits (diplopia, sensory deficits) may be treated by observation (17). Indications for ORIF include aesthetic and functional impairment such as facial asymmetry, enophthalmos $> 3\,\text{mm}$, anesthesia or paresthesia in the distribution of the infraorbital nerve (V_2), orbital floor defects, and entrapment of orbital soft tissues with or without limitations in eye movement (127,128). Surgical treatment is also indicated in comminuted fractures (129). ORIF with microplates should be performed as soon as the initial edema has resolved, i.e., after 3–5 days. Postponing of orbital repair may result in higher rates of posttraumatic enophthalmos and the need for additional orbital or muscle surgery (128).

As in adults, exposure of the lines of fracture can be achieved via the lateral eyebrow, or lateral upper eyelid incision (frontozygomatic suture line), the lower eyelid, infraciliary, or transconjuctival incision (infraorbital rim and orbital floor), and the transoral buccal sulcus approach (zygomatic buttress). Contrary to adults, one-point fixation at the frontozygomatic suture may suffice in children, because of shorter lever arm forces from the frontozygomatic suture to the infraorbital rim (94). If unstable, further reduction and fixation may be achieved via a transoral approach using a Carol-Girard screw at the zygomatic buttress. Plating at the zygomatic buttress may carry the risk of traumatizing maxillary tooth buds, particularly in children below age 6 (130). Therefore, a microplate at the infraorbital rim may be preferred to achieve two-point fixation. When soft tissue is entrapped at the orbital floor, or when sensory deficits suggest involvement of the infraorbital nerve, exploration of the infraorbital rim and orbital floor may be required.

Primary reconstruction of the orbital floor in isolated blowout fractures or zygomatic complex fractures is indicated when unretrievable bony fragments have disappeared into the maxillary sinus leaving a defect. Autologous calvarial bone grafts are preferred over alloplastic materials in children.

For zygomatic complex fractures as well as isolated zygomatic arch fractures, a Gillies temporal approach can be used to elevate the zygoma. Zygomatic arch fractures are usually stable without further fixation (36).

In the fortunately rare more complex cases of frontonasoethmoid or Le Fort III fractures, the zygomatic arch can be approached via a coronal incision behind the hairline, which simultaneously gives the opportunity for harvesting split cranial bone grafts.

D. Orbital Fractures

Clinical signs and symptoms of orbital wall fractures may include periorbital swelling, monocular hematoma, and hyposphagma, painful limited eye mobility, diplopia, and enophthalmos. Sensory abnormalities in the distribution of the infraorbital nerve may be missing. Indications for early open reduction via a transconjunctival (94), infraciliary (36), or infraorbital incision are identical to those for zygomatic complex fractures: enophthalmos > 3 mm, orbital floor defects, and entrapment of orbital soft tissues with or without limitations in globe mobility. The overall goal is to restore orbital volume and free incarcerated soft tissues. Primary orbital floor reconstruction with autogenous calvarial bone may be necessary in large orbital floor defects. Severely displaced orbital roof fractures may need an interdisciplinary neurosurgical (transcranial) approach (17).

E. Frontal Skull and Frontonasoethmoid Fractures

Clinical signs of frontal skull and frontonasoethmoid fractures may include swelling, hematoma, and symmetry of the frontonasal and periorbital region, mobility of the nose, epistaxis, and telecanthus.

Most patients require surgical treatment to reestablish sinus anatomy. A coronal approach behind the hairline offers wide exposure including the orbital rims, zygomatic arches, and nasal root for reduction and microplate fixation of the often comminuted fractures. When severely disrupted, the sinus mucosa should be ablated and the cavity obliterated. Alternatively, if possible, drainage via the natural ostium and nasofrontal duct should be established by means of a tracheal spiral catheter for several weeks to prevent mucocele formation (131). In posterior frontal sinus wall involvement, and interdisciplinary neurosurgical approach is necessary.

In frontonasoethmoid fractures the medial canthal ligament, usually still attached to a bony fragment at its insertion, needs to be repositioned and fixed with (132) or without (129) microplates or transnasal wire fixation to avoid telecanthus. Clavarial bone grafts and primary stenting of the nasolacrimal duct may be necessary in severely comminuted fractures.

F. Le Fort Fractures

Clinical signs of Le Fort fractures depend on the level of injury and may include mobility, malocclusion, and symptoms seen in zygomatic complex fractures.

Treatment of unstable or displaced low Le Fort fractures consists of intermaxillary fixation and suspension from the zygomatic arches or piriform aperture for 2–3 weeks (36,94), or stabilization with plates and screws in the older child without risk of damaging tooth germs or erupting teeth (17).

G. Nasal Fractures

Nasal fractures in children are easily missed, because of edema, missing crepitation of the resilient bones, and difficult examination of the young patient (e.g., intranasal examination with a spectrum to exclude septal deviation or hematoma). The diagnosis of a pediatric nasal fracture is made clinically and based on the history, which often includes a fall on the face. While a blow from the front may produce a fracture of both nasal bones with impaction, a lateral blow will cause displacement and deviation to the contralateral side. Standard x-rays (lateral nasal projection, Waters view) in children are of limited value (15).

In the case of a displaced fracture, treatment should be carried out within 7 days (36). Accurate anatomical reduction has to be achieved. However, unlike in adults, radical surgical reconstruction is contraindicated in the growing child (75). In most cases, anatomical realignment, hemostasis, and fixation is achieved under general anesthesia by closed reduction (17), bilateral intranasal packing or splinting for 3 days, and an external splint for 10–12 days. The use of bilateral nasal packing should be avoided in newborns, because they are obligatory nasal breathers. As facial swelling decreases, the external splint may have to be renewed to provide sufficient stabilization. In the rare case that requires open reduction, tissue injury must be minimal (133).

Septal hematoma constitutes a medical emergency, beeause it requires immediate drainage to prevent septal cartilage necrosis with subsequent saddle nose deformity and potential midface growth retardation.

H. Complications

Compared to adults, postoperative infection, malunion, or nonunion is rare in children owing to their greater osteogenic potential, higher healing rates, and the greater number of fractures that can be treated without an operation. These complications usually only occur in severely comminuted fractures (18,58,69,75).

Malocclusion is also less common than in adults (75). Minimal malocclusion may be self-limited and corrected as deciduous teeth shed and permanent teeth erupt (134). Malocclusion has been attributed to inadequate fixation times in alveolar fractures (66) and may be caused by growth alternation after condylar fracture (18,22).

Growth abnormalities, reported in 15% of condylar fractures (78), are more likely to occur in intracapsular crush injuries of the condyle, particularly below age 2.5 years (72). Condylar fractures sustained during the growth period may lead to mandibular asymmetry by compensatory growth with overgrowth in 30% or dysplastic (under-) growth in 22% of patients, particularly in fractures that are required during puberty (84,135). In the remaining 48% of patients, compensatory overgrowth on the affected side will lead to a symmetrical mandible (84).

Ankylosis of the TMJ with or without growth retardation is reported to occur in 1–7% of condylar fractures (29,31,136). The risk for ankylosis is higher in bilateral condylar fractures, in children between 2 and 5 years of age, if treatment is delayed (63), or MMF is prolonged (31). Severe facial deformities will occur if ankylosis develops at any early age (e.g., before age 3), because they will become progressively worse with growth (19). Growth disturbances requiring surgical correction are rare in fractures occurring after age 12 (82). With short immobilization and consecutive active mobilization of the joint remarkable restitution is seen and the incidence of ankylosis is very low (84,85).

Complications in midface fractures including adverse effects on midfacial growth, even in severe nasoethmoid and orbital fractures, are rare, when early and adequate surgical treatment is performed (40,69,111). Possible complications in midface fractures include interorbital widening, nasolacrimal obstruction, telecanthus, and nasal collapse, in nasoethmoidal fractures; encephalocele and globe protrusion, in orbital roof fractures;

enophthalmos, persistent diplopia from orbital soft-tissue entrapment, and scarcicatrization of hemiated orbital contents, in orbital floor fractures.

Growth disturbances after nasal trauma have been attributed to involvement of the nasoethmoid and/or septovomerine sutures (137,138). Other potential complications after a nasal fracture include nasal deformity, septal deviation, and nasal airway obstruction (139), mandating secondary rhinoplasty for aesthetic and/or functional reasons (29). Strictly cosmetic rhinoplasty may be delayed until after completion of growth.

III. SUMMARY AND CONCLUSION

The incidence of facial fractures in the pediatric population is much lower than in adults. Nevertheless, the clinician should be suspicious of CMF injury, particularly when obvious injury in other body locations is noted. The overall fracture patterns are similar, but diagnosis and treatment in children differ from adults. In children, clinical diagnosis is confirmed best by CT scans. Because of higher osteogenic potential and faster healing rates, treatment should be initiated as soon as possible, can be non-operative in nondisplaced and minimally displaced fractures, and immobilization by MMF should be shorter than in adults. Surgical treatment should be least invasive, giving consideration to the stage of dental development. Microplates may be used for stabilization and their interval removal may be considered. Primary reconstruction should be preferred over secondary reconstruction, and autogenous bone grafts should be favored over alloplastic materials. Long-term follow-up is essential for timely detection of complications and alterations in growth pattern that may require additional conservative or surgical management.

REFERENCES

1. Adams CD, Januszkiewcz JS, Judson J. Changing patterns of severe craniomaxillofacial trauma in Auckland over eight years. Aust NZ J Surg 2000; 70:401–404.
2. Transportation USDo. Status of Occupant Protection in America: National Highway Traffic Safety Administration, 2001.
3. Carroll SM, O'Connor TP. Trends in the aetiology of facial fractures in the south of Ireland (1975–1993). Irish Med J 1996; 89:188–189.
4. Beck RA, Blakeslee DB. The changing picture of facial fractures: 5-year review. Arch Otolaryngol Head Neck Surg 1989; 115:826–829.
5. Telfer MR, Jones GM, Shepherd JP. Trends in aetiology of maxillofacial fractures in the United Kingdom (1977–1987). Br J Oral Maxillofac Surg 1991; 29:250–255.

6. van Beek GJ, Merkx CA. Changes in the pattern of fractures of the maxillofacial skeleton. Int J Oral Maxillofac Surg 1999; 28:424–428.
7. Marciani RD, Caldwell GT, Levine HJ. Maxillofacial injuries associated with all-terrain vehicles. J Oral Maxillofac Surg 1999; 57: 119–123.
8. De Gioanni PP, Mazzeo R, Servadio F. [Sports activities maxillofacial injuries: current epidemiologic and clinical aspects relating to a series of 379 cases (1982–1998)]. Minerva Stomatol 2000; 49:21–26.
9. Emshoff R, Schoning H, Rothler G, Waldhart E. Trends in the incidence and cause of sport-related mandibular fractures: a retrospective analysis. J Oral Maxillofac Surg 1997; 55:585–592.
10. Garri JI, Perlyn CA, Johnson MJ, Mobley SR, Shatz DV, Kirton OC, Thaller SR. Patterns of maxillofacial injuries in powered watercraft collisions. Plast Reconstr Surg 1999; 104:922–927.
11. Gassner R, Ulmer H, Tuli T, Emshoff R. Incidence of oral and maxillofacial skiing injuries due to different injury mechanisms. J Oral Maxillofac Surg 1999; 57:1068–1073.
12. Gassner R, Tuli T, Emshoff R, Waldhart E. Mountainbiking—a dangerous sport: comparison with bicycling on oral and maxillofacial trauma. Int J Oral Maxillofac Surg 1999; 28:188–191.
13 Litwan M, Fliegel C. [Roentgen diagnosis of midfacial fractures]. Radiologe 1986; 26:421–426.
14. Pogrel MA, Podlesh SW, Goldman KE. Efficacy of a single occipitomental radiograph to screen for midfacial fractures. J Oral Maxillofac Surg 2000; 58:24–26.
15. Maniglia AJ, Kline SN. Maxillofacial trauma in the pediatric age group. Otolaryngol Clin North Am 1983; 16:717–730.
16. Holland AJ, Liang RW, Singh SJ, Schell DN, Ross FI, Cass DT. Driveway motor vehicle injuries in children. Med J Aust 2000; 173:192–195.
17. Posnick JC, Wells M, Pron GE. Pediatric facial fractures: evolving patterns of treatment. J Oral Maxillofac Surg 1993; 51:836–844; discussion 844–835.
18. Graham GG. The management of mandibular fractures in children. J Oral Surg Anesth Hosp D Serv 1960; 18:416–423.
19. Rowe NL. Fractures of the jaws in children. J Oral Surg 1969; 27:497–507.
20. Schuchardt K, Schwenzer N, Rottke B, Lentrodt J. [Causes, frequency, and localization of craniofacial fractures]. Fortschr Kiefer Gesichtschir 1966; 11:1–6.
21. MacLennan WD. Fractures of the mandible in children under the age of six years. Br J Plast Surg 1956; 9:125–128.
22. McGraw BL, Cole RR. Pediatric maxillofacial trauma: age-related variations in injury. Arch Otolaryngol Head Neck Surg 1990; 116:41–45.
23. Carroll MJ, Mason DA, Hill CM. Facial fractures in children. Br Dent J 1987; 163:289.
24. Frazer JE. The skull: general account. In: Breathnach AS, ed. Anatomy of the Human Skeleton. London: J&A Churchil Ltd, 1965:161–181.

25. Meier K, Barsekow F, Hausamen JE. [Problems associated with fractures of the visceral cranium involving multiple injuries in children]. Dtsch Zahnarztl Z 1990; 45:806–807.
26. Yarington CT Jr. Maxillofacial trauma in children. Otolaryngol Clin North Am 1977; 10:25–32.
27. Holland AJ, Broome C, Steinberg A, Cases DT. Facial fractures in children. Pediatr Emerg Care 2001; 17:157–160.
28. Anderson PJ. Fractures of the facial skeleton in children. Injury 1995; 26: 47–50.
29. Kaban LB, Mulliken LB, Murray JE. Facial fractures in children: an analysis of 122 fractures in 109 patients. Plast Reconstr Surg 1977; 59: 15–20.
30. Lukas J, Rambousek P. [Injuries of the upper and middle thirds of the face: analysis of the cause of injury]. Cas Lek Cesk 2001; 140:47–50.
31. Oji C. Fractures of the facial skeleton in children: a survey of patients under the age of 11 years. J Craniomaxillofac Surg 1998; 26:322–325.
32. Jaber MA, Porter SR. Maxillofacial injuries in 209 Libyan children under 13 years of age. Int J Paediatr Dent 1997; 7:39–40.
33. Porter SR. Facial fractures in children. Br Dent J 1987; 163:144.
34. Zachariades N, Papavassiliou D, Koumoura F. Fractures of the facial skeleton in children. J Craniomaxillofac Surg 1990; 18:151–153.
35. Ramba J. Fractures of facial bones in children. Int J Oral Surg 1985; 14: 472–478.
36. Kaban LB. Facial trauma I: midface fractures. In: Kaban LB, ed. Pediatric Oral and Maxillofacial Surgery. Philadelphia: WB Saunders, 1990: 209–232.
37. Benoit R, Watts DD, Dwyer K, Kaufmann C, Fakhry S. Windows 99: a source of suburban pediatric trauma. J Trauma 2000; 49:477–481; discussion 481–472.
38. Zerfowski M, Bremerich A. Facial trauma in children and adolescents. Clin Oral Invest 1998; 2:120–124.
39. Shinya K, Taira T, Sawada M, Isshiki N. Facial injuries from falling: age-dependent characteristics. Ann Plast Surg 1993; 30:417–423.
40. Lizuka T, Thoren H, Annino DJ Jr, Hallikainen D, Lindqvist C. Midfacial fractures in pediatric patients: frequency, characteristics, and causes. Arch Otolaryngol Head Neck Surg 1995; 121:1366–1371.
41. Kotilainen R, Karja J, Kullaa-Mikkonen A. Jaw fractures in children. Int J Pediatr Otorhinolaryngol 1990; 19:57–61.
42. Ghosh A, Di Scala C, Drew C, Lessin M, Feins N. Horse-related injuries in pediatric patients. J Pediatr Surg 2000; 35:1766–1770.
43. Shorter NA, Jensen PE, Harmon BJ, Mooney DP. Skiing injuries in children and adolescents. J Trauma 1996; 40:997–1001.
44. Shorter NA, Mooney DP, Harmon BJ. Snowboarding injuries in children and adolescents. Am J Emerg Med 1999; 17:261–263.
45. Smith GA. Injuries to children in the United States related to trampolines, 1990–1995: a national epidemic. Pediatrics 1998; 101:406–412.

46. Powell EC, Tanz RR. Cycling injuries treated in emergency departments: need for bicycle helmets among preschoolers. Arch Pediatr Adolesc Med 2000; 154:1096–1100.
47. Brudvik C. Child injuries in Bergen, Norway. Injury 2000; 31:761–767.
48. Bamjee Y, Lownie JF, Cleaton-Jones PE, Lownie MA. Maxillofacial injuries in a group of South Africans under 18 years of age. Br J Oral Maxillofac Surg 1996; 34:298–302.
49. Ambrose JB. Orofacial signs of child abuse and neglect: a dental perspective. Pediatrician 1989; 16:188–192.
50. Becker DB, Needleman HL, Kotelchuck M. Child abuse and dentistry: orofacial trauma and its recognition by dentists. J Am Dent Assoc 1978; 97:24–28.
51. Worlock P, Stower M, Barbor P. Patterns of fractures in accidental and non-accidental injury in children: a comparative study. Br Med J (Clin Res Ed) 1986; 293:100–102.
52. Naidoo S. A profile of the oro-facial injuries in child physical abuse at a children's hospital. Child Abuse Negl 2000; 24:521–534.
53. da Fonseca MA, Feigal RJ, ten Bensel RW. Dental aspects of 1248 cases of child maltreatment on file at a major county hospital. Pediatr Dent 1992; 14: 152–157.
54. Jessee SA. Physical manifestations of child abuse to the head, face and mouth: a hospital survey. ASDC J Dent Child 1995; 62:245–249.
55. Statistics NCfH. National Vital Statistics Report. Vol. 49, 2001:16–29.
56. Down KE, Boot DA, Gorman DF. Maxillofacial and associated injuries in severely traumatized patients: implications of a regional survey. Int J Oral Maxillofac Surg 1995; 24:409–412.
57. Murphy RX Jr., Birmingham KL, Okunski WJ, Wasser TE. Influence of restraining devices on patterns of pediatric facial trauma in motor vehicle collisions. Plast Reconstr Surg 2001; 107:34–37.
58. Stylogianni L, Arsenopoulos A, Patrikiou A. Fractures of the facial skeleton in children. Br J Oral Maxillofac Surg 1991; 29:9–11.
59. Hartel J, Sonnenburg I. [Fractures in childhood]. Zahntechnik (Berl) 1982; 23:81–84.
60. Hartel J, Pohl A, Greve JW. [Fractures of the facial skull in the growth period and concomitant injuries]. Unfallchirurg 1994; 97:991–993.
61. Meier K, Barsekow F. [Fractures of the facial skull in multiple injuries in childhood]. Z Kinderchir 1998; 43:11–14.
62. Denloye OO, Fasola AO, Arotiba JT. Dental emergencies in children seen at University College Hospital (UCH), Ibadan, Nigeria—5 year review. Afr J Med Med Sci 1998; 27:197–199.
63. Adekeye EO. Pediatric fractures of the facial skeleton: a survey of 85 cases from Kaduna, Nigeria. J Oral Surg 1980; 38:355–358.
64. Bamjee Y. Paediatric maxillofacial trauma. J Dent Assoc S Afr 1996; 51: 750–753.
65. Sherick DG, Buchman SR, Patel PP. Pediatric facial fractures: a demographic analysis outside an urban environment. Ann Plast Surg 1997; 38:578–584; discussion 584–575.

66. Tanaka N, Uchide N, Suzuki K, Tashiro T, Tomitsuka K, Kimijima Y, Amagasa T. Maxillofacial fractures in children. J Craniomaxillofac Surg 1993; 21:289–293.
67. Sherick DG, Buchman SR, Patel PP. Pediatric facial fractures: analysis of differences in subspecialty care. Plast Reconstr Surg 1998; 102:28–31.
68. Bataineh AB. Etiology and incidence of maxillofacial fractures in the north of Jordan. Oral Surg Oral Med Oral Pathol Oral Radiol Endodont 1998; 86: 31–35.
69. McCoy FJ, Chandler RA, Crow ML. Facial fractures in children. Plast Reconstr Surg 1966; 37:209–215.
70. Rowe NL. Fractures of the facial skeleton in children. J Oral Surg 1968; 26:505–515.
71. Haug RH, Foss J. Maxillofacial injuries in the pediatric patient. Oral Surg Oral Med Oral Pathol Oral Radiol Endodont 2000; 90:126–134.
72. MacLennan WD. Consideration of 180 cases of typical fractures of the mandibular condylar process. Br J Plast Surg 1952; 5:122–128.
73. Fortunato MA, Fielding AF, Guernsey LH. Facial bone fractures in children. Oral Surg Oral Med Oral Pathol 1982; 53:225–230.
74. Thoren H, Iizuka T, Hallikainen D, Nurminen M, Lindqvist C. An epidemiological study of patterns of condylar fractures in children. Br J Oral Maxillofac Surg 1997; 35:306–311.
75. Gussack GS, Luterman A, Powell RW, Rodgers K, Ramenofsky ML. Pediatric maxillofacial trauma: unique features in diagnosis and treatment. Laryngoscope 1987; 97:925–930.
76. Hartel J. [Facial bone fractures and their accompanying injuries during growth]. Stomatol DDR 1985; 35:247–253.
77. Morgan WC. Pediatric mandibular fractures. Oral Surg Oral Med Oral Pathol 1975; 40:320–326.
78. Selle A, Thieme V. [Injuries to the facial portion of the skull and their late effects in children and juveniles—a 10-year analysis (author's transl)]. Zahn Mund Kieferheikd Zentralbl 1979; 67:377–385.
79. Powell EC, Tanz RR, DiScala C. Bicycle-related injuries among preschool children. Ann Emerg Med 1997; 30:260–265.
80. Acton CH, Nixon JW, Clark RC. Bicycle riding and oral/maxillofacial trauma in young children. Med J Aust 1996; 165:249–251.
81. Kaban LB. Facial trauma II: dentoalveolar injuries and mandibular fractures. In: Kaban LB, ed. Pediatric Oral and Maxillofacial Surgery. Philadelphia: WB Saunders, 1990:233–260.
82. Demianczuk AN, Verchere C, Phillips JH. The effect on facial growth of pediatric mandibular fractures. J Craniofac Surg 1999; 10:323–328.
83. Berthouze E, Sagne D, Momege B, Achard R. [Treatment of mandibular fractures in children: our therapeutic approach (author's transl)]. Rev Stomatol Chir Maxillofac 1980; 81:285–288.
84. Lund K. Mandibular growth and remodelling processes after condylar fracture: a longitudinal roentgencephalometric study. Acta Odontol Scand Suppl 1974; 32:3–117.

85. Lindahl L, Hollender L. Condylar fractures of the mandible. II. A radiographic study of remodeling processes in the temporomandibular joint. Int J Oral Surg 1977; 6:153–165.
86. Raflo GT. Blow-in and blow-out fractures of the orbit: clinical correlations and proposed mechanisms. Ophthalm Surg 1984; 15:114–119.
87. Messinger A, Radkowski MA, Greenwald MJ, Pensler JM. Orbital roof fractures in the pediatric population. Plast Reconstr Surg 1989; 84:213–216; discussion 217–218.
88. Koltai PJ, Amjad I, Meyer D, Feustel PJ. Orbital fractures in children. Arch Otolaryngol Head Neck Surg 1995; 121:1375–1379.
89. Wright DL, Hoffman HT, Hoyt DB. Frontal sinus fractures in the pediatric population. Laryngoscope 1992; 102:1215–1219.
90. Weiglein AH. Development of the paranasal sinuses in humans. In: Koppe T, Nagai H, Alt KW, eds. The Paranasal Sinuses of Higher Primates: Development, Function, and Evolution. Chicago, Berlin, London, Tokyo, Paris, Barcelona, Sao Paulo, Moscow, Prague, Warsaw: Quintessence Publishing Co. Inc., 1999:35–50.
91. Nahum AM. The biomechanics of maxillofacial trauma. Clin Plast Surg 1975; 2:59–64.
92. Muraoka M, Nakai Y, Nakagawa K, Yoshioka N, Nakaki Y, Yabe T, Hyodo T, Kamo R, Wakami S. Fifteen-year statistics and observation of facial bone fracture. Osaka City Med J 1995; 41:49–61.
93. Regel G, Tscheme H. [Fractures of the facial bones—second most frequent concomitant injury in polytrauma]. Unfallchirurg 1997; 100:329.
94. Mulliken JB, Kaban LB, Murray JE. Management of facial fractures in children. Clin Plast Surg 1977; 4:491–502.
95. Lee D, Honrado C, Har-El G, Goldsmith A. Pediatric temporal bone fractures. Laryngoscope 1998; 108:816–821.
96. Tyroch AH, Kaups KL, Sue LP, O'Donnell-Nicol S. Pediatric restraint use in motor vehicle collisions: reduction of deaths without contribution to injury. Arch Surg 2000; 135:1173–1176.
97. Reath DB, Kirby J, Lynch M, Maull KI. Injury and cost comparison of restrained and unrestrained motor vehicle crash victims. J Trauma 1989; 29:1173–1176; discussion 1176–1177.
98. Johnston C, Rivara FP, Soderberg R. Children in car crashes: analysis of data for injury and use of restraints. Pediatrics 1994; 93:960–965.
99. Margolis LH, Wagenaar AC, Liu W. The effects of a mandatory child restraint law on injuries requiring hospitalization. Am J Dis Child 1988; 142:1099–1103.
100. Agran PF, Dunkle DE, Winn DG. Effects of legislation on motor vehicle injuries to children. Am J Dis Child 1987; 141:959–964.
101. Sewell CM, Hull HF, Fenner J, Graff H, Pine J. Child restraint law effects on motor vehicle accident fatalities and injuries: the New Mexico experience. Pediatrics 1986; 78:1079–1084.
102. Wagenaar AC, Webster DW. Preventing injuries to children through compulsory automobile safety seat use. Pediatrics 1986; 78:662–672.

103. Wagenaar AC, Wiviott MB. Effects of mandating seatbelt use: a series of surveys on compliance in Michigan. Public Health Rep 1986; 101:505–513.
104. Dodson TB, Kaban LB. California mandatory seat belt law: the effect of recent legislation on motor vehicle accident related maxillofacial injuries. J Oral Maxillofac Surg 1988; 46:875–880.
105. Shelness A, Charles S. Children as passengers in automobiles: the neglected minority on the nation's highways. Pediatrics 1975; 56:271–284.
106. Thompson DC, Nunn ME, Thompson RS, Rivara FP. Effectiveness of bicycle safety helmets in preventing serious facial injury. JAMA 1996; 276:1974–1975.
107. Bayliss T, Bedi R. Oral, maxillofacial and general injuries in gymnasts. Injury 1996; 27:353–354.
108. Kaban LB. Diagnosis and treatment of fractures of the facial bones in children 1943–1993. J Oral Maxillofac Surg 1993; 51:722–729.
109. Cawood JI, Stoelinga PJ. Facial trauma. Int J Oral Maxillofac Surg 1990; 19:193.
110. Denny AD, Rosenberg MW, Larson DL. Immediate reconstruction of complex cranioorbital fractures in children. J Craniofac Surg 1993; 4:8–20.
111. Heitsch M, Mohr C, Schettler D. [Indications for the surgical treatment of midfacial fractures in children]. Dtsch Zahnarztl Z 1990; 45:803–805.
112. Rowe NL, Killey HC. Fractures of the Facial Skeleton. Edinburgh, London: E&S Livingstone Ltd, 1968:896.
113. Zachariades N, Papademetriou I, Rallis G. Complications associated with rigid internal fixation of facial bone fractures. J Oral Maxillofac Surg 1993; 51:275–278; discussion 278–279.
114. Costantino P, Wolpoe ME. Short- and long-term outcome of facial plating following trauma in the pediatric population. Facial Plast Surg 1999; 7:231–242.
115. Berryhill WE, Rimell FL, Ness J, Marentette L, Haines SJ. Fate of rigid fixation in pediatric craniofacial surgery. Otolaryngol Head Neck Surg 1999; 121:269–273.
116. Becelli R, Renzi G, Frati R, Iannetti G. [Maxillofacial fractures in children]. Minerva Pediatr 1998; 50:121–126.
117. Marschall MA, Chidyllo SA, Figueroa AA, Cohen M. Long-term effects of rigid fixation on the growing craniomaxillofacial skeleton. J Craniofac Surg 1991; 2:63–68; discussion 69–70.
118. Eppley BL, Platis JM, Sadove AM. Experimental effects of bone plating in infancy on craniomaxillofacial skeletal growth. Cleft Palate Craniofac J 1993; 30:164–169.
119. Polley JW, Figueroa A, Hung KF, Cohen M, Lakars T. Effect of rigid microfixation on the craniomaxillofacial skeleton. J Craniofac Surg 1995; 6:132–138.
120. Wong L, Richtsmeier JT, Manson PN. Craniofacial growth following rigid fixation: suture excision, miniplating, and microplating. J Craniofac Surg 1993; 4:234–244; discussion 245–236.
121. Mooney MP, Losken HW, Siegel MI, Tsachakaloff A, Losken A, Janosky J. Plate fixation of premaxillomaxillary suture and compensatory midfacial growth changes in the rabbit. J Craniofac Surg 1992; 3:197–202.

122. Laurenzo JF, Canady JW, Zimmerman MB, Smith RJ. Craniofacial growth in rabbits: effects of midfacial surgical trauma and rigid plate fixation. Arch Otolaryngol Head Neck Surg 1995; 121:556–561.
123. Connelly SM, Smith RJ. Effects of rigid plate fixation and subsequent removal on craniofacial growth in rabbits. Arch Otolaryngol Head Neck Surg 1998; 124:444–447.
124. Schliephake H, Berten JL, Neukam FW, Bothe KJ, Hausamen JE. [Growth disorders following fractures of the midface in children]. Dtsch Zahnarztl Z 1990; 45:819–822.
125. Dahlstrom L, Kahnberg KE, Lindahl L. 15 years follow-up on condylar fractures. Int J Oral Maxillofac Surg 1989; 18:18–23.
126. Troulis MJ, Kaban LB. Endoscopic approach to the ramus/condyle unit: clinical applications. J Oral Maxillofac Surg 2001; 59:503–509.
127. Perrott DH. Controversies in the management of orbital floor fractures. In: Worthington P, Evans JR, eds. Controversies in Oral and Maxillofacial Surgery. Philadelphia: WB Saunders, 1994:258–266.
128. Dulley B, Fells P. Long-term follow-up of orbital blow-out fractures with and without surgery. Mod Probl Ophthalmol 1975; 14:467–470.
129. Posnick JC. Craniomaxillofacial fractures in children. In: Kaban LB, ed. Oral and Maxillofacial Surgery in Children and Adolescents. Philadelphia: WB Saunders, 1994:169–185.
130. Beirne OR, Myall RWT. Rigid internal fixation in children. In: Kaban LB, ed. Oral and Maxillofacial Surgery in Children and Adolescents. Vol. 6. Philadelphia: WB Saunders, 1994:6:153–167.
131. Smoot EC III, Bowen DG, Lappert P, Ruiz JA. Delayed development of an ectopic frontal sinus mucocele after pediatric cranial trauma. J Craniofac Surg 1995; 6:327–331.
132. Winzenburg SM, Imola MJ. Internal fixation in pediatric maxillofacial fractures. Facial Plast Surg 1998; 14:45–58.
133. McGraw-Wall BL. Facial fractures in children. Facial Plast Surg 1990; 7:198–205.
134. Siegel MB, Wetmore RF, Potsic WP, Handler SD, Tom LW. Mandibular fractures in the pediatric patient. Arch Otolaryngol Head Neck Surg 1991; 117:533–536.
135. Proffit WR, Vig KW, Turvey TA. Early fracture of the mandibular condyles: frequently an unsuspected cause of growth disturbances. Am J Orthod 1980; 78:1–24.
136. Amaratunga NA. Mandibular fractures in children—a study of clinical aspects, treatment needs, and complications. J Oral Maxillofac Surg 1988; 46: 637–640.
137. Precious DS, Delaire J, Hoffman CD. The effects of nasomaxillary injury on future facial growth. Oral Surg Oral Med Oral Pathol 1998; 66:525–530.
138. Ousterhout DK, Vargervik K. Maxillary hypoplasia secondary to midfacial trauma in childhood. Plast Reconstr Surg 1987; 80:491–499.
139. Mustoe TA, Kaban LB, Mulliken JB. Nasal fractures in children. Eur J Plast Surg 1987; 10:135–138.

18

Reconstruction of Avulsive Maxillofacial Injuries

Robert E. Marx and Mark Stevens
University of Miami, Miami, Florida, U.S.A.

I. HISTORICAL PERSPECTIVE

Prior to World War I, maxillofacial injuries in the United States were relatively uncommon, and most were not very avulsive. This was largely due to low-velocity bullets and the gentlemanly attitude of "aim for the heart" that prevailed during the Revolutionary and Civil wars and even in the well-publicized shootouts of the American West. However, owing to the development of trench warfare and the use of helmets (1), World War I saw a dramatic increase in the number of maxillofacial injuries. For the first time, the face was the only exposed portion of the body and therefore became the obvious target (1,2). Although severe, the projectiles of that day were less avulsive than the high-velocity missiles developed during the Vietnam War and thereafter. Consequently, the majority of maxillofacial injuries suffered during World War I can be classified as fractures. Although World War II, and later the Korean War, witnessed a similar number, type, and proportion of maxillofacial injuries as World War I, by this time the advantages of field resuscitation and transport to local field hospitals for early definitive management had been realized. Along with these advances came the principles of airway management, wound debridement, fracture stabilization, primary closure in certain situations, and delayed primary closure in other situations. These time-honored principles significantly improved the chances for survival and introduced the need for secondary reconstructions (3). Later, during the Vietnam War, the widespread use of high-velocity missiles led to an exponential increase in the degree of maxillofacial tissue loss. Surgeons of that era began treating individuals who had lost large segments of bone and soft tissue and thus required wider debridements than ever before. The increased avulsiveness of maxillofacial injuries coupled with the increased number of survivors afforded by the introduction of helicopter evacuations created a demand for even more and improved reconstructive techniques (1).

While certainly regrettable, all of these wars have immeasurably advanced our understanding of the surgical wound management and reconstructive principles discussed in this chapter. However, equally regrettable is the fact that the same numbers and types of high-velocity and low-velocity avulsive maxillofacial injuries suffered during the Vietnam War are now commonplace among the civilian population. As a result, surgeons today who specialize in the maxillofacial area have a responsibility to master the resuscitative, stabilization, and definitive reconstruction principles that can return these individuals to their families, friends, and the workplace.

II. PRESERVATION OF LIFE: INITIAL TREATMENT OF GUNSHOT WOUNDS "THE ABC"

Reconstruction can be accomplished only on the living. Therefore, as obvious and as axiomatic as this sounds, preservation of life and of as much native soft tissue as possible is the first step in the reconstruction process. All deaths secondary to trauma have a trimodal distribution: immediate, early, and late (4). Those classified as immediate occur within the first few minutes and involve direct injuries to the heart, brain, or vital structures such as the spinal cord or major blood vessels. Respiratory compromise secondary to airway obstruction is the next most common cause of death. Gunshot wounds to the maxillofacial area can lead to airway obstruction for a variety of reasons, including mechanical causes, but the number one cause is loss of consciousness associated with adverse positioning whereby the tongue and other oral tissues prolapse into the airway. One surgeon was quoted during World War I as saying that "a soldier who has suffered a maxillofacial injury and is positioned facing the heavens, may soon be there" (5).

A. Airway Control

Primary assessment of the compromised airway must be accomplished within the first few seconds. Patients who present with signs of respiratory distress, stridor, cyanosis, anxiety, or tachypnea >25/min require immediate attention and treatment (4,5). The most common causes of airway obstruction secondary to gunshot wounds of the maxillofacial region are:

1. Hemorrhage into the airway.
2. Foreign bodies displaced into the airway (teeth, bone, and/or dental prostheses).
3. Tongue prolapse, especially in those injuries involving the anterior mandible.
4. Edema (especially in wounds in the posterior pharyngeal area and base of the tongue). This situation can occur rapidly, and preplanning for probable airway obstruction secondary to edema should be followed. The rule is: "When in doubt, intubate or trach."
5. Lacerations extending into the soft palate.

Although airway control is a top priority, the surgeon should also keep in mind the possibility of a concomitant cervical spine injury. A 10% incidence of cervical spine injury is found in unconscious patients who present with injuries resulting from a motor vehicle accident or a fall (6). Initial standard neck extension procedures to access and open the airway can injure the spinal cord and result in paralysis. Cephalic traction and jaw thrust maneuvers can be accomplished to secure the airway while maintaining the long axis of the spine and body. Initial measures should consist of cleaning the oropharynx with suction under appropriate lighting. Foreign bodies and/or blood clots and mucus not only lead to direct obstruction but can also precipitate laryngospasms. Loss of anterior tongue support can be immediately corrected with forward positioning of the tongue using a towel clamp or large suture. Oral or nasal airways can be inserted to temporarily maintain an airway. Supplemental oxygen, 100% at a 6-L flow, should always be given. If ventilation is not achieved within minutes with these maneuvers, or if there is massive injury, access to the airway must be achieved from below via a tracheostomy. Indications for trachesotomy in maxillofacial gunshot wounds are:

1. Failed local airway techniques or massive soft-tissue and bone injury with impending edema
2. Probable need for prolonged intubation
3. Need for multiple staged surgical procedures
4. Maxillomandibular fixation or other postoperative recovery procedure

The simplest and fastest way to access the trachea is through a cricothyrotomy and is preferred over the traditional tracheostomy in most airway emergency situations (7–9). This procedure is accomplished by palpating the cricothyroid membrane between the thyroid and cricothyroid cartilages and incising in a transverse fashion (4). The opening can then be intubated with a small-sized endotracheal tube no. 5 or 6. Complications such as laryngeal nerve damage, vocal cord injuries, and/or stenosis have been shown to be minimal. Conversion to a standard tracheostomy can be performed when the patient is more stable.

Once the airway is secured, by this or some other means, appropriate ventilation should be continuously assessed. Clinical examination by thorough auscultation and radiological methods is essential. Concomitant pneumothorax or hemothorax will need to be treated by placement of thoracostomy tubes to maintain adequate ventilation.

B. Circulation Control

After the airway is secured and adequate ventilation is maintained, the next priority is hemorrhage control. Patients presenting to the hospital emergency room usually arrive with some form of direct pressure dressing to the wounds and bleeding sites. The uncomplicated gunshot wound usually will not require urgent fluid or blood replacement. This can be assessed by simply examining the patient and evaluating capillary refill. Pale, cool extremities with poor capillary refill (> 2 s) are evidence of shock (10). In cases where there is impending shock, intravenous lines must be established immediately. Blood should also be drawn for typing and cross match as well as for laboratory values (Hgb/Hct/platelets).

The severity of clinical signs arising from hemorrhagic shock determines the number of intravenous lines, locations (peripheral vs. central), volumes, and types of replacements administered. The standard protocol in the use of fluid resuscitation consists of a balanced salt solution such as Ringer's lactate followed by whole blood and packed red blood cells. If transfusions are immediately required, they should not be delayed because of the time needed for a type and cross match. The use of several million units of the universal donor O-negative blood during the Vietnam War was without a reaction and is a safe and effective urgent blood replacement. Patients in shock are best managed by a comprehensive multispecialty trauma team.

Local hemorrhage control is best accomplished by the following:

1. Direct pressure. This can slow active bleeding and is effective during transportation.
2. Direct clamping or ligation through the wound. However, adequate visualization is mandatory because blind clamping can injure nearby structures such as nerves and ducts.

3. Control of midfacial gunshot wound bleeding with anterior and/or posterior nasal packs.
4. Angiography and embolization for control of bleeding not amenable to direct ligation and clamping.
5. Low external-carotid ligation in cases when angiographic embolizations are not available.

Most maxillofacial gunshot wounds do not cause acute circulatory failure. However, significant blood loss over time can lead to compromised would healing of traumatized tissues and a delay in the patient's readiness for future surgical procedures. Therefore, adequate blood replacement and stabilization are essential for minimizing complications.

C. Control of Infection

By their very nature, all gunshot wounds to the maxillofacial region are contaminated owing to their cavitation effect and devitalizing adjacent tissues and direct bacterial contamination.

To prevent serious infections such as tetanus, all patients should receive tetanus immune globulin (250 units intramuscularly per dose) and tetanus toxoid, 0.5 mL intramuscularly for two doses, 4–8 weeks apart. Prophylactic antibiotics must be administered as soon as possible. A combination of intravenous penicillin (2,000,000 U) and/or a cephalosporin (2 g) with a gram-negative-spectrum antibiotic such as gentamicin 1.2 mg/kg will likely provide comprehensive initial coverage. Equally important are local debridement of obviously dead tissues and the placement of protective dressings. Once bony coverage is achieved and soft-tissue wounds appear normal in color, the risk of active infection during subsequent reconstructive procedures is minimized.

D. Basic Principles of Initial Gunshot Wound Management

Despite the additional complexities of soft tissue treatment of gunshot wounds in the maxillofacial region, they follow the basic principles similar to the initial management of blunt trauma (11): (1) perform thorough clinical assessments and accurate diagnosis with computed tomography (3-D); (2) expose, explore, and evaluate all wounds and bony fracture lines or tissue loss (the "three e's"); (3) accomplish anatomical reduction and stabilization with rigid internal fixation in the maxilla and midface and selected use of reconstruction plates in the mandible; (4) perform immediate bone grafting of the nasal, orbital, and midface areas and secondary but early bone grafting of the mandible; cranial bone is the first choice followed by grafts from the ilium, if cranial bone grafting is not feasible; (5) debride obviously nonvital and detached bone and foreign bodies such as teeth, bullet fragments, wadding, dental materials, etc.; (6) achieve closure of mucosa to mucosa, skin to skin, or mucosa to skin as well as adjacent tissue transfers if primary closure is not possible; (7) time treatments in the maxillofacial area as early as possible. Early reconstruction allows for optimal results by preventing collapse and secondary scarring of the overlying soft-tissue envelope.

III. RECONSTRUCTING THE MANDIBLE

A. Assessment of Hard and Soft Tissue

Most reconstructive maxillofacial surgeons receive many referrals of patients who were initially managed elsewhere, and usually several weeks or months will have elapsed since their original injury. Even if the initial management was accomplished by the definitive reconstructive surgeon, he/she should not assume that the tissues of the patient are ready for reconstructive surgery and should resist the temptation to immediately begin extensive bone grafting.

Three keys factors in achieving a successful definitive bony reconstruction of the mandible are: (1) an adequate vascular soft-tissue cover, (2) a stabilized and immobile graft, and (3) an infection-free, contamination-free tissue bed into which a bone graft can be placed (12). Therefore, the soft tissue should be assessed in terms of its adequacy of vascularity and size for covering a planned bone graft; the presence of contracted scar tissue and foregin bodies; and the presence of fistulae or periodic episodes of swelling, which sould alert one to the possible presence of a focus of infection such as necrotic bone or tooth fragments.

The assessment of the mandible should also focus on the alignment of residual bone segments and the presence of exposed bone. An avulsion of the body of the mandible will usually cause the proximal segment, consisting of the ramus, condyle, and coronoid process, to be contracted superiorly and medially owing to the force vector of the temporalis, masseter, and pterygoid muscle groups on this segment. This may in turn produce a perforation of bone through the mucosa in the molar region or cause the patient to ulcerate the mucosa by biting it. The distal segment will collapse into the defect and rotate medially from the pull of the mylohyoid muscle. This displacement will produce malocclusion, compromise speech and swallowing, and if severe, compromise the airway.

An avulsion of the symphysis area, such as is commonly seen in self-inflicted gunshot wounds, will of course sever the attachment of the tongue to the mandible via the genioglossus muscle. This creates the possibility of immediate or future airway obstruction and almost always necessitates a short-term or long-term tracheostomy. In this type of injury, both proximal segments of the mandible are displaced superiorly and medially by the masseter, pterygoid, and temporalis muscle groups. These individuals also may develop perforations of bone through a thinned mucosa or via the process of biting the displaced bony segment.

Avulsion of only the ramus or condyle is less common but occasionally does occur. Because the parotid gland and duct and the facial nerve are frequently injured in such cases as well, assessment for sialoceles and facial muscle paralysis must be performed. The mandible will deviate to the injured side to some degree, depending on the amount of bone lost. This collapse, the concomitant muscle injury, the anticipated scarring, and the loss of the temporomandibular joint disc will predispose the individual to a fibrous and/or bony ankylosis.

The greatest obstacle to a successful bone graft reconstruction of the mandible is posed by the presence of unrecognized infection or of nonvital and contaminated bone or tooth fragments. A careful clinical assessment must be undertaken to identify granulation tissue, fistulae, areas of drainage, and areas of unresolved swelling. Each of these findings points to a focus of infection that can adversely affect reconstructive efforts. Similarly, radiographs and computed tomography scans should be assessed for bone and tooth fragments and even for dental filling materials, bullet fragments, bullet wadding, and embedded pieces of clothing. In addition, the edges of each main bone segment should be carefully evaluated for viability. Viable bone edges will show radiographic signs of rounding off within at least 3 months owing to remodeling. If bone segments remain pointed or jagged, they are most likely nonviable.

B. Setup Surgery

Definitive bone grafting should not be done during the first reconstructive surgery even if the bone graft technique transfers soft tissue as well. The purpose of the first surgery, referred to as a "setup surgery," is to provide debridement, bony alignment, bone stabilization, and soft-tissue cover. It "sets up" the tissues to receive a graft that will not become infected or resorbed, will be correctly aligned for optimal dental rehabilitation, and will achieve a stable, functional, and cosmetic outcome. The goal of this surgery is to debride nonvital bone, teeth, and foreign-body fragments to create well-defined bleeding bone ends (i.e., viable bone ends), to align the segments back into their correct anatomical position, and to reorient and reattach displaced and retracted muscles.

The most common setup surgery for an avulsive defect of the mandible approaches the mandible with a submandibular midneck crease incision; the same type will be used later to place the bone graft. The bone ends of the defect should be excised about 0.5–1.0 cm to create a right-angled cut surface and to eliminate jagged edges. Removing this amount of host bone will not make the graft significantly larger or more complex, whereas leaving even a small portion of nonvital bone or a sharp edge, which can protrude through the mucosa, can easily result in an infection.

After dissection of the tissue, all nonvital bone segments, bullet fragments, previously placed wires, plates, or screws, and tooth fragments should be removed and cultures should be taken. The proximal bone fragment should undergo a coronoidectomy so that it can be repositioned correctly, that is, with the condyle in the fossa and the angle of the mandible aligned to the inferior border of the distal segment. The temporalis muscle will reattach to the mandible at the coronoid resection edge and reestablish its function. The distal segment is then aligned into its preinjury position using maxillomandibular fixation or Gunning splints. In this position, the proximal and distal segments are rigidly fixated with a sturdy 2.4- or 2.7-mm titanium reconstruction plate, which will stabilize the mandible throughout the healing process, maintain jaw position, provide contour, and serve as a containment crib for a bone graft at the next stage. This reconstruction plate must therefore be placed with great precision. It should be placed at the inferior border of the mandible and along the posterior border of the ramus and should ideally be fixated with four bicortical screws in each segment (three screws in each segment is the minimum number acceptable). The screw closest to the edge of each segment (mean screw) should be at least 1 cm from the edge to avoid devitalization of this bone. Following these principles will prevent plate exposures, loosening, and breakages and will ensure long-term stability in most cases.

With the bony segments aligned and the reconstruction plate correctly positioned, the surgeon should take advantage of the opportunity to dissect out muscles that may be contracted and enmeshed in scar, such as the anterior digastric, mylohyoid, and masseter, and to suture them to the mandibular segments or to the plate using transosseous bur holes or unused plate holes, respectively. By this means the muscles will regain their original length and functions and will attach to the bone graft when it is placed.

This setup surgery also is the appropriate time to correct the soft-tissue loss in avulsive maxillofacial injuries. In many cases only a minimum amount of soft tissue has been lost, thus requiring only a primary closure or local skin or mucosal flaps. The various local flaps that may be used in cases of small to medium soft-tissue loss over the mandible are too numerous to describe here; however, one flap the authors have found to be reliable, straightforward, and well matched in thickness and color is the bipedicled skin platysma flap. This flap is accomplished by making an incision over the clavicles parallel to the neck incision and connecting the two incisions with a dissection deep to the platysma but superficial to the strap muscles. This skin platysma composite can then be superiorly advanced to cover small to medium-sized defects around the inferior border of the mandible and upper neck.

Larger tissue losses require not only skin cover and perhaps oral lining but a volume of vascular tissue as well. In these situations, pedicled myocutaneous flaps and/or free vascular transfers are indicated. The choice of flap depends on the size and location of the defect as well as the training and experience of the surgeon. However, some flaps are more appropriate for particular areas. For instance, large tissue volumes in the chin and floor of the mouth area are well served by a pectoralis major myocutaneous flap or a free vascular rectus abdominis flap. Areas of the tongue, cheek, and floor of the mouth that have undergone mucosal surface loss are well suited to a free vascular fasciocutaneous flap from either the radial forearm or the circumflex scapular systems. Soft tissue needs around the angle of the mandible and parotid regions are well served by the excellent thickness and color match of the trapezius myocutaneous flap. For those defects requiring the largest surface areas of coverage, the latissimus dorsi flap, either as a pedicled myocutaneous flap or as a free vascular transfer, is a good choice.

C. Definitive Bony Reconstruction

As a result of recent advancements in bone science, reconstruction of the mandible can now be straightforward, permanent, predictable, and have a low morbidity (12). After the setup surgery just described, the authors recommend using condensed autogenous cancellous marrow grafts with platelet-rich plasma (PRP) growth factor additions in place of free vascular bone transfers. Although the free vascular transfer of soft tissue is a valuable technique for soft-tissue reconstruction, free vascular bone transfers of fibula are too small and straight and transfers of ilium are too bulky and have an unacceptably high rate of morbidity. Neither bone aligns the arch form of the jaws or is readily amenable to dental implants in their proper trajectory for denture support or for other types of dental rehabilitation.

The rigid reconstruction plates used in the setup surgery serve as the containment crib for the graft, as noted above. Earlier concerns about the negative effects of stress shielding on bone grafts have been proven to be clinically insignificant and today the plates are left permanently in place once the graft has been placed. The plate is uncovered and the tissue bed developed using the same incision used for the setup surgery. Autogenous cancellous marrow is harvested from the posterior ilium, which represents the greatest reservoir of cancellous bone marrow and allows for the lowest degree of discomfort and earliest ambulation. The marrow is first condensed into 5-mL syringes to compact the bone and thereby increase its cellular density. The tips of the syringes are then cut off and the graft material expressed and further compacted into the recipient site using bone packers. PRP is added to the cancellous marrow during the compaction process and then as a final layer over the compacted graft.

The PRP is developed from approximately 50 mL of autogenous blood drawn in 7 mL of ACD-A anticoagulant immediately before surgery and then sterile-processed in the Smart PReP PRP device (Harvest Technologies, Boston, MA), where it undergoes a double-centrifugation process of approximately 11,000 g minutes to separate the platelets from the other components of blood. The platelets are then activated by adding two drops of a mixture of 10% calcium chloride and 5000 units of bovine thrombin to initiate a clotting process causing the concentrated platelets to actively secrete at least seven growth factors shown to support bone regeneration and soft-tissue healing: three platelet-derived growth factors (PDGFaa, PDGFbb, and PDGFab); two transforming growth factor betas (TGF-β and TGF-β_2); a vascular endothelial growth factor (VEGF); and an epithelial growth factor (EGF) (13). Since the PRP contains four to seven times the number of platelets found in the normal blood clot around a graft, the bone regenerates more quickly, producing a much greater degree of bone density. Studies have shown that grafts treated with PRP mature in one half the usual time and contain 19% enhanced bone content (14). Such grafts are placed into the developed tissue bed and closed primarily. The use of such cancellous marrow grafts does not prolong recovery and does not require intensive care, transfusions, adjuvant systemic anticoagulation, or volume expansion. With the combined use of rigid plate fixation and the PRP, such grafts can be released from maxillomandibular fixation after just 3 weeks rather than the 6-week average. After just 3 months, the graft is sufficiently mature to undergo placement of dental implants and oral scar releases (vestibuloplasty procedures) in preparation for dental rehabilitation. Because the bone density is enhanced, the dental implants can be activated after just 3 months rather than waiting the usual 6 months, thus allowing the patient to proceed to dental rehabilitation much sooner.

Such reconstructions are functional and permanent because the graft produces a sufficient height and arch contour for dental rehabilitation and becomes part of the skeletal bone mass complex that responds positively to functional loading to maintain its content.

IV. INITIAL MANAGEMENT AND ASSESSMENT OF HARD AND SOFT TISSUES

A. Upper Facial Area

The superiormost zone where injuries occur is the anterior cranium and lateral orbital regions. These regions are generally approached from a lateral vector and are among the most common injury sites in the midface area. The vast majority are suicide attempts and require a team approach to treatment with other specialists such as a neurosurgeon and an ophthalmologist.

Because of the formation of secondary missiles and the delicate nature of tissues (brain and globes), extensive excision and exenteration, respectively, are often needed. Initial management consists of evacuation of intracranial hematomas and debridement of necrotic tissues. Because of the danger of infection (meningitis), most neurosurgeons perform a very thorough soft-tissue and bony debridement. Consequently, original defects are often much larger from a reconstructive standpoint than initially anticipated. In most of these cases, immediate bone grafting has been highly predictable and is therefore preferred. The proximity and availability of large amounts of cranial bone make it an excellent source for reconstruction of this region. Split calvarial gaps are harvested through an extended bicoronal flap employed to manage these injuries. The outer table calvarial segments are then fixated to adjacent stable bone to redefine the skull shape and contours. Bur holes and calvarial graft donor sites may be reconstructed with hydroxyapatite cement. When the frontal sinus is involved, a thorough sinusotomy with a bur to remove all the invaginated sinus mucosa and obliteration of both the sinus and ducts are required (15). Fat is used to obliterate the sinus and Surgicel with Bacitracin is used in a rolled fashion to seal the frontal ducts.

Scalp and forehead soft-tissue defects usually can be closed primarily with adjacent tissue transfer techniques. More challenging to reconstruct are cases where there is loss of tissue in the perioral eyelid structures. These are usually staged revisional surgeries. Oculoplastic surgeons are best qualified to manage these soft-tissue injuries. If exenteration of the globe is necessary, internal spacers can be used for an ocular prosthesis. Residual dead space should be obliterated. Split temporalis flaps provide an excellent soruce of intense soft-tissue bulk to eliminate dead space.

B. Lateral Midface Region

The lateral midface is the second most common region affected by gunshot wounds usually as a result of assault. Although they are somewhat less morbid than injuries to the upper face, severe loss of the structural pillars of the maxilla and orbital rim result in significant deformity. In such cases, bone grafts and tenting of the soft tisssues with cranial bone struts and blocks are required to prevent collapse of the facial envelope and/or orbital displacement. One specific structure of anatomical concern in this region is the lacrimal system. If the canaliculi are involved, primary repair followed by internal stinting should be performed (16). Loss of medial eyelid tissue and/or canaliculi structures will require Jones tube placement for lacrimal drainage. Soft tissue reconstruction begins with adjacent local tissue transfers from the paramedian forehead and/or lateral midface. Defects of less than 3 cm are most often closed primarily without major distortion of the surrounding area. In cases where extensive loss of soft tissue occurs, closure over the exposed bone can be accomplished by suturing skin to internal mucosal lining. If a stable mandible is present, the use of the teeth for positioning the maxilla is extremely helpful to obtain the correct spatial relationship to the midface. Oral antral or nasal fistulas may require unique local flaps, such as the split temporalis muscle, tongue, or buccal fat, to provide adequate closure. These are usually accomplished in secondary staged revisional procedures.

C. Central MidFace

Gunshot injuries in this region are among the most challenging to treat. The facial structure most commonly involved in avulsive gunshot wounds in this region is the nose. Because of its shape, specificity, and unique function, nasal region reconstruction is often less than optimal. In these cases, delayed prosthetic rehabilitation with root-form dental implants may provide retention and stability for aesthetic nasal prosthesis. When extensive loss of structural framework occurs, plates may be used initially to support the overlying soft tissue in this region, to prevent secondary scarring, and to minimize the difficulty of achieving soft-tissue facial projection in secondary or delayed procedures. The paramedian forehead here is used as a midline soft-tissue donor site because of its accessibility, soft-tissue bulk, texture, and skin color similar to that of the nose. If distant flaps are planned, they should include enough skin tissue for internal lining requirements.

The split temporalis flap is the most reliable and predictable flap for midface and maxillary oral mucosa reconstruction. It is particularly useful for closing large communications between the oral cavity and nose or sinuses related to gunshot wounds and for adding vascular soft tissue to the midface and orbital areas. The temporalis flap derives its predictability from its vascularity, which is supplied by two deep temporal arteries that are proximal early branches of the internal maxillary artery and rarely lost in maxillofacial injuries. The authors prefer the split temporalis muscle flap because only one half of the muscle is needed for most defects, only one deep temporal artery and a concomitant vein are required to maintain viability, and a concave deformity of the donor site can be prevented by advancing the unused posterior half of the muscle into the anterior temporal defect.

The temporalis muscle flap is approached with the standard bicoronal flap for access. Once the muscle and temporal fascia are exposed, an incision is made through the temporal fascia in a line from the height of the pinna to 1 cm superior to the zygomatic frontal sutures. A dissection deep to the temporal fascia and superficial to the temporal muscle from this point to the zygomatic arch will permit a reflection of periosteum from the zygomatic arch and infratemporal surface of the zygoma without risking facial nerve injury. With the zygomatic arch exposed, an incision to bone around the origin of the temporalis muscle is accomplished. The entire muscle is then reflected from the parietal, temporal, and sphenoid bones as well as from the infratemporal surface of the zygoma so that its only remaining attachment is its tendinous insertion into the coronoid process. With the muscle's deep surface in view, a sterile Doppler sounding of the deep temporal arteries is outlined with a marking pen or with a methylene blue stain. The two deep temporal arteries can then be seen to course parallel to each other and 1.5 cm apart. The muscle is split between these two vessels into anterior and posterior segments. The anterior segment is transferred into the oral cavity through a wide soft-tissue tunnel between the zygomatic arch and the greater wing of the sphenoid. The posterior segment is advanced into the original space of the anterior segment, which is the anterior temporal recess visible to the casual observer. The posterior muscle segment is sutured to the pericranium in this area and to serve as a soft-tissue reconstruction and thereby prevent a visible deformity. The anterior segment is both fanned out and inset into tissues surrounding an oroantral or oronasal defect or inset into the cheek substance or over the anterior maxillary wall for contour.

The temporalis muscle flap is not a myocutaneous flap and therefore will not transfer a skin surface. However, neither a skin paddle nor skin grafting is required if the flap is transferred into the oral cavity. If left exposed to the oral environment, the muscle surface will undergo an epithelialization within 1 month. Therefore, this flap can be used reliably to close large oral defects, to obtain a vascular tissue that will support a bone graft, and to reline the oral cavity.

D. Definitive Bony Reconstruction

Whereas corticocancellous blocks and cancellous marrow are most often used in the denture-bearing portions of the maxillary alveolus, autogenous split calvarial grafts are more appropriate for the maxilla nasal bones and orbits as they are not under direct load. Instead, since their purpose is to provide soft-tissue support and facial contours, they are thinner and have unique convex-concave contours. Calvarial bone has similar thickness and contours to the facial bones. In addition, it undergoes a more rapid revascularization than other cortical bone, and therefore its volume loss due to remodeling is only 15–25% compared to 30–40% for the iliac crest. It was once thought that the midface and the cranium shared a similar embryology and this type of bone was termed "ectomysenchymal." However, it is now recognized that all bone is mesenchymal and that the advantageous difference in calvarial bone is actually its rich diplopic vascular network. The diplopic system is an evolutionary process of venting heat from cerebral metabolism by connecting cerebral veins to scalp veins through the diplopic network of the calvarium. Therefore, the numerous haversian systems and Volkmann canals in calvarial bone permit this early revascularization and hence greater bone survival and less bone-volume reduction.

While definitive bony reconstruction of the skull, orbits, nasal bones, and non-tooth-bearing areas of the maxilla is accomplished at the time of the injuries, bony reconstruction of the tooth-bearing or dental-appliance-bearing alveolar bone is often accomplished secondarily.

The sinus membrane will regenerate in maxillary injuries where the sinus has been entered and teeth avulsed but where no oral-antral fistula has developed the sinus membrane will regenerate. In such situations, classic sinus lift bone grafting can be accomplished to accommodate dental implants. A 2 cm × 2 cm portion of the lateral sinus wall is removed in a standard Caldwell-Luc approach. The intact sinus membrane is elevated and cancellous marrow placed between the bony sinus floor and the elevated sinus membrane within 4 months; the abundant blood supply of the bony maxilla and the elevated sinus membrane, together with the rich osteogenic potential of autogenous cancellous marrow, will result in a consolidated bone into which dental implants can be placed.

For maxillary injuries in which this entire maxillary alveolar process is missing or where large segments have been avulsed, it is best to use corticocancellous blocks from the posterior or anterior ilium. These blocks of bone will incorporate into the mature maxilla but will remodel to lose some of their volume. This volume reduction can be reduced by lagscrew fixation to gain absolute immobilization of the graft, by supplementing the blocks with cancellous marrow, by using PRP, and by covering the graft with a tissue-guided membrane, which inhibits the fibrous ingrowth into the graft from the scarred periosteum. The graft subsequently becomes revascularized from the native maxilla. This is advantageous because blood vessels growing into a graft from a source in bone bring osteoprogenitor cells along with these blood vessels whereas blood vessels that grow in from soft tissues, particularly areas of scarred periosteum, bring in fibroblasts and fibrous tissue.

Block bone grafts to the maxilla require 4 months to consolidate and fuse to the native maxilla. At that time, both the maxillary reconstruction and any mandibular reconstruction can be modified to accept a functional dental prosthesis or a facial unit restoration (eye, ear, or nose).

V. POSTRECONSTRUCTION PREPROSTHETIC SURGERIES

A. Vestibuloplasties

Once mature bone has been established in the jaws (about 3 months after grafting) the soft tissues must be revised and scars released to shape an alveolar ridge. This is usually accomplished by means of a split-thickness skin graft vestibuloplasty. The best results are obtained by a supraperiosteal dissection along the buccal surface of the alveolar ridge. This must be done sharply because the scar tissue in the area will be adherent to the bone. The residual soft tissue against the bone should be thinned as much as possible. Then an acrylic tray made from self-setting polymethylemthacrylate is adapted directly on the tissues. As it sets, the exothermic polymerization will generate heat, which will necessitate cooling by irrigation. Once the acrylic is set, a finer layer of a soft-tissue liner (Coesoft) is used to more precisely adapt to the tissue bed. This will create a tray into which the split-thickness skin graft of 0.014–0.018 in. (average 0.016 in.) can be adapted. The inner surface of the tray is painted either with a skin adhesive or with rubber base cement both of which will "glue" the epithelial surface of the graft to the inner lining of the tray. The tray is then inserted over the alveolar ridge. In the mandible the tray is fixated with two circummandibular sutures and in the maxilla it is fixated with a palatal screw. Leaving this tray in place for a full 3 weeks will protect the graft and adapt it to the ridge so that a near 100% take is the rule. This fixed keratinized tissue is the desired tissue to interface with a denture appliance. The ridge form and the vestibular depth created by this procedure allow for the denture to provide lip and cheek support as well as dental rehabilitation.

B. Dental Implants

Dental implants have been the single greatest advance in converting a mere reconstruction into rehabilitation. Dental implants are placed with the guidance of a prosthodontist. However, the surgeon must consider the following important aspects about dental implants. The best dental implants have a textured surface. This actually stimulates bone ingrowth for osseointegration. Implants should be placed parallel to each other to permit a perfect fit of the denture superstructure, and they should be placed about 1 cm apart to allow self-cleaning and prevent peri-implantitis. The implants should be at least 3.5 mm in diameter and as a long as the bone will accommodate. The prosthetic surface should be a simple design such as an external or internal hexagonal to adapt to common prosthetic systems. The implants should remain beneath the mucosa unloaded for 4 months to gain maximum osseointegration before functional loading.

Short-span defect of two to six teeth may be restored with a cemented fixed prosthesis using one implant each to support two crowns (Fig. 16). For edentulous jaws a minimum of four implants are needed and up to eight may be used. In such cases, a cast Hader bar for a clip retained over denture is a simple and time-honored means of gaining full dentures with easy cleaning and good retention (Fig. M). Otherwise, swing-lock retention or a spark erosion precision fit may also be used.

VI. FACIAL UNIT RESTORATIONS

Facial unit restorations today are not retained by the unreliable and messy adhesives of a decade ago. Instead modified titanium implants of 3-mm, 4-mm, or 6-mm lengths are used. These implants, like dental implants, become osseointegrated into bone local to the defect and will serve as anchors for either a nose, ear, or eye prosthesis. In some cases the implants are connected by a Hader bar so that the facial unit prosthesis is retained by a clip-bar arrangement. In other cases the exposed implants are connected and gold-samarium magnets are placed so that the prosthesis is retained by magnetic force. In either situation, the patient will enjoy a morphological and cosmetic prosthesis, which will not fall off during even strenuous activities.

A. Nasal Prostheses

For a nasal prosthesis, three implants are placed in the shape of an isosceles triangle. One implant is placed at the nasal bridge area and two are placed at the alar base. The two at the alar base must be within the anticipated alar flare of the nasal prosthesis to keep the implant heads hidden from view. To add further function to his type of prosthesis we have often opened the nasal passages and placed a tracheostomy cannula adapted to a Hader Bar. This will conveniently allow nasal breathing and be hidden from view. In most cases, it has allowed permanent removal of the tracheostomy cannula in the neck.

B. Ear Prostheses

For an ear prosthesis, three implants are placed into the mastoid bone along a 110° arc from the actual or anticipated external ear canal. These implants are usually 3 mm or 4 mm in length to avoid perforating the dura. A computerized-tomography scan can be used to measure the bone thickness at the planned placement site as well. These implants are also allowed to osseointegrate for 4 months after which they are connected by a Hader bar. Ear prostheses are usually retained with magnets.

C. Eye Prostheses

For an eye prosthesis, implants of 6–8 mm are placed in either the lateral superior orbital rim or the inferior lateral orbital rim contributed to by the zygoma. Here it is important to place the implants from an agle inside the orbit. In this manner the superstructure, which usually contains several magnets, is unseen and is covered by the prosthesis. These implants are also allowed to osseointegrate for about 4 months before they are uncovered and loaded with the prosthesis. All external facial unit prostheses undergo wear and fading of their original color. This process can be slowed by limiting their direct exposure to sunlight and heat. They should also not be allowed to come into contact with strong chemicals. Simple light soap solutions are best to clean these prosthesis. On a yearly basis these prostheses need to be examined and, often, refitted with new clips, material added to frayed edges, and partly repainted to restore their natural-appearing colors.

REFERENCES

1. Triplett RG, Kelly JF, eds. Management of War Injuries to the Jaws and Related Structures. Washington, DC: US Government Printing Office, 1977: 1–15.
2. Blair VP. Relation of the early care to the final outcome of major face wounds in war surgery. Milit Surg 1943; 92:12–17.

3. Ogilbie WH. General Introduction. Surgery in War Time. History of the Second World War: Surgery. London: Her Maj Stat Off, 1953.
4. Fonseca RJ, Walker RV, eds. Oral and Maxillofacial Trauma. Vol 2. 2d ed. PA. 1997:949–981, 1101–1203..
5. Fonseca RJ, Walker RV, eds. Oral and Maxillofacial Trauma. Vol 1. 2d ed. 1997:103–134.
6. DeeMuth WE, Smith JM. High velocity missile wounds of muscle and bone: the basis of rational early treatment. J Trauma 1966; 6:744.
7. Khall AF. Civilian gunshot injuries to the face and jaws. Br J Oral Surg 1980; 18:205.
8. Iantin T, Ivantury PR, Simm RJ, et al. Early management of civilian gunshot wounds to the face. J Trauma 1993; 35:569.
9. Rowe NL, Williams JW. Maxillofacial Injuries. Edinburgh: Churchill Livingstone, 1985:2:560–595.
10. Key JM, Tami T, Donald PJ. Gunshot wounds of the frontal sinus. Head Neck 1990; 4:357–361.
11. Robertson BC, Manson PN. High-energy ballistic and avulsive injuries: a management protocol for the next millennium. Surg Clin North Am 1999; 79: 1489–1502.
12. Marx RE. Mandibular reconstruction. J Oral Maxillofac Surg 1993; 51: 466–479.
13. Marx R. Platelet-rich plasma (PRP): what is PRP and what is not PRP?. Implant Dent 2001; 10.
14. Marx RE, Carlson ER, Schimmele SR, Eichstaedt RM, Strauss JE, Georgeff K. Platelet rich plasma: growth factor enhancement for bone grafts. Oral Surg 1998; 85:638–646.
15. Stevens, MR, Kline SN. Management of frontal sinus fractures. J Cranio Maxillofac Trauma 1995; 1:29–37.
16. MacGillirray RF, Stevens MR. Primary surgical repair of traumatic lacerations of the lacrimal canaliculi. Oral Surg Oral Med Oral Pathol Oral Radiol Endodont 1996; 81:157–163.

Index